School Health
Policy and Practice

7TH EDITION

AUTHOR:

American Academy of Pediatrics
Council on School Health

EDITORS:

Rani S. Gereige, MD, MPH, FAAP
Elisa A. Zenni, MD, FAAP

American Academy of Pediatrics
141 Northwest Point Blvd
Elk Grove Village, IL 60007-1019
www.aap.org

Library of Congress Control Number: 2013948801
ISBN: 978-1-58110-844-6
eBook: 978-1-58110-845-3

The recommendations in this publication do not indicate an exclusive course of treatment or serve as a standard of medical care. Variations, taking into account individual circumstances, may be appropriate.

The American Academy of Pediatrics is not responsible for the content of the resources mentioned in this publication. Web site addresses are as current as possible but may change at any time.

This book has been developed by the American Academy of Pediatrics. The authors, editors, and contributors are expert authorities in the field of pediatrics. No commercial involvement of any kind has been solicited or accepted in the development of the content of this publication.

The publishers have made every effort to trace the copyright holders for borrowed materials. If they have inadvertently overlooked any, they will be pleased to make the necessary arrangements at the first opportunity.

MA0698
3-234/0316

1 2 3 4 5 6 7 8 9 10

American Academy of Pediatrics
Council on School Health
2015-2016

Executive Committee Members
Breena Welch Holmes, MD, FAAP, Chairperson
Mandy A. Allison, MD, MSPH, MEd, FAAP, Chairperson-Elect
Richard C. Ancona, MD, FAAP
Elliott S. Attisha, DO, FAAP
Nathaniel S. Beers, MD, MPA, FAAP
Cheryl Duncan De Pinto, MD, MPH, FAAP
Peter A. Gorski, MD, MPA, FAAP
Chris L. Kjolhede, MD, MPH, FAAP
Marc A. Lerner, MD, FAAP
Adrienne Weiss-Harrison, MD, FAAP
Thomas L. Young, MD, FAAP

Liaisons
Nina R. Fekaris, MS, BSN, RN, NCSN
Linda M. Grant, MD, MPH, FAAP
Veda Charmaine Johnson, MD, FAAP
Sheryl Kataoka, MD, MSHS
Sandra Leonard, DNP, RN, FNP

Former Executive Committee Members/Reviewers (2011–2015)
Cynthia DiLaura Devore, MD, MS, FAAP, Past Chairperson
Robert Gunther, MD, MPH, FAAP
Jeffrey Lamont, MD, FAAP
Mark Minier, MD, FAAP
Jeffrey K. Okamoto, MD, FAAP, Immediate Past Chairperson
Lani S. M. Wheeler, MD, FAAP, FASHA

Staff
Madra Guinn-Jones, MPH
Florence Rivera, MPH

Editors and Contributors

Editors

RANI S. GEREIGE, MD, MPH, FAAP
Director of Medical Education
Designated Institutional Official
Nicklaus Children's Hospital – Miami Children's Health System
Clinical Professor, Department of Pediatrics
Florida International University
Herbert Wertheim College of Medicine
Miami, FL

ELISA A. ZENNI, MD, FAAP
Associate Dean for Educational Affairs
Professor, Department of Pediatrics
University of Florida College of Medicine – Jacksonville
Jacksonville, FL

Contributors

OXIRIS BARBOT, MD
First Deputy Commissioner
New York City Department of Health and Mental Hygiene
Queens, NY

SERAPHINE PITT BARNES, PHD, MPH, CHES
Health Scientist, Division of Population Health, School Health Branch
National Center for Chronic Disease Prevention and Health Promotion
US Centers for Disease Control and Prevention
Atlanta, GA

NATHANIEL S. BEERS, MD, MPA, FAAP
Chief Operating Officer
District of Columbia Public Schools
General and Developmental Pediatrician
Children's National Health System
Washington, DC

CAPT STEPHANIE BRYN, MPH
US Public Health Service (Ret.)
Director, Injury and Violence Prevention
US Department of Health and Human Services
Health Resources and Services Administration
Rockville, MD

SHARON DABROW, MD, FAAP
Professor of Pediatrics
Program Director, Residency Program
University of South Florida
Tampa, FL

WILLIAM POTTS-DATEMA, MS, FASHA, FAAHE
Chief, Program Development and Services Branch
Division of Adolescent and School Health
US Centers for Disease Control and Prevention
Atlanta, GA

CYNTHIA DILAURA DEVORE, MD, MS, FAAP
Pediatrician, school physician
Williamsburg, VA

JOYCE L. EPSTEIN, PHD
Director, Center on School, Family, and Community Partnerships
Johns Hopkins University
Baltimore, MD

ROBERT J. GELLER, MD, FAAP, FACMT
Professor of Pediatrics
Emory University School of Medicine
Atlanta, GA

LINDA M. GRANT, MD, MPH, FAAP
Associate Professor of Pediatrics
Boston University School of Medicine
Director, Medical Services
Boston Public Schools
Boston, MA

MANUEL E. JIMENEZ, MD, MS, FAAP
Assistant Professor and Chancellor's Scholar
Departments of Pediatrics & Family Medicine and Community Health
Director of Developmental and Behavioral Pediatrics Education
Rutgers Robert Wood Johnson Medical School
Attending Developmental and Behavioral Pediatrician
Children's Specialized Hospital
New Brunswick, NJ

VEDA C. JOHNSON, MD, FAAP
Associate Professor, Department of Pediatrics
Emory University School of Medicine
Executive Director, Partners for Equity in Child and Adolescent Health
Atlanta, GA

LLOYD J. KOLBE, PHD
Emeritus Professor of Applied Health Science
Indiana University School of Public Health
Bloomington, IN

CLAIRE MA LEBLANC, MD, FAAP, FRCPC
Associate Professor of Pediatrics
McGill University Health Centre
Division Head, Rheumatology
Montreal Children's Hospital
Montreal, Quebec, Canada

SUSAN P. LIMBER, PHD, MLS
Dan Olweus Professor
Department of Youth, Family, and Community Studies
Clemson University
Clemson, SC

DAVID K. LOHRMANN, PHD, MA, MCHES
Professor and Chair, Department of Applied Health Science
Indiana University School of Public Health – Bloomington
Bloomington, IN

ERIN D. MAUGHAN, PHD, MS, RN, APHN-BC
Director of Research
National Association of School Nurses
Robert Wood Johnson Foundation Executive Nurse Fellow
Silver Spring, MD

ROBERT D. MURRAY, MD, FAAP
Professor of Human Nutrition
Department of Human Services
The Ohio State University
Columbus, OH

BLAISE A. NEMETH, MD, MS, FAAP
Associate Professor, Department of Orthopedics and Rehabilitation
University of Wisconsin School of Medicine and Public Health
Pediatric Orthopedics and Pediatric Fitness
American Family Children's Hospital
Madison, WI

JEFFREY K. OKAMOTO, MD, FAAP
Medical Director, Developmental Disabilities Division
Hawaii State Department of Health
Assistant Professor of Pediatrics, John A. Burns School of Medicine
University of Hawaii at Manoa
Honolulu, HI

JANETH CEBALLOS OSORIO, MD, FAAP
Assistant Professor of Pediatrics
University of Kentucky
Lexington, KY

JOY A. OSTERHOUT, MS, MCHES
Principal, Health & Education Consultants
Augusta, ME

OLGA ACOSTA PRICE, PHD
Associate Professor, Department of Prevention and Public Health
Director, Center for Health and Health Care in Schools
Milken Institute School of Public Health
The George Washington University
Washington, DC

CATHERINE N. RASBERRY, PHD, MCHES
Health Scientist, Division of Adolescent and School Health
National Center for HIV/AIDS, Viral Hepatitis, STD, and TB Prevention
US Centers for Disease Control and Prevention
Atlanta, GA

SHIRLEY SCHANTZ, EDD, ARNP
Director of Nursing Education
National Association of School Nurses
Silver Spring, MD

DAVID J. SCHONFELD, MD, FAAP
Director, National Center for School Crisis and Bereavement
University of South California School of Social Work
USC Department of Pediatrics
Children's Hospital Los Angeles
Los Angeles, CA

KENNETH TELLERMAN, MD, FAAP
Clinical Assistant Professor of Pediatrics
University of Maryland School of Medicine
Chairman, Emotional Health Committee
Maryland Chapter American Academy of Pediatrics
Baltimore, MD

WEIJUN WANG, PHD
Post-doctoral Fellow of Education and Psychology
Faculty of Education, University of Ottawa
Ottawa, Ontario, Canada

HOWELL WECHSLER, EDD, MPH
Chief Executive Officer
Alliance for a Healthier Generation
New York, NY

LANI S. M. WHEELER, MD, FAAP, FASHA
School Health Consultant
Naples, FL

YURI OKUIZUMI-WU, MD
Assistant Professor
Emory University School of Medicine
Atlanta, GA

THOMAS L. YOUNG, MD, FAAP
Jim and Suzanne Elliot and Family Professor of Pediatrics
University of Kentucky Department of Pediatrics
Lexington, KY

Table of Contents
. . . .

Preface

More than 50 million children and adolescents from kindergarten through 12th grade spend every school day in 130,000 public and private schools, usually for 13 of the most developmentally sensitive years of their lives. Throughout successive generations, these schools indelibly weave the fabric and the future of our nation—substantively shaping the health and education of our children and, consequently, the adults they will become. During the past several decades, efforts to respectively reform our education system and our health system sometimes have neglected the great potential for carefully designed school health programs to improve both the health and education of all young people; especially young people most likely to suffer health and education problems.

The American Academy of Pediatrics (AAP) was established in 1930; today it is an organization of 64,000 pediatricians committed to the optimal physical, mental, and social health and well-being for all infants, children, adolescents, and young adults. Since its inception, the AAP purposefully has been working to help our nation's schools protect and improve the health and education of children and youth. Since its scientific journal, *Pediatrics*, first was published in 1948, the AAP has regularly provided expert information about practical means schools could use to ensure the health of students. The AAP Council on School Health (formerly the Committee on School Health) has provided a wide array of continuously evolving resources that can be used to inform and implement effective school health policies, programs, and practices. These resources can be reviewed or acquired at **http://www2.aap.org/sections/schoolhealth/**. Paramount among them is *School Health: Policy and Practice*, the 7th edition of which follows this Preface. Since 60% of public schools have pre-K children (< 5 years of age), the reader may refer to "Caring for Our Children: National Health and Safety Performance Standards" for policies and best practices related to the pre-K age group.

School Health: Policy and Practice purposefully has been written not solely for school physicians. Rather, it has been written for a broader complement of health, education, and social service professionals as well as others who care about school children and youth; who might work together as a team—with physicians as crucial partners—to improve the lives of young people.

Certainly, *School Health: Policy and Practice* has been written for school physicians and for all pediatricians, as well as family practitioners, to help them understand specific means by which schools—more than any other institution—profoundly influence the short- and long-term health of children and youth. Indeed, in our current era of expanding private, independent, and charter schools—and of increasingly more parents who are providing home-schooling for their children—health care providers must be ever more informed and vigilant about recommended health interventions that may not be provided for those children who do not attend public schools. *School Health: Policy and Practice*, thus, can serve as a priceless in-service training tool for pediatricians who are committed to staying up-to-date about ever-changing health hazards among young people as well as ever-changing means that could be used by schools to mitigate those hazards. Equally important, *School Health: Policy and Practice* also can serve as a text and curriculum for preservice pediatrician training and residency programs. Such preservice training could do much to expand the informed participation and leadership of pediatricians across our nation in improving school health programs, and, thus, might help precipitate a more robust national public health strategy to protect and improve the health of school-aged populations.

However, *School Health: Policy and Practice* was also written for school teachers, who bear close witness to often insidious health threats; for school nurses, to whom everyone first turns when health threats emerge; and for school administrators—principals as well as district, city, and state superintendents—who ultimately are responsible for protecting and fostering the health of children in schools and who (perhaps uniquely) can help establish healthy psychosocial climates in schools. It was written for school counselors, psychologists, and social service workers, who often help students with difficult life circumstances and emotional health problems—and who sometimes can help when others cannot. It was written for school food service personnel, physical educators, and coaches, who shape early if not longer-lived habits of eating and physical activity that we now know affect short- and long-term health and education outcomes. It was written for school health educators, who help young people develop the skills they will need to cultivate their own health, the health of families for which they will become responsible, and the health of the communities and the world in which they will live. It was written for school custodial staff, who protect students from school environmental hazards, and for school safety officers, who protect students from school-wide emergencies. It was written for teachers' unions and other organizations that strive to secure the health of all school employees. It was written for parent teacher associations and for governmental and nongovernmental agencies that serve youth. It was written for local and state education agencies, boards of education, health departments, and boards of health. It was written for local, state, and federal legislators, whose support sometimes is required to help schools implement good health policies and practices. It was written for school health coordinators appointed by schools, districts, and states to garner efficiency and synergy by integrating otherwise independent and scattered efforts of the many individuals listed previously. And it was written as a unifying text to help otherwise disconnected faculties across colleges of medicine, education, public health, and social work to provide more integrated training for various professionals so they consequently might work together with schools to improve the health and education of young people.

School Health: Policy and Practice aims to help these individuals and agencies answer the fundamental question: How might schools most effectively improve the health and education of students in a rapidly changing world? More specifically, how might schools most effectively manage administration of many different medications required by students? What mental health services might schools provide? On which priorities might school health education programs focus? How might schools be made safe for students acutely sensitive to peanuts and other allergens? What might schools do to reduce student exposures to toxic molds, pesticides, and cleaning solutions? How might schools protect students from bullying, cyber-bullying, and other violence? What might schools do to help the increasing number of students who have asthma, diabetes, attention-deficit/hyperactivity disorder, autism spectrum disorders, and other special health care needs? How might schools employ school nurses, school-based clinics, and other community health services to meet the needs of their students? What kind of food and physical activity might schools provide? What might schools do to preserve the health of school employees? How might school health policies and programs increase educational achievement, especially among students who live in poverty? Why and how might schools establish means to coordinate their plans and procedures to efficiently address each of these discrete questions? Indeed, these questions are merely a few of many fundamental health policy and practice questions that each school must address—questions carefully answered by *School Health: Policy and Practice*. How each of our nation's 130,000 schools answers these questions will greatly affect the lives of students in each school. How schools across the nation collectively answer these questions will shape the health and education of successive generations of Americans.

The AAP, its Council on School Health, and those who collaboratively produced this text have codified into one source the disparate technical information that could enable our nation's schools to markedly improve the health and education of our young people. What remains is for this information to be used—that is, for the wide and varied institutions and professions named above to come together and collaboratively exert the political will needed to implement those school health policies, programs, and practices so well explained in the pages that follow.

Lloyd J. Kolbe, PhD

Emeritus Professor of Applied Health Science
Indiana University School of Public Health—Bloomington
Founding Director (1988-2003), Division of Adolescent and School Health
US Centers for Disease Control and Prevention

CHAPTER

1

An Overview of School Health in the United States

William Potts-Datema, MS , FASHA, FAAHE[a]
Howell Wechsler, EdD, MPH

Introduction

When asked why he robbed banks, renowned thief Willie Sutton is often credited with saying, "Because that's where the money is." Although Mr. Sutton often denied uttering the famous phrase, the urban legend remains, along with its obvious logic.

Pediatricians, educators, other professionals, and community members interested in improving health and wellness will understand this obvious logic when considering how to reach children and youth. Schools are a critical setting for health promotion and disease prevention efforts, because the vast majority of youth attend school. In the United States, schools have direct contact with more than 50 million students for at least 6 hours a day during 13 key years of their social, physical, and intellectual development.[1] After the family home, schools are one of the primary entities responsible for the development of young people.

Establishing healthy behaviors during childhood and adolescence is easier and more effective than trying to change unhealthy behaviors during adulthood. Schools can influence students' likelihood of risk of a variety of conditions through a variety of approaches, including health education, provision of or referral to physical and mental health services, and establishment of a safe and supportive environment that provides social and emotional support to young people.

[a] The findings and conclusions in this chapter are those of the authors and do not necessarily represent the official position of the CDC.

> In the United States, schools have direct contact with more than 50 million students for at least 6 hours a day during 13 key years of their social, physical, and intellectual development.[1]

Schools have been a site for health programming in the United States since the early colonial period. In the 1890s, the focus was on protecting the school environment, whereby physicians and nurses were hired in both Boston and New York City schools to exclude potentially contagious students. In the early 1900s, the focus of school health shifted to protecting students. During this era, school health services spread and we saw the blossoming of the first schools to provide full clinical services on site, leading to multiple and new possibilities. When public education became compulsory in the mid-19th century, the strategic role that schools could play in promoting and protecting health became recognized; schools soon became the front line in the fight against infectious disease and the hub for providing a wide range of health and social services for children and families.[2] School health in the 1950s and 1960s involved health education, immunization documentation, screenings, treatment for minor injuries, and referrals for diagnosis and treatment of certain problems; however, services did not include treatment of acute conditions. Health education and physical education have been staples of public education for well over a century. Schools and school systems have played central roles in providing health services, improving nutrition, fostering mental health promotion, and slowing the spread of disease across the nation.

In addition to students, school faculty and staff members present another important and large population that can be reached through schools. In 2008, public school systems employed more than 4.7 million people as administrators, classroom teachers, other professional staff, clerical workers, and service workers.[3] School systems are often among the largest employers in cities and counties across the nation. School districts are like businesses in the private sector when it comes to employee-related expenses: they must pay for employee absenteeism, health care costs, workers' compensation, lost productivity, and disability. Reaching school faculty and staff affects not only individual staff members but also their students, families, and the community at large. Enlisting faculty and staff members in healthy school initiatives can have a powerful influence on students through modeling and supporting healthy behavior.

Schools and school systems have played central roles in providing health services, improving nutrition, fostering mental health promotion, and slowing the spread of disease across the nation.

School Health Programs

School health programs and policies in the United States have resulted, in large part, from a wide variety of federal, state, and local mandates, regulations, initiatives, and funding streams. The result, in many schools, is a "patchwork" of policies and programs with differing standards, requirements, and populations to be served. The most comprehensive summary of the different federal, state, and local laws and policies that affect school health programs can be found in a 2008 supplement to the *Journal of School Health* titled "A CDC Review of School Laws and Policies Concerning Child and Adolescent Health" (**http://onlinelibrary.wiley.com/doi/10.1111/j.1746-1561.2007.00272_4.x/pdf**).[4] The most comprehensive summary of current state laws and policies on school health topics can be found in the State School Health Policy Database, managed by the National Association of State Boards of Education (**http://nasbe.org/healthy_schools/hs**).[5] Work in the field of school health is further complicated by the fact that the professionals who oversee the different pieces of the patchwork come from multiple disciplines: education, nursing, social work, psychology, nutrition, and school administration, each bringing specialized expertise, training, and approaches.

The Whole School, Whole Community, Whole Child Approach

The Whole School, Whole Community, Whole Child (WSCC) approach is the new standard framework that has been developed to bring order and cohesion to the patchwork that is school health. Released in 2014, the WSCC was developed through a partnership of the Centers for Disease Control and Prevention (CDC) and one of the largest education associations, ASCD, in collaboration with key leaders from the fields of health, public health, education, and school health.[6]

The WSCC approach responds to calls from the education, public health, and school health sectors for greater alignment, integration, and collaboration between education and health to improve each child's cognitive, physical, social, and emotional development. Public health and education serve the same children, often in the same settings. The WSCC focuses on the child to align the common goals of both sectors.[7] The approach builds on lessons learned from collaborative partnerships between education and health[8] and evidence of connections between health and learning.[9]

The WSCC model (see Figure 1.1) combines and builds on the ASCD's Whole Child framework[10] and an expanded version of the Coordinated School Health approach first described by Allensworth and Kolbe in a 1987 article for the *Journal of School Health*.[11] The WSCC incorporates the 5 tenets of the

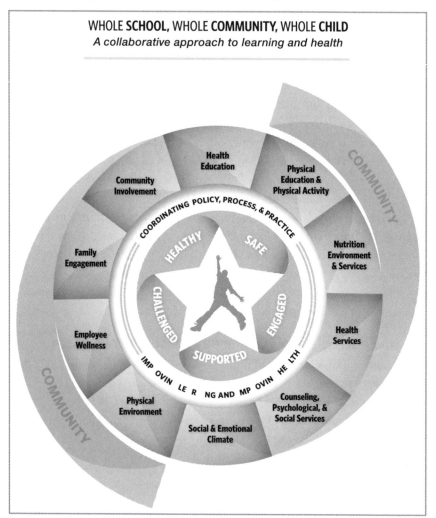

Figure 1.1: The Whole School, Whole Community, Whole Child Model (WSCC). Retrieved November 13, 2015 from http://www.ascd.org/programs/learning-and-health/wscc-model. aspx. Reproduced with permission of ASCD and the U.S. Centers for Disease Control and Prevention (CDC). Learn more about WSCC at www.ascd.org.

Whole Child model by putting the student at the center and making him or her the focal point.[6] The inner ring represents the tenets:

- Each student enters school **healthy** and learns about and practices a healthy lifestyle.[12]
- Each student learns in an environment that is physically and emotionally **safe** for students and adults.[13]
- Each student is actively **engaged** in learning and is connected to the school and broader community.[14]
- Each student has access to personalized learning and is **supported** by qualified, caring adults.[15]
- Each student is **challenged** academically and prepared for success in college or further study and for employment and participation in a global environment.[16]

Surrounding the child/student is a ring that stresses the need for coordination among policy, process, and practice. This ring also describes the critical role of day-to-day practices and process and the essential role of policy in sustaining a school environment that supports both health and learning.[6]

The outer ring of the WSCC model reflects greater integration and alignment between health and education by incorporating the components of the Coordinated School Health approach and emphasizing the school as an integral part of the community.[17] As part of the development of the WSCC model, components of the Coordinated School Health approach were expanded and modified to better reflect current evidence and practice.[18] Definitions and descriptions were also updated and revised.[19] These expanded and modified components include:

- health education;
- physical education and physical activity;
- nutrition environment and services;
- health services;
- counseling, psychological, and social services;
- social and emotional climate;
- physical environment;
- employee wellness;
- family engagement; and
- community involvement.

Under the WSCC approach, each of these components needs to be guided by well-qualified and appropriately prepared staff who implement policies and practices supported by the strongest scientific evidence available. However, the key contribution made by WSCC is its emphasis on bringing together leaders from each of the components into a team that works together to strategically plan, implement, and monitor school health activities.

Coordinating the many parts of school health into a systematic approach can enable schools to:

- eliminate gaps, reduce redundancies, and reinforce efforts across different initiatives and funding streams;
- build partnerships and teamwork among school health and education professionals in the school; and
- present a unified approach to potential community partners that makes it a great deal easier for schools to access community-based health and safety resources.[20]

States and local school districts have been successful in creating greater alignment between health and education using WSCC.[21] More information about the WSCC approach is available on the Web sites of the CDC (**http://www.cdc.gov/healthyyouth/wscc/index.htm**) and ASCD (**http://www.ascd.org/programs/learning-and-health/wscc-model.aspx**).

Local Infrastructure

In local school districts, a coordinated approach to school health includes two critical, interconnected leadership structures:

❶ A team approach to guide programming and facilitate collaboration between the school and the community. At the district level, this group may be called a school health council, and at the school level, it is typically called a school health team. Ideally, the district school health council includes at least one representative from each of the components and school administrators, parents, students, and community representatives involved in the health and well-being of students, such as a representative from the local health department and the school district's medical consultant. School health teams generally include a site administrator, an identified school health leader, teachers and other staff representing the components, parents, students, and community representatives when appropriate. A comprehensive guide to organizing and maintaining school health councils is available from the American Cancer Society: **http://www.cancer.org/acs/groups/content/@nho/documents/document/guidetocommunityschoolhealhcou.pdf**.[22]

❷ A full-time or part-time school health coordinator, who may be a physician, school nurse, teacher, counselor, or another individual with interest and training in health matters. The school health coordinator helps maintain active school health councils, facilitates health programming in the district and school, and leads efforts to obtain health-related resources from the community. The coordinator organizes the components of school health and facilitates actions to achieve a successful, coordinated system, including policies, programs, activities, and resources.[23]

Assessing school health needs and existing school health policies and practices is a critical, early, and ongoing activity for school health councils, under the leadership of a school health coordinator. A number of tools exist to help schools assess health needs and existing health policies and practices, including the CDC's School Health Index: A Self-Assessment and Planning Tool[24] (**http:// www.cdc.gov/healthyyouth/shi**) and ASCD's Healthy School Report Card (**http://www.healthyschoolcommunities.org/HSRC/pages/reportcard/ index.aspx**).[25] School health councils also can play a critical role in integrating health-related goals, objectives, language, and data into school mission statements and improvement plans that guide school management decisions.

Priority Health Issues

Another key task for school health councils is to decide which of the many different health problems that can affect the health and academic achievement of young people will be addressed by their school health policies and programs. Prioritizing is essential, because the primary mission of schools is to educate young people, and schools typically do not have the time in the school day or the resources to address a broad spectrum of health issues.

On the basis of an epidemiologic analysis, the CDC has identified 6 clusters of health risk behaviors as the highest priority health issues for schools to address.[26] They are:

- behaviors that result in injuries, whether unintentional (eg, car crashes) or intentional (eg, homicide, suicide);
- sexual behaviors that increase risk of infection with human immunodeficiency virus (HIV) and other sexually transmitted diseases (STDs), as well as unintended pregnancy;
- alcohol and other drug use;
- tobacco use;
- physical inactivity; and
- unhealthy dietary choices.

Federal agency efforts to support school health programs have largely focused on collecting data, sponsoring evaluations of school-based health and safety promotion interventions, issuing evidence-based guidance on effective policies and practices, and providing funding for state and local school health programs.

Injuries are, by far, the leading cause of death among young people, and young people 15 to 24 years of age account for approximately half of all new cases of STDs and a growing proportion of HIV cases. Use of alcohol and other drugs is a major contributing factor to social delinquency as well as injury-related mortality and morbidity and unsafe sexual behavior. Tobacco use, physical inactivity, and unhealthy dietary choices are behaviors that are established in childhood and adolescence and contribute greatly to the chronic diseases (eg, cardiovascular disease, cancer, diabetes) that account for most of the nation's deaths and health care costs. The CDC also has urged schools to address other critical health issues, such as mental health, management of asthma and other chronic diseases, food allergies, noise-induced hearing loss, skin cancer prevention, and insufficient sleep.[27]

The Campaign for Educational Equity at Teachers College/Columbia University, the nation's oldest college of education, has argued that low-income, urban schools should focus their attention on addressing health problems that are the most important barriers to student academic achievement. The Campaign used 3 criteria—prevalence and extent of health disparities, evidence of causal effects on educational outcomes, and feasibility of implementing proven or promising school-based programs and policies—to identify the following 7 most critical health priorities: vision; asthma; teen pregnancy; aggression and violence; physical activity; breakfast; and inattention and hyperactivity.[28]

Support for School Health Programs

Federal Support

Federal agency support for school health programs has been limited by the role that the federal government plays in education decision making. Education is primarily a state and local responsibility in the United States, with less than 13% of the funds for elementary and secondary education coming from federal sources.[29] Federal influence on state and local education decision making has dramatically increased in recent years with new federal education initiatives. However, these initiatives have not emphasized addressing health-related barriers to learning. Federal agency efforts to support school health programs have largely focused on collecting data, sponsoring evaluations of school-based health and safety promotion interventions, issuing evidence-based guidance on effective policies and practices, and providing funding for state and local school health programs.

Many units within federal agencies provide funding and support for research and implementation of state and local school health and safety programs. The primary unit addressing health and safety issues at the US Department of Education is the Office of Safe and Healthy Students. Within the US Department of Health and Human Services, a number of different agencies provide support for school-based health and safety promotion research and program efforts, including the Office of Adolescent Health in the Office of the Assistant Secretary for Health, the Administration for Children and Families, the CDC, the Food and Drug Administration, the Health Resources and Services Administration; the Indian Health Service, the National Institutes of Health, and the Substance Abuse and Mental Health Services Administration. Other federal agencies that provide support for school health and safety research and program efforts include the Department of Agriculture, Department of Defense, Environmental Protection Agency, Department of Justice, and Department of Transportation.

Several federal agencies collect data that provide critical information about what schools are doing to address student health and safety problems. The CDC collects data about school health policies and practices related to many different school health program components and many different health issues through 2 ongoing surveillance systems: the School Health Policies and Practices Study collects data on a nationally representative sample of school districts, schools, and health education and physical education classrooms[30;] and the School Health Profiles system collects data that are representative of school health policies and practices in states and selected large urban school districts.[31] The US Department of Agriculture collects extensive data related to the school meal programs that it administers. The National Cancer Institute maintains the Classification of Laws Associated with School Students Web site, which summarizes and evaluates state

---

The AAP Council on School Health works to establish standards of best practice for school health for children and adolescents beginning in prekindergarten and continuing through 12th grade.[33]

laws that affect school nutrition and physical activity programs (**http://class. cancer.gov**).[32]

Support From National Organizations

National nongovernmental organizations (NGOs), such as the American Academy of Pediatrics (AAP), provide valuable support for school health efforts in education agencies and other agencies that serve youth. NGOs have access to a wide range of highly trained experts who know how to appropriately tailor and disseminate guidance and tools for school board members, administrators, teachers, and parents and have the capacity to use a wide range of media to transmit critical information and skills across the nation. For example, the AAP Council on School Health works to establish standards of best practice for school health for children and adolescents beginning in prekindergarten and continuing through 12th grade.[33] In addition, NGOs help education agencies develop strategic partnerships and collaborations, including coalitions, to advance school health work.

Other highly active national NGOs include:

- Professional associations that represent health professionals who work in the school setting. The broadest cross-section of different types of school health professionals can be found in the American School Health Association. Other relevant associations include the American School Counselor Association, National Association of School Nurses, National Association of School Psychologists, School Nutrition Association, School Social Work Association of America, SHAPE America, and Society for Public Health Education.
- A number of professional associations that represent education professionals have played active roles in supporting school health initiatives. These include the American Association of School Administrators, ASCD, Council of Chief State School Officers, National Association of State Boards of Education, National Education Association, National School Boards Association, and Society of State Leaders of Health and Physical Education.
- Public health associations that have engaged in supporting school health initiatives include the American Public Health Association, Association of Maternal and Child Health Programs, Directors of Health Promotion and Education, National Association of Chronic Disease Directors, National Association of County and City Health Officials, National Association of State and Territorial AIDS Directors, and National Coalition of STD Directors.

Other national NGOs that provide support to school health initiatives include the American Cancer Society, which has been a supporter of school health education and implementation of coordinated approaches to school health, and the American Heart Association, which has encouraged federal and state policies that support school-based efforts to promote cardiovascular health. A number of strong national NGOs have emerged in the past decade to bolster school-based efforts to prevent obesity. These include Action for Healthy Kids, which has a national network of more than 11,000 volunteers working in every state to make school environments healthier; the Alliance for a Healthier Generation, which provides expert advice, resources, and an award program for schools that meet rigorous health policy and practice benchmarks; and Mission: Readiness, an organization of senior retired military leaders that argues that childhood obesity is a threat to national security and encourages investments in school health programs to improve the health and fitness of our nation's young people.

A number of foundations have provided funding to support a variety of school health programs across the nation. Among the most prominent are the Robert Wood Johnson Foundation, W. K. Kellogg Foundation, and Michael and Susan Dell Foundation.

State Support

State health departments lead many health promotion and disease prevention efforts, which sometimes include school-based activities. However, health agencies do not determine school curricula, policies, and services; that is the role of state education agencies and districts. Education agencies are government agencies responsible for providing policy guidance, curricula, information, resources, and technical assistance on educational matters to schools.

Most states have staff employed in a state agency to provide technical assistance and, when available, resources to support local school health programs. These staff are most often situated in the state education agency but are sometimes found in the state health department and are typically supported by either state or federal funding. Many, although not all, states have one official who serves as the overall lead of all school health program efforts. Other positions often found in state agencies include staff who lead school-based efforts related to child nutrition services, violence and drug abuse prevention programs, physical education programs, nursing or other health service delivery programs, and sexual health promotion (ie, prevention of HIV/AIDS, other STDs, and teen pregnancy).

Tennessee has established the strongest state-supported infrastructure to support school health programs of any state. Legislation passed in 2006 established authority and appropriated $15 million in annual funding that is largely used

> Only 4% of elementary schools, 8% of middle schools, and 2% of high schools provide daily physical education or its equivalent for the entire school year for students in all grades in the school[49]; and only 30% of elementary schools, 40% of middle schools, and 44% of high schools had a full-time school nurse.[50]

to cover the costs of having school health coordinators who focus on implementing the coordinated approach to school health in every school district in the state.[34]

The Role of Schools in Promoting Health

A strong and growing body of evidence has emerged in recent decades that documents the positive impact that school policies and practices can have on youth health behaviors and outcomes. A number of school-based policies and practices are recommended by the Task Force on Community Preventive Services,[35-39] and a series of evidence-based, school health guidance documents have been released by Institute of Medicine panels,[2,40-42] the CDC,[43-46] and a collaboration of multiple federal agencies and national NGOs.[47]

Despite increasing evidence of the effectiveness of school health programs and growing concern over critical health problems affecting youth, such as obesity, the CDC School Health Policies and Practices Study has found that less than one third of high schools require health education in a particular grade[48]; only 4% of elementary schools, 8% of middle schools, and 2% of high schools provide daily physical education or its equivalent for the entire school year for students in all grades in the school[49]; and only 30% of elementary schools, 40% of middle schools, and 44% of high schools had a full-time school nurse.[50]

Educational accountability pressures have created a wave of significant change that has diverted time and financial resources from areas viewed as support services (such as health promotion and disease prevention programs) to pursuits seen as "core" educational activities. Rigorous state and local testing programs have intensified and become the central focus of school systems across the nation.[51] These changes have increased classroom performance pressure on administrators and teachers, especially in English language arts and mathematics. In many local areas, class time for other subjects (eg, science, social studies, health education, physical education, fine arts) has been reduced.[52]

The Common Core Standards were developed by the National Governors Association Center for Best Practices and the Council of Chief State School Officers to define the knowledge and skills students should have within their K-12 education careers. They have been adopted by 43 states, the District of Columbia, 4 territories, and the Department of Defense Education Activity. However, to date, the only standards developed have addressed English language arts and mathematics. Common Core Standards do not address other academic areas, including health education and physical education.[53]

Basch argued that the many different, failed strategies used to date to improve academic achievement are likely to continue to be futile until addressing health-related barriers to learning is included as one of the fundamental components of school reform.[54] A growing body of scientific evidence documents the impact of health behaviors and school health programs on academic achievement. A comprehensive and authoritative summary of this evidence was presented in a series of articles by Basch published in an October 2011 supplement to the *Journal of School Health,* which delineated the causal pathways by which specific health problems are linked to critical educational risks and poor educational outcomes.[54]

One of the largest education associations, ASCD, has called for a "new compact to educate the whole child" that identifies health promotion as one of the essential components of the new compact for our schools.[10] A strong emphasis on health promotion is evident in the educational frameworks of a number of prominent school reform coalitions, including the Partnership for 21st Century Skills, which is supported by some of the nation's largest technology corporations.[55] This integration of health promotion into the fundamental mission of schools is not a new idea; in fact, it is entirely consistent with the vision of early leaders of the public school movement in the United States. The 19th century education advocate Horace Mann, considered "the father of American public education," wrote, "In the great work of education, our physical condition, if not the first step in point of importance, is the first in order of time. On the broad and firm foundation of health alone can the loftiest and most enduring structures of the intellect be reared."[56]

> The 19th century education advocate Horace Mann, considered the father of American public education, wrote, "In the great work of education, our physical condition, if not the first step in point of importance, is the first in order of time. On the broad and firm foundation of health alone can the loftiest and most enduring structures of the intellect be reared."[56]

> Pediatricians can be highly credible experts for integrating health strategies and objectives into the school improvement plan and other documents that guide the overall functioning of the school.

Recommendations for Pediatricians

Pediatricians have long engaged with schools in important health care delivery roles as clinicians and health care consultants. Following are suggestions regarding additional areas of influence and impact for pediatricians and related health professionals.

Serving on School Health Councils and Teams

Pediatricians are ideal candidates to serve as community representatives on a school health council or team. They can bring to these bodies expert knowledge of the consequences of failing to prevent critical health problems and skills in accessing data and scientific evidence that can guide the decision-making process. As highly respected members of the community, pediatricians can have an enormous degree of influence on the priorities established by the health council or team; they also can be highly persuasive in motivating school administrators, school board members, and local office holders to support the implementation of health council or team plans. Furthermore, pediatricians can be highly credible experts for integrating health strategies and objectives into the school improvement plan and other documents that guide the overall functioning of the school.

Assessment and Planning

Pediatricians can play an active role in school health assessment and planning processes. For example, they may serve on a small group that reviews and identifies areas for improvement in a school's existing health service policies and practices through an assessment tool, such as the CDC *School Health Index*, which:

- enables schools to identify strengths and weaknesses of health and safety policies and programs;
- enables schools to develop an action plan for improving student health, which can be incorporated into the school improvement plan; and
- engages teachers, parents, students, and the community in promoting health-enhancing behaviors and better health.[24]

Furthermore, many schools have found that implementation of a rigorous assessment and planning tool, such as the *School Health Index*, is often easier to do when the entire process is facilitated by a respected community member who is not part of the school staff; a pediatrician could make an extraordinary contribution to his or her local school health program by serving in this facilitation role.

Pediatricians also may serve on committees that select health education and physical education curricula for school districts. With their expertise and prestige, pediatricians could make a strong case for the district employing a rigorous, evidence-based approach to curriculum selection, such as the use of the CDC's *Health Education Curriculum Analysis Tool*[57] and *Physical Education Curriculum Analysis Tool*.[58] During the analysis process, they can assist with data interpretation and later help to conceptualize and implement initiatives the are developed to address deficiencies identified in current practices and curricula.

Program Implementation

Pediatricians can play an important role in influencing the nature and quality of the school health programs that are established at the state, county, city, school district, and school building levels. Policies at various levels guide program implementation, such as the selection of health education curricula, the amount of time available for physical education, the nutritional quality of foods and beverages available on campus, the health and mental health services schools are required to deliver, the discipline schools must administer for offenses related to substance use and bullying, the professional preparation required of school health professionals, and countless other factors that influence the quality of a school's health and safety programs. With their obvious concern for the well-being of young people and their credibility as scientific experts, pediatricians can play a unique role in development of policies to support school health programs and goals.

This 7th edition of *School Health: Policy and Practice* can serve as a guide to the types of health-related initiatives that might have a positive impact on student health outcomes. The National Association of State Boards of Education publishes *Fit, Healthy, and Ready to Learn*,[59] a series of guides to school health policy that feature model policy language; the *State School Health Policy Database*,[5] which highlights relevant policies in every state; and *How Schools Work and How to Work with Schools*,[60] which can guide community-based pediatricians in understanding how to advise the educational policy-making process.

> Pediatricians' existing relationships with community-based organizations and businesses might be helpful to secure support for school health initiatives.

Procedure Development

As trusted clinicians, pediatricians can play a vital role in helping school health service programs develop standard procedures for addressing critical problems that affect not only the health and quality of life of students but also their ability to attend school and remain productive in the classroom. These typically include common health problems, such as asthma, allergies, and injuries. However, increasing concerns over pandemic influenza and other serious emerging infectious diseases have renewed interest in development of mitigation procedures. Issues such as school closure, mass immunization, and disaster mitigation may be addressed proactively to ensure prevention and preparedness for such events.

Accessing Community Resources

Pediatricians can provide expert technical assistance to school health coordinators in the development of proposals for funding that are to be submitted to foundations, businesses, or government agencies. They also can advise school health coordinators on the development of collaborative relationships with community-based organizations, such as a provider of after-school programming or a health care provider that can deliver services in the school. Pediatricians' existing relationships with community-based organizations and businesses might be helpful to secure support for school health initiatives.

Pediatricians also can serve as a key link between school districts and schools and local public health agencies. This is particularly important with the recent growth in federal investments in community health promotion. For example, the CDC Community Transformation Grants program supports and enables awardees to design and implement community-level programs that prevent chronic diseases such as cancer, diabetes, and heart disease. The program is expected to improve the health of more than 4 out of 10 US citizens—about 130 million Americans.[61] Pediatricians can provide essential guidance to schools to assist them in linking to these programs and others to maximize their benefits for students.

Recommendations for Program Directors and Trainees

Trainees can best learn about school health by observing the work of, and engaging in dialogue with, pediatricians who deliver health care in schools and pediatricians who play a broader role in supporting school health programs. They would benefit greatly from discussions with these pediatricians about the unique rewards and challenges experienced by those who promote health in the school setting. Trainees need to be well grounded in how to influence school health-related policies; the National Association of State Boards of Education's primer, *How Schools Work and How to Work with Schools*,[60] would be an invaluable reference text. A basic understanding of the WSCC approach is essential knowledge for all school health professionals. Program directors could bring this model to life for trainees and help them gain a deep understanding of critical school health practices by requiring them to read and master the content of the CDC's *School Health Index: A Self-Assessment and Planning Guide*. Trainees with strong interests in school health and excellent interpersonal communication skills can demonstrate their mastery of this content by volunteering to facilitate the *School Health Index* process for a local school.

In addition, trainees can use the *School Health Index* as a base for their quality improvement project by assisting schools in their communities to address areas of improvements based on their *School Health Index*. When possible, program directors can make available to interested trainees an elective experience in school health whereby the trainee would spend time with the school district physician learning the promotion of school health. Public Health and Nursing students can benefit with similar experiences through participation on School Health Advisory Councils and school board meetings.

Take-Home Points

- Schools are a critical setting for health promotion and disease prevention, because the vast majority of youth attend school, and more than 4.7 million adults work in schools.
- The WSCC approach brings together leaders from each component area to work together as a team to strategically plan, implement, and monitor school health activities.

- The school health council at the school district level and the school health team at the school building level, guided by a school health coordinator, are the critical, interconnected leadership structures that shape school health policies and programs.
- School health programs need to prioritize the key health issues they will address; key criteria for prioritization include health impact and the extent to which the health problem is a barrier to learning.
- Support for school health is provided by a number of federal and state agencies, national NGOs, and foundations.
- A growing body of evidence documents the impact that health problems and school health programs have on student academic achievement and attendance.
- In addition to delivering health care to students, pediatricians can support school health programs through service on school health councils and teams, participating in assessment and planning activities, program implementation, procedure development, and accessing community resources.

Resources

For additional school health related resources, visit www.aap.org/schoolhealthmanual.

References

1. National Center for Education Statistics. Enrollment for the 100 largest school districts, by enrollment size in 2009: Fall 2009, 2008-09, and federal fiscal year 2011. Table 97. Available at: http://nces.ed.gov/programs/digest/d11/tables/dt11_097.asp. Accessed April 13, 2015
2. Institute of Medicine. *Schools and Health: Our Nation's Investment*. Washington, DC: National Academies Press; 1997
3. US Census Bureau. Statistical abstract of the United States: 2012. Table 260. Available at: https://www.census.gov/library/publications/2011/compendia/statab/131ed.html. Accessed April 13, 2015
4. Centers for Law and the Public's Health: A Collaborative at Johns Hopkins and Georgetown Universities. A CDC review of school laws and policies concerning child and adolescent health. *J Sch Health*. 2008;78(2):69-128
5. National Association of State Boards of Education. State School Health Policy Database. Available at: http://nasbe.org/healthy_schools/hs. Accessed April 13, 2015
6. Lewallen T, Hunt H, Potts-Datema W, Zaza S, Giles W. The Whole School, Whole Community, Whole Child Model: A new approach for improving educational attainment and healthy development for students. *J Sch Health*. 2015; 85(11): 729–739
7. Centers for Disease Control and Prevention. Whole School, Whole Community, Whole Child (WSCC). Atlanta, GA: Centers for Disease Control and Prevention; February 2015. Available at: http://www.cdc.gov/healthyyouth/wscc/index.htm. Accessed April 13, 2015
8. Kolbe LJ, Allensworth DD, Potts-Datema WH, White DR. What have we learned from collaborative partnerships to concomitantly improve both education and health? *J Sch Health*. 2015; 85(11): 766–774

9. Michael S, Merlo C, Basch C, Wentzel K, Wechsler H. Critical connections: health and academics. *J Sch Health*. 2015; 85(11): 740–758

10. ASCD. The whole child approach. 2015. Available at: http://www.wholechildeducation.org/. Accessed April 13, 2015

11. Allensworth DD, Kolbe LJ. The comprehensive school health program: exploring an expanded concept. *J Sch Health*. 1987;57(10):409–412

12. ASCD. The whole child initiative: healthy. 2015. Available at: http://www.ascd.org/programs/The-Whole-Child/Healthy.aspx. Accessed April 13, 2015

13. ASCD. The whole child initiative: safe. 2015. Available at: http://www.ascd.org/programs/The-Whole-Child/Safe.aspx. Accessed April 13, 2015

14. ASCD. The whole child initiative: engaged. 2015. Available at: http://www.ascd.org/programs/The-Whole-Child/Engaged.aspx. Accessed April 13, 2015

15. ASCD. The whole child initiative: supported. 2015. Available at: http://www.ascd.org/programs/The-Whole-Child/Supported.aspx. Accessed April 13, 2015

16. ASCD. The whole child initiative: challenged. 2015. Available at: http://www.ascd.org/programs/The-Whole-Child/Challenged.aspx. Accessed April 13, 2015

17. ASCD, Centers for Disease Control and Prevention. Whole School, Whole Community, Whole Child: A Collaborative Approach to Learning and Health. Alexandria, VA: ASCD; 2014

18. Centers for Disease Control and Prevention. Expanding the Coordinated School Health Approach. Atlanta, GA: Centers for Disease Control and Prevention; 2015. Available at: http://www.cdc.gov/healthyyouth/wscc/approach.htm. Accessed April 13, 2015

19. Centers for Disease Control and Prevention. Components of the Whole School, Whole Community, Whole Child (WSCC). Atlanta, GA: Centers for Disease Control and Prevention; January 2015. Available at: http://www.cdc.gov/healthyyouth/wscc/components.htm. Accessed April 13, 2015

20. Centers for Disease Control and Prevention. The Case for Coordinated School Health: Why Coordinate School Health? Atlanta, GA: Centers for Disease Control and Prevention; February 2015. Available at: http://www.cdc.gov/healthyyouth/cshp/case.htm. Accessed April 13, 2015

21. Johnsson Chiang R, Meagher W, Slade S. How the Whole School, Whole Community, Whole Child Model works: creating greater alignment, integration, and collaboration between health and education at the state and local levels. *J Sch Health*. 2015; 85(11): 775–784

22. American Cancer Society. Promoting Healthy Youth, Schools, and Communities: A Guide to Community-School Health Councils. Atlanta, GA: American Cancer Society; January 2003. Available at: http://www.cancer.org/acs/groups/content/@nho/documents/document/guidetocommunityschoolhealhcou.pdf. Accessed April 13, 2015

23. Centers for Disease Control and Prevention. How Schools Can Implement Coordinated School Health. Atlanta, GA: Centers for Disease Control and Prevention; February 2015. Available at: http://www.cdc.gov/healthyyouth/cshp/schools.htm. Accessed April 13, 2015

24. Centers for Disease Control and Prevention. School Health Index: A Self-Assessment and Planning Guide. Atlanta, GA: Centers for Disease Control and Prevention; September 2014. Available at: http://www.cdc.gov/healthyyouth/shi. Accessed April 13, 2015

25. ASCD. Healthy school report card. Alexandria, VA: ASCD; 2010. Available at: http://www.healthyschoolcommunities.org/HSRC/pages/reportcard/index.aspx. Accessed April 13, 2015

26. Centers for Disease Control and Prevention. Youth Risk Behavior Survey 2013 Standard Questionnaire Item Rationale. Available at: http://www.cdc.gov/healthyyouth/yrbs/pdf/questionnaire/2013_standard_itemrationale.txt. Accessed April 13, 2015

27. Centers for Disease Control and Prevention. Health topics. Available at: http://www.cdc.gov/healthyyouth/healthtopics/index.htm. Accessed April 13, 2015

28. Basch CE. Healthier students are better learners: a missing link in school reforms to close the achievement gap. New York, NY: Campaign for Educational Equity, Teachers College, Columbia University; March 2010

29. US Department of Education. The Federal Role in Education. Washington, DC: US Department of Education; February 2012. Available at: http://www2.ed.gov/about/overview/fed/role.html. Accessed April 13, 2015

30. Centers for Disease Control and Prevention. School Health Policies and Practices Study. Atlanta, GA: Centers for Disease Control and Prevention; March 2015. Available at: http://www.cdc.gov/healthyyouth/shpps/index.htm. Accessed April 13, 2015

31. Centers for Disease Control and Prevention. School Heath Profiles. Atlanta, GA: Centers for Disease Control and Prevention; April 2014. Available at: http://www.cdc.gov/healthyyouth/profiles/index.htm. Accessed April 13, 2015

32. National Cancer Institute. Classification of Laws Associated with School Students. Available at: http://class.cancer.gov/. Accessed April 13, 2015

33. American Academy of Pediatrics, Council on School Health Web site. Available at: http://www2.aap.org/sections/schoolhealth/. Accessed April 13, 2015

34. Tennessee Government. The Coordinated School Health (CSH) Approach: CSH History. Available at: http://tennessee.gov/education/schoolhealth/aboutcsh.shtml. Accessed April 13, 2015

35. Elder RW, Nichols JL, Shults RA, Sleet DA, Barrios LC, Compton R; Task Force on Community Preventive Services. Effectiveness of school-based programs for reducing drinking and driving and driving and riding with drinking drivers: a systematic review. *Am J Prev Med.* 2005;28(5 Suppl):288-304

36. The Community Guide. Prevention of HIV/AIDS, other STIs and pregnancy: group-based comprehensive risk reduction interventions for adolescents. Atlanta, GA: The Community Guide; June 2009. Available at: www.thecommunityguide.org/hiv/riskreduction.html. Accessed April 13, 2015

37. Centers for Disease Control and Prevention. The effectiveness of universal school-based programs for the prevention of violent and aggressive behavior: a report on recommendations of the Task Force on Community Preventive Services. *MMWR Recomm Rep.* 2007;56(RR-7):1-16

38. The Community Guide. Preventing dental caries: dental school-based or -linked sealant delivery programs. Atlanta, GA: The Community Guide; April 2013. Available at: www.thecommunityguide.org/oral/schoolsealants.html. Accessed April 13, 2015

39. The Community Guide. Behavioral and social approaches to increase physical activity: enhanced school-based physical education. Atlanta, GA: The Community Guide; December 2013. Available at: www.thecommunityguide.org/pa/behavioral-social/schoolbased-pe.html. Accessed April 13, 2015

40. Food and Nutrition Board, Institute of Medicine. *School Meals: Building Blocks for Healthy Children.* Washington, DC: National Academies Press; 2009

41. Food and Nutrition Board, Institute of Medicine. *Nutrition Standards for Foods in Schools: Leading the Way Toward Healthier Youth.* Washington, DC: National Academies Press; 2007

42. Food and Nutrition Board, Institute of Medicine. *Preventing Childhood Obesity: Health in the Balance.* Washington, DC: National Academies Press; 2004

43. Centers for Disease Control and Prevention. School health guidelines to prevent unintentional injuries and violence. *MMWR Recomm Rep.* 2001;50(RR-22):1-73

44. Centers for Disease Control and Prevention. Guidelines for school and community programs to promote lifelong physical activity among young people. *MMWR Recomm Rep.* 1997;46(RR-6):1-36

45. Centers for Disease Control and Prevention. Guidelines for school health programs to promote lifelong healthy eating. *MMWR Recomm Rep.* 1996;45(RR-9):1-41

46. Centers for Disease Control and Prevention. Guidelines for school health programs to prevent tobacco use and addiction. *MMWR Recomm Rep.* 1994;43(RR-2):1-18

47. American Academy of Pediatrics, National Association of School Nurses. *Health, Mental Health, and Safety Guidelines for Schools.* Taras H, Duncan P, Luckenbill D, Robinson J, Wheeler L, Wooley S, eds. Elk Grove Village, IL: American Academy of Pediatrics; 2004. Available at: www.nationalguidelines.org. Accessed April 13, 2015

48. Kann L, Telljohann SK, Wooley SF. Health education: results from the School Health Policies and Programs Study 2006. *J Sch Health.* 2007;77(8):408-434

49. Lee SM, Burgeson CR, Fulton JE, Spain CG. Physical education and physical activity: results from the School Health Policies and Programs Study 2006. *J Sch Health.* 2007;77(8):435-463

50. Brener ND, Wheeler L, Wolfe LC, Vernon-Smiley M, Caldart-Olson L. Health services: results from the School Health Policies and Programs Study 2006. *J Sch Health.* 2007;77(8):464-485

51. Rothstein R, Jacobsen R, Wilder T. *Grading Education: Getting Accountability Right.* New York, NY: Teachers College Press and Economic Policy Institute; 2008

52. Dillon S. Schools cut back subjects to push reading and math. *New York Times.* March 26, 2006. Available at: http://www.nytimes.com/2006/03/26/education/26child.html. Accessed April 13, 2015

53. Common Core State Standards Initiative. About the Standards. 2015. Available at: http://www.corestandards.org/about-the-standards. Accessed April 13, 2015

54. Basch CE. Healthier students are better learners. *J Sch Health.* 2011; 81(10):591-662

55. Partnership for 21st Century Skills. Framework for 21st century learning. Available at: http://www.p21.org/index?hp?option=com_content&task=view&id=254&Itemid=120. Accessed April 13, 2015

56. Mann H. Annual reports of the Secretary of the Board of Education of Massachusetts for the years 1839-1844 by Horace Mann. In: Mann H, Mann MTP, Mann GC, Pécant F, eds. *Life and Works of Horace Mann.* Vol III. Boston, MA: Lee and Shepard; 1891:229

57. Centers for Disease Control and Prevention. Health Education Curriculum Analysis Tool. Atlanta, GA: Centers for Disease Control and Prevention; July 2013. Available at: http://www.cdc.gov/healthyyouth/hecat/index.htm. Accessed April 13, 2015

58. Centers for Disease Control and Prevention. Physical Education Curriculum Analysis Tool. Atlanta, GA: Centers for Disease Control and Prevention; September 2014. Available at: http://www.cdc.gov/healthyyouth/pecat/index.htm. Accessed April 13, 2015

59. National Association of State Boards of Education. *Fit, Healthy, Ready to Learn.* Arlington, VA: National Association of State Boards of Education; 2000

60. National Association of State Boards of Education. *How Schools Work and How to Work with Schools.* Arlington, VA: National Association of State Boards of Education; 2003

61. Centers for Disease Control and Prevention. Community Transformation Grants. Atlanta, GA: Centers for Disease Control and Prevention; October 2014. Available at: http://www.cdc.gov/communitytransformation. Accessed April 13, 2015

CHAPTER

2

School Health and Medical Education

Rani S. Gereige, MD, MPH, FAAP

Sharon Dabrow, MD, FAAP

"All physicians specializing in the care of children and adolescents must have the knowledge and skills to identify and manage school problems"

"School health should be part of residency programs"

⮞ The American Academy of Pediatrics ⮜

Introduction

The American Academy of Pediatrics (AAP) Council on School Health recommends all physicians specializing in the care of children and adolescents have the knowledge and skill to identify and manage school problems and that school health be a part of residency programs.

Historical Perspective

Physicians and other health care professionals have been involved in schools at various levels for many centuries. In the 1930s, the emphasis on improved physical examination and the detection of physical defects lead to the expansion of the scope of the school physician to include health education that could result from the detection of physical defects.[1]

Linking health practices to schools, particularly in the areas of health promotion and disease prevention, has resulted in successful outcomes that support the medical home.

In the 1970s, school health witnessed the expansion of service provisions by new provider types (eg, nurse practitioners) in the setting of school-based health centers (SBHCs). During this time, the focus was on individual student health, health care of poor children, and the incorporation of services mandated by federal law for students with disabilities. Most recently, in the 1990s, health policies helped shape school health into what it now is through the spread of the SBHCs, the focus on education for academic success, accountability, standardized testing, and the integration of school health as part of overall health systems. During that time, medical education began to use SBHCs as potential rotation sites for training Pediatric and Family Medicine residents, and Adolescent Medicine fellows. It is worth noting that linking health practices to schools, particularly in the areas of health promotion and disease prevention, has resulted in successful outcomes that support the medical home. A perfect example is immunization rates, which did not significantly increase until immunizations were linked to school entry.[2]

> Pediatricians who practice in rural areas are 3.6 times more likely to be involved in school health (especially sports-related school health activities).

Background

Despite the evolution of school health to its current state, pediatric medical education curricula and residency training have not kept pace with the evolution of school health to meet the needs of children and the demands of practice. With the national emphasis on ambulatory care and preventive medicine, pediatricians are increasingly involved in school health; however, most of them do not feel prepared to provide these services, as documented by the Task Force on Pediatric Education.[3]

In addition, the pressures of managed care result in less time for community activities such as school health.[4] School health, according to the AAP, should be part of a residency program. The emphasis on community experiences for residents has led residency programs to include this training into their curricula. In a 1996 survey of residency programs, 34% (52/154) of the surveyed programs required a defined clinical experience in school health and 43% (66/154) offered the experience.[3] Another study by Zenni et al[5] showed a positive effect of a school health experience during residency on residents' knowledge of school structure, child development, communication with children, school-related problems, and special education together with a positive effect on residents' attitudes about teamwork between teachers and pediatricians and the role of pediatricians in schools. Only 19% of practicing pediatricians surveyed by Black et al[6] in 1991 reported clinical or didactic education in school health during residency, yet 77% reported some involvement with school health in their practice. In a survey of pediatric residency programs' school health educational activities, Nader et al[4] compared the results of the survey conducted in 2001 with a similar one from 1991. They reported that 50% to 70% of surveyed pediatricians reported involvement in school health; however, only 20% reported having had training in school health (19% in 1991 and 20% in 2001). Pediatricians who practice in rural areas are 3.6 times more likely to be involved in school health (especially sports-related school health activities). Offering education in school health during residency was found to be associated with a higher likelihood (2.9 times) of pediatricians' involvement in school health later in practice (observed in both 1991 and 2001 surveys). There was little change reported in didactic content or practical experiences between 1991 and 2001. In this study, respondents from 1991 reported that school health during residency was required 51% of the time versus 45% in 2001. This shows the need for better training of residents in school health if we are to address the new morbidities such as childhood obesity, school environmental problems, and violence.

Preparing residents for school health will improve overall child health and increase involvement as future practicing physicians. Chilton, in 1979, reported that in a survey of board-certified practicing pediatricians in New Mexico, the majority felt ill prepared to deal with school health issues. Despite the fact that only 22.4% of respondents had any training in the area of school health, 76% of these physicians were providing school health services.[7]

Barnett et al[8] published the results of a self-administered questionnaire mailed to a randomized representative sample of 1602 AAP members, which had a 65% response rate.[9] The following was the level of awareness reported about the school health services: curriculum on risky adolescent behavior: more than 50%; counseling services: 58%; nursing services: 63%; and screening services: 71%. More than half of respondents were not aware of curricula on injury/violence prevention or fitness or whether a school health advisory council (SHAC) is present. However, respondents supported comprehensive school health education and services. Among respondents, only 22% are currently working with schools, but more than 70% wanted to become more involved and needed information on how they may be able to participate and only 25% believed they were adequately prepared for that role in residency.[8]

An overwhelming majority of pediatricians agreed that schools are an appropriate setting for health education in HIV prevention (91%) and human sexuality/pregnancy prevention (87%), that pediatricians should serve as a resource for school health education programs (85%), and that medical schools and residency programs should train pediatricians in school health (79%).[9]

School Health in the New Millennium

Medical education should prepare learners to assist schools and provide them with the skills needed to link the medical and the educational homes. This can occur at all levels of medical education (undergraduate, graduate, subspecialty, and continuing medical education) as well as interprofessional education with learners from other disciplines (eg, public health, nursing, social work, physical therapy, nutrition, psychology). Schools are an important yet underutilized training setting for health and its related fields, because:

- Children spend most of their time in school.
- School health is a natural environment for wellness (education and practice).
- Children with chronic diseases routinely attend school and are mainstreamed.
- Rapid social change and biomedical advances have created new sets of developmental, behavioral, and social challenges for the schools.
- Many of the problems caused by the new morbidities are best handled by focusing on disease prevention and health promotion and can only be addressed by partnering with the schools.

In regard to children's well-being, the new millennium has presented schools with new challenges:

- More children with nondisabling chronic diseases (eg, asthma, diabetes, allergies, attention-deficit/hyperactivity disorder [ADHD]) attend school, and more children and youth with special health care needs are in regular classrooms. Because of this, a significant number of medications are administered by schools each day.
- More than 3.5 million children take medication at school every day. This includes 200 types of prescription drugs, which is about 3 times the number taken in the 1980s.
- Schools are asked more than ever to address the morbidities in the millennium, such as obesity, asthma, ADHD, etc.
- Sicker children with more complex diseases are hospitalized and often discharged earlier than in the past. They often return to require home-bound education services or to their previous school where at-school services are frequently needed.

- High risk behavior among youth often starts in middle school (earlier than before) and continues through adolescence.
- There is a new era of resistant infections (eg, methicillin-resistant *Staphylococcus aureus*, vancomycin-resistant enterococci), bullying, school violence, and natural and man-made disasters. These increase the need that schools have to rely on health care providers for emergency preparedness at the student level, the school, and the community.

The Value of School Health Experiences in Medical Education

The AAP recognizes the important role physicians play in promoting the optimal biopsychosocial well-being of children in the school setting.[10] The discrepancy between physician education and later patient care needs is the best justification for the inclusion of school health content in medical school, residency, and continuing education curricula. A structured curriculum has proven more effective than an unstructured approach. Training in school health should begin during medical school and should be across the continuum of pediatric education.

Medical Student Education

The medical students' curriculum should cover normal child growth and development as well as developmental factors that might affect school performance. During the clinical years, medical students should sharpen their interviewing skills and elicit concerns from parents and children related to school issues. The curriculum is expected to expose the students to effective communication with schools and provide them with basic knowledge of developmental and behavioral problems (eg, learning disabilities, ADHD, intellectual disabilities, school refusal, and school readiness). It should also expose them to chronic medical conditions managed in school and their impact on school achievement. This can be achieved through course work and community-based clerkships in pediatrics and family medicine.

Resident Education

At the residency level, pediatric and family medicine residents should have a good understanding of the school system, federal laws, and the coordinated school health model. They should have educational opportunities and clinical experiences that allow them to achieve competence in the Accreditation Council for Graduate Medical Education-related core competencies and related milestones to be able to effectively work with schools to manage and/or coordinate the health care of a school-aged child. This can be achieved through a multitude of both required and elective clinical exposures, such as ambulatory pediatrics, adolescent medicine, developmental and behavioral pediatrics, and elective subspecialty rotations. Pediatric medical subspecialists in practice may deal with school-related issues, like primary care providers. It is important for subspecialty faculty to highlight the impact of the diseases specific to their specialty on school performance and attendance and ways to work with schools on coordinating the care of the child with complex medical needs. In some residency programs, a stand-alone elective rotation in school health might be offered for interested residents who want to sharpen their school health skills and knowledge.

Residency program curricula should provide residents with the basic understanding of psychometric tests, screening tools, and their interpretation. Residents should be familiar with their local school systems as a whole and the various federal and state laws that relate to school health. In addition, school health experiences can be an excellent venue for interprofessional team experiences (eg, care coordination, action plans, staffing) and advocacy venues (eg, SHACs, school boards), in addition to care provision. Residents may have a role in supplementing and supporting the schools' health education programs by serving as speakers on various topics. Finally, residency programs should expose residents (particularly those interested in primary care) to the various roles that physicians can play in linking the medical home to the educational home,[10] including:

- school consultant;
- school physician/care provider (in the context of SBHCs);
- educator (providing health education to students, staff, parent-teacher associations [PTAs], etc);
- athletic events team coverage; and
- multidisciplinary team member in the context of the local SHAC.

> Getting started with schools on the topic of medical education may vary depending on the community, the readiness, established partnerships with the training institution/university, and the relationships with the community.

Education of Fellows

School health experiences may be a resource for many fellowship programs to meet the curricular goals and objectives as a way to reach the milestones in related topics. School health could be a site for training fellows in adolescent medicine, sports medicine, developmental and behavioral pediatrics, emergency medicine, and general academic pediatric/community pediatrics. Schools can be excellent sites for fellows to conduct projects and help establish programs in advocacy, public health, healthy nutrition, physical activity, emergency preparedness, and exceptional education programs. Fellows can have leadership roles in schools by leading teams, building partnerships, getting involved in community-based research projects.

Continuing Medical Education

School health topics should be well represented in continuing medical education programs designed for faculty and practicing physicians. Also, self-education through resources, such as this manual, will allow the pediatric generalist and subspecialist to broaden their horizons and provide their patients and their communities with expertise and advocacy.

How to Work With Schools

Leaders in medical education should reach out to their local school districts to engage school health professionals. It is important for the relationship to be mutually beneficial to both schools and training programs. On one hand, schools benefit tremendously from physicians' involvement at various levels and on the other hand involvement with schools can benefit training programs by helping trainees achieve several milestones related to key competencies in systems-based practice, professionalism, communication skills. Getting started with schools on the topic of medical education may vary depending on the community, the readiness, established partnerships with the training institution/ university, and the relationships with the community. Some ideas include the following: the program director could deliver a presentation at a school board meeting, a school district meeting, or a meeting for the supervisors of the school health services. The presentation might highlight the value of partnerships to both parties attending to the needs of the schools while illustrating how schools can meet the needs of the training programs. Some educational institutions have already established strong ties with the schools and the community through area health education centers, SBHCs, departments of health, or other programs. Others might need more grassroots work at the level of the training program to build these relationships.

Models That Work

There is no one single way to infuse the medical education curriculum with school health topics and experiences. Various training programs across the country have adopted different models to allow their trainees to achieve a certain degree of competency in school health topics. The following are suggestions to incorporate school health into the medical education curriculum.

❶ Teaching Tools
   a. Self-study Web-based modules
   b. Didactics/case discussions
   c. Self-directed learning with self-reflection/journaling
   d. Structured longitudinal experience (throughout residency)
   e. Community-based advocacy or quality improvement projects based in schools
   f. A combination of the above

❷ Clinical Experiences
   a. Stand-alone school health rotation block
   b. School health experience integrated with other general rotations (adolescent medicine, developmental-behavioral pediatrics, ambulatory pediatrics, sports medicine)
   c. Integration into other rotations by addressing school health issues in every rotation (including subspecialty rotations)
   d. Longitudinal experience whereby resident(s) adopt school(s):
      i. This could involve a single resident, a specific residency class or level, or an entire residency could adopt a school or several schools. This can allow several residents to work as a team on adopting a particular school in their community.
      ii. Adopting a school could entail as little or as much involvement as the resident/groups want, such as giving talks, tutoring, book drives, or acting as school consultant. Other episodic involvement, such as giving talks ad hoc, like the Great American Teach In, or participation in school health fairs, athletic events, and education to athletes.
   e. Participation on committees such as SHACs
   f. A combination of the above

Recommendations for Pediatricians

- The pediatrician should be prepared to act as a resource to parents and schools when it comes to child health-related issues.
- The primary care pediatrician and the pediatric medical subspecialist should reinforce the training they received in school health during residency through continuing education. Pediatricians can get involved in schools in 3 different roles[10] (see Table 2.1).

  ❶ **School consultant:** In this role, the pediatrician does not provide direct patient care in schools but serves as a resource to the school district for policy and administrative health issues and may serve on the local or regional SHAC or school board.

  ❷ **School physician:** In this role, the pediatrician provides care in the school through an established or periodic school-based or school-linked health center. The physician may be employed by the school district or the Department of Education or Department of Health.

  ❸ **The primary care physician:** The primary care physician provides a medical home for students who attend school and interacts with schools to link the medical home to the educational home.

- Pediatricians with interest in school health issues may get involved at the community level through volunteer participation on school boards or local or school district SHACs.
- The AAP state chapter is an excellent avenue to get involved in statewide school health activities.
- Pediatricians interested in national school health issues should consider joining the AAP Council on School Health, which serves as an educational forum to enhance their school health knowledge as well as a venue to put their skills into practice at the national level.

Table 2.1. Roles That Pediatricians Can Assume as They Get Involved in School Health[10]

The School Consultant	The School Physician	The PCP (Medical Home) +/- Subspecialist
1. Administration and planning (policies, emergency preparedness)	1. Limited function to provision of care in a school setting in the context of a SBHC	1. Link to schools in the context of an individual student's health needs
2. Liaison to community physicians		2. Action plans (eg, emergency action plans, asthma action plan)
3. Direct service (school/sports physicals)	2. Provides primary care in the school setting	3. Individualized education programs (IEPs), 504 plans
4. Clinical consultation with school personnel	3. Health fairs	
5. Policy consultation (through local SHAC)	4. Team coverage/ sports medicine	4. Children with special health care needs in the schools
6. Health education (fairs, athletic events)		5. Medication administration
7. Public relations (media representation on health issues)		6. Extension of the medical home concept
8. Advocacy (public hearings, etc)		
9. Systems development consultation		

PCP indicates primary care physician; SHAC, school health advisory council; SBHC, school-based health center.

Recommendations for Program Directors and Trainees

- Program directors should view school health as an integral part of the ambulatory/community pediatric training curriculum. This manual serves as a guide for program directors and trainees. The Academic Pediatric Association's Educational Guidelines for Pediatric Residency (**https://www.mededportal.org/publication/1736**) provide a framework for curricular goals and objectives and evaluation tools for community-based experiences including school health.[11]

- Program directors may reach out to their community/school district and build partnerships with the schools as a training site for residents and fellows as well as an opportunity for interprofessional education.

- School health experiences allow program directors to assess some the trainees' hard-to-assess competencies in the areas of professionalism, communication skills, and systems-based practice. School health staff working with the trainees can be a valuable source of assessment for the newly developed milestones for such competencies.
- With the new ACGME pediatric requirements that allow the "individualized mentored learning experiences," a school health experience might be an excellent opportunity for an individualized experience for trainees interested in community pediatrics or school health as a career. Program directors might make use of the school health activity companions posted on this manual's resource Web site to direct the residents' experiences and document their school health activities in their portfolio.
- For the trainees, a school health experience allows them to view their patients in a different environment outside the hospital/clinic walls.
- School health may be a great opportunity for trainees to complete community-based, quality improvement, and advocacy projects, including health education and other related activities.

Take-Home Points

- For many years, schools have been a valuable resource for medical education.
- The morbidities of the new millennium (eg, childhood obesity, ADHD, autism), the increased number of children with special health care needs who are mainstreamed, and the school-related problems of bullying, violence, and natural and man-made disasters have necessitated more than ever before that pediatric providers be competent in school health. Hence, the need to reinforce the medical education curricula with school health-related milestones and competencies.
- There are multiple ways to infuse the medical education curricula with school health topics at various levels of training depending on the individual community and the institutional resources.
- Pediatricians who receive school health training and experience in their residency are more likely to continue to be involved in schools throughout their career both as primary care pediatricians and pediatric medical subspecialists.

> **Resources**
>
> For additional school health related resources, visit www.aap.org/
> schoolhealthmanual.

References

1. Senn MJE. The role, prerequisites and training of the school physician. *Pediatr Clin North Am.* 1965;12(4):1039–1056

2. Horlick G, Shaw FE, Gorji M, Fishbein DB; Working Group on Legislation, Vaccination and Adolescent Health. Delivering new vaccines to adolescents: the role of school-entry laws. *Pediatrics.* 2008;121(Suppl 1):S79–S84

3. Bradford BJ. School health in pediatric residency training: 1994. *Arch Pediatr Adolesc Med.* 1996;150(3):315–318

4. Nader PR, Broyles SL, Brennan J, Taras H. Two national surveys on pediatric training and activities in school health: 1991 and 2001. *Pediatrics.* 2003;111(4 Pt 1):730–734

5. Zenni EA, Sectish TC, Martin BN, Prober CG. Pediatric resident training in a school environment: a prescription for learning. *Arch Pediatr Adolesc Med.* 1996;150(6):632–637

6. Black JL, Nader PR, Broyles SL, Nelson JA. A national survey on pediatric training and activities in school health. *J Sch Health.* 1991;61(6):245–248

7. Chilton LA. School health experience before and after completion of pediatric training. *Pediatrics.* 1979;63(4):565–568

8. Barnett S, Duncan P, O'Connor KG. Pediatricians' response to the demand for school health programming. *Pediatrics.* 1999;103(4):e45

9. American Academy of Pediatrics, Division of Child Health Research. Periodic Survey No. 26. Pediatricians' Participation and Interest in School Health Programs. Elk Grove Village, IL: American Academy of Pediatrics; August 1995

10. American Academy of Pediatrics, Council on School Health. Role of the school physician. *Pediatrics.* 2013;131(1):178–182. Available at: http://pediatrics.aappublications.org/content/131/1/178.full.html. Accessed April 13, 2015

11. Academic Pediatric Association. Educational Guidelines for Pediatric Residency Training. Available at: www.academicpeds.org/egwebnew. Accessed April 13, 2015

CHAPTER

3

Health Services

SECTION 1
Guidance for School-Based Screenings

Lani S. M. Wheeler, MD, FAAP, FASHA
Oxiris Barbot, MD

Background

Screening detects previously unrecognized conditions or preclinical illnesses and offers an opportunity for early intervention to limit disability and negative effects on learning. The scope and nature of a school-based screening program should be based on the documented health needs of a student population, state law, evidence base that screenings are useful, availability of a reliable and valid screening tool, and effective referral mechanisms.[1]

For all school screening programs, specific procedures for notifying and informing families and students about normal and abnormal results should be developed. Screenings should be carried out by trained individuals who follow clearly written protocols. Appropriate referrals should be made to students' health care providers when needed.[1]

The value of schools' screening programs should be regularly assessed. First, the extent to which families follow through with school referrals should be determined. Next, the outcome of community-based assessments that occur as a result of school referrals of students with positive screens should be ascertained. If results of such assessments show that a screening program is inadequate, school health personnel should work with public health officials and community health practitioners to update screening techniques, redesign screening procedures, and/or reexamine current mandates. Finally, jurisdictions should consider incorporating family input in the process of adopting screening programs and designing the screening process.[1]

The American Academy of Pediatrics (AAP) considers 8 specific criteria to be essential features of a successful screening program (Table 3.1.1). Failure in any one of these criteria is likely to reduce or eliminate the benefit of the program.[3]

Table 3.1.1. Criteria for Successful Screening

Program Aspect	Criterion
Disease	High prevalence or high incidence
Treatment	Available and able to prevent or reduce morbidity
Screening test	High sensitivity and specificity
Screener	Well trained, skilled, and experienced
Target population	Highest prevalence or most beneficial
Referral and treatment	Definitive evaluation and appropriate treatment following all positive screens
Cost-benefit ratio	Cost is less than the benefit of early intervention
Program maintenance	Improvement of quality and assessment of efficiency and effectiveness[2]

Disease: Undetected cases of the disease must be common (high prevalence), or new cases must occur frequently (high incidence). The disease must be associated with adverse consequences (morbidity), either physical or psychological.

Treatment: Treatment must be available that will effectively prevent or reduce morbidity from the disease. There must be some benefit from this treatment before the disease would have become obvious without screening; that is, there must be an early intervention benefit.

Screening test: The ideal test detects all subjects who have the disease (high sensitivity) and correctly identifies all who do not (high specificity). A good test is sensitive, specific, simple, brief, and acceptable to the students being screened (and their families). The test must also be highly reliable; that is, repeated testing will yield the same results.

Screener: The screener must be well trained and monitored for quality assurance.

Target population: To reduce inefficiency, the screening should be focused on groups in which the undetected disease is most prevalent or in which early intervention will be most beneficial.

Referral and treatment: All students with a positive screening result must receive a more definitive evaluation and, if indicated, appropriate treatment. Community links for referrals and evaluation resources must be in place before screening is conducted.

Cost-benefit ratio: Costs include all expenses of screening, referral, and treatment, including administrative costs and the cost and anxiety that result from false-positive results. The benefit is the reduction in morbidity from early intervention among students with true-positive results who are in need of treatment. This benefit is difficult to quantify in dollars and can vary among communities. Greater efficiency at any level will improve this ratio.

Program maintenance: The need for improvements in program efficiency should be determined by a periodic review of research on the value of each screening program and an assessment of program effectiveness within a community. Local review also permits community leaders to make reasonable decisions about the allocation of limited resources for screening. School screenings that are no longer necessary in a community should be discontinued.[1]

These criteria apply to most screening programs. There are additional issues to consider when a school is the screening site. Not all proven, cost-effective screenings may be appropriate or cost-effective if performed in a school setting. Parents should receive ample notification of all screening schedules and encouraged to be present during screening. In jurisdictions where screening programs are not conducted by employees indemnified by the local government authority, school-based screenings should have at least passive parental consent. Any invasive screening procedures should have signed parental permission. The parent should be notified of all screening results whether positive or negative. Compared with a physician's office, where most children are accompanied by a parent, schools may have difficulty effectively reaching parents in person in a cost-effective manner. Telephone and mail contact with parents are only slightly better, particularly with older students and working parents and when English is only one of multiple languages understood at home. Some conditions (eg, obesity, signs of type 2 diabetes mellitus, asthma) are confounded with emotional issues, making telephone or mailed information less appropriate.

Not all screening is appropriate for all school settings. Evaluation and appropriate treatment for students with positive screening results is much easier when screenings are performed by the medical home. Unfortunately, children and adolescents may not be seen in their medical home when screening is most appropriate. School-based screenings may be more necessary where access to a medical home is limited.

School-based screening programs are, themselves, subject to a number of inefficiencies that can significantly reduce or eliminate their utility. The value of a particular screening program should be regularly reassessed to ensure that it is worth the valuable school resources that are being devoted to it. Whenever screening is considered or conducted, schools should work closely with local public health officials to determine the local prevalence or incidence of each condition. Up-to-date early intervention treatment information should be obtained from pediatricians and evaluated by public health and school health physicians. Screening test costs, validity, sensitivity, specificity, and reliability need periodic reassessment, along with education programs for screeners.[1] Program evaluation should compile data on positive, negative, and false-positive screening results based on student population (grade and gender) as well as by screener or school. These data will enable the school/district to determine the need for additional training and focus on appropriate target populations. Advocates can use deidentified compiled data to support appropriate screening programs, improve weak ones, and reduce or eliminate inappropriate programs. Documentation of follow-up evaluation should be obtained for at least 90% of positive screening results. Appropriate allocation of resources for follow up should be in place prior to implementing any new screening programs. When inappropriate screening programs are mandated by legislature, pediatricians can work with public health and school nurse colleagues to revise or remove them. Appropriate school-based screening must be a complete program, not just the act of doing the screening test.

RED FLAGS FOR SCHOOL-BASED SCREENING—SOMETHING IS PROBABLY WRONG IF:

Prevalence of positive screening results are +2 or -2 standard deviations from the district or state levels (by screener, school, and district)

Prevalence of false-positive screening results are +2 or -2 standard deviations from the district or state levels (by screener, school, and district)

Percentage of positive screening results with follow-up evaluation is less than 90% (by school or district)

Evidence Base for Childhood Screenings

The US Preventive Services Task Force (USPSTF) is an independent panel of nonfederal experts in prevention and evidence-based medicine and is composed of primary care providers (such as internists, pediatricians, family physicians, gynecologists/obstetricians, nurses, and health behavior specialists).[4]

The USPSTF conducts scientific evidence reviews of a broad range of clinical preventive health care services (such as screening, counseling, and preventive medications) and develops recommendations for primary care clinicians and health systems. These recommendations are published in the form of "Recommendation Statements." The USPSTF strives to make accurate, up-to-date, and relevant recommendations about preventive services in primary care.

For the USPSTF to recommend a service, the benefits of the service must outweigh the harms. The USPSTF focuses on maintenance of health and quality of life as the major benefits of clinical preventive services and not simply the identification of disease. The USPSTF has published 30 recommendations on child and adolescent screening or counseling.[5] Most of them have no relevance to school health programs.

Evidence Base for School Screenings

The USPSTF has not made any school screening recommendations. Despite a long history of school screening dating back to early 1900s,[6] there are very few well-designed studies of school-based screening programs. In the past, schools have been mandated to screen for various diseases without a public health evaluation or recommendation. Too often, screenings are mandated by legislatures as a result of pressure from lobbyists or others. For example, in the 1960s, suburban junior high students had urine dipstick screenings for diabetes. Although several feasibility studies have been published, there are even fewer studies of the effectiveness of school-based screening programs. Evidence is needed that shows that the screening program makes a difference, not simply that it can be performed. Education is the primary responsibility of schools. Staff and student time should not be diverted to school-based screenings unless they are known to be effective and are monitored and evaluated to ensure benefits in each school.

Screenings in a school-based health center (SBHC) should follow the recommendations for primary care providers. The availability of evaluation and treatment resources enable clinics to ensure a more complete process.

Issues and Evidence for Specific Conditions

Asthma

Child and adolescent asthma screening programs have not been shown to improve student health, despite being promoted by some national organizations[7] and the subject of several published feasibility studies.[8-12] They are not recommended by the American Thoracic Society[13] and most other national health organizations.

Dental

Dental caries are very common and may be the most common chronic condition among school-aged children. Several states have mandated oral health screenings,[14] but no published studies have documented improved student health.[15, 16]

Depression/Mental Health

Mental health screening is recommended for adolescents, and screening in schools has been promoted[17] and shown to be feasible,[18] but no published studies have documented improved student health.[19]

- The USPSTF recommends screening of adolescents (12–18 years of age) for major depressive disorder when systems are in place to ensure accurate diagnosis, psychotherapy (cognitive-behavioral or interpersonal), and follow-up.
- The USPSTF concludes that the current evidence is insufficient to assess the balance of benefits and harms of screening of children (7–11 years of age).[20]
- The USPSTF concludes that the evidence is insufficient to recommend for or against routine screening by primary care clinicians to detect suicide risk in the general population.[21]

Hearing

The USPSTF recommends newborn hearing screening.[22] Most states mandated hearing screening before newborn screenings were available. Most school-based hearing screening programs are not evaluated for their ability to improve student health. When access to primary health care is good, school health programs may benefit from limiting school-based screening to those students not already screened and those with academic problems.

Overweight/Obesity

Although many schools are developing obesity screening and prevention programs, no published studies have documented improved student health.[23]

The USPSTF recommends that clinicians screen children 6 years and older for obesity and offer them or refer them for comprehensive, intensive behavioral interventions to promote improvement in weight status.

Scoliosis

The USPSTF recommends against the routine screening of asymptomatic adolescents for idiopathic scoliosis.[24] In recent years, several states have repealed this mandate.[25,26]

Vision

The USPSTF recommends vision screening for all children at least once between the ages of 3 and 5 years to detect the presence of amblyopia or its risk factors.[27] Most states mandated vision screening before preschool screenings by pediatricians were widely available. Most school-based vision screening programs are not evaluated for their ability to improve student health. When access to primary health care is good, school health programs may benefit from limiting school-based screening of those students not already screened and those with academic problems.

How to Work With Schools

Most screening programs are state mandated, and most states have a state-level council or advisory committee. Pediatricians are critical members of these groups and have led successful efforts to remove inappropriate school screening requirements and strengthen appropriate ones.

AAP chapters often have formal representation on these groups. By helping to set evidence-based policies at the state level, pediatricians can then promote effective implementation in districts and schools.

District and school health advisory councils or committees should have input into screening programs and be actively involved in annual program evaluations. Pediatricians can often share their experience with specific screening tools and can help problem-solve if evaluation and treatment resources are limited.

Recommendations for Pediatricians

Pediatricians can contribute to improving the quality of screening programs in schools in several ways. Nationally, the AAP and its Council on School Health contribute policy statements and advocacy positions that have helped to promote strong national school policies related to school screening. Through participation on school wellness councils, pediatricians can bring to schools a holistic view of child development, health, fitness, and social-emotional well-being. In daily practice, pediatricians can ensure good communication back to schools when evaluating or treating a patient with as positive school screening result. Lastly, many physicians serve as medical directors, consultants, team physicians, and advisors to schools.

Recommendations for Program Directors

Schools are complex systems that are able to offer students and residents a unique perspective on how we seek to optimize child health through policies, programs, practices, education, and measures. The school nurse is the appropriate link between health professionals and school children. Review of school district screening policies, compared with national "best practices," can be enlightening for trainees. The benefit and cost-benefit of school screenings, the challenges of implementing screening programs at the school, as well as difficulties with obtaining feedback information from parents and community providers are all topics that trainees can experience. Examining the pros and cons of the many controversial issues surrounding schools is an exercise that sharpens a student's sensitivity to the nuances of public health issues and policy making for schools. Program directors can arrange for trainees to work directly with school and school districts. Group discussions of on-site observations can expand learning for a group of trainees.

Recommendations for Trainees

To gain a better understanding of the issues, trainees can view school screenings from multiple perspectives:

- students and families;
- school nurses;
- medical home pediatricians;
- local public health;
- local school and school district; and
- state departments of health and education.

Trainees can learn to apply principles of sensitivity, specificity, reliability, and validity in real, public health settings. They can learn to assess effectiveness and cost-effectiveness.

Take-Home Points

- The scope and nature of a school-based screening program should be based on the documented health needs of a student population, state law, availability of a reliable and valid screening tool, and effective referral and treatment mechanisms.
- Successful screening programs meet 8 essential criteria.
- Not all proven, cost-effective screenings are appropriate in school or cost-effective if performed in school.
- Many screenings are more effective when performed in the medical home. School-based screenings may be more necessary where access to a medical home is limited.
- If schools or districts have insufficient resources for effective referrals and follow-up, screening programs should not be implemented. Appropriate school-based screening must be a complete program, not just the act of performing the screening test.
- Pediatricians can work to improve, add appropriate or eliminate ineffective screening programs in their local public schools.

Resources

For additional school health related resources, visit www.aap.org/schoolhealthmanual.

References

1. American Academy of Pediatrics, National Association of School Nurses. *Health, Mental Health, and Safety Guidelines for Schools*. Taras H, Duncan P, Luckenbill D, Robinson J, Wheeler L, Wooley S, eds. 4-18: School health screening programs. Available at: http://www.nationalguidelines.org/guideline.cfm?guideNum=4-18. Accessed April 13, 2015

2. Committee on School Health, American Academy of Pediatrics. *School Health: Policy and Practice*. 6th ed. Elk Grove Village, IL: American Academy of Pediatrics; 2004;35-39

3. Committee on School Health, American Academy of Pediatrics, Nader PR, ed. *School Health: Policy and Practice*. 5th ed. Elk Grove Village, IL: American Academy of Pediatrics; 1993:88

4. US Preventive Services Task Force. Available at: http://www.uspreventiveservicestaskforce.org. Accessed April 13, 2015

5. US Preventive Services Task Force. Special Populations. Focus on Children and Adolescents. Available at: http://www.uspreventiveservicestaskforce.org/tfchildcat.htm. Accessed April 13, 2015

6. Gulick LH, Ayers LP. *Medical Inspection of the Schools*, 2nd ed. New York, NY: Survey Associates/Russell Sage Foundation; 1913

7. American College of Allergy, Asthma and Immunology. ACAAI asthma and allergy screening information. Available at: http://www.acaai.org/allergist/asthma/screening-for-asthma/Pages/default.aspx. Accessed April 13, 2015

8. Galant SP, Crawford LJ, Morphew T, Jones CA, Bassin S. Predictive value of a cross-cultural asthma case-detection tool in an elementary school population. *Pediatrics*. 2004;114(3):e307–316

9. Yawn BP. Asthma screening, case identification and treatment in school-based programs. *Curr Opin Pulm Med*. 2006;12(1):23–27

10. Gerald LB, Grad R, Turner-Henson A, et al. Validation of a multistage asthma case-detection procedure for elementary school children. *Pediatrics*. 2004;114(4):e459–468

11. Gerald JK, Grad R, Bailey WC, Gerald LB. Cost-effectiveness of school-based asthma screening in an urban setting. *J Allergy Clin Immunol*. 2010;125(3):643–650, 650.e1–650.e12

12. Yawn BP, Wollan P, Scanlon P, Kurland M. Are we ready for universal school-based asthma screening? An outcomes evaluation. *Arch Pediatr Adolesc Med*. 2002;156(12):1256–1262

13. Gerald LB, Sockrider MM, Grad R, et al. An official ATS workshop report: issues in screening for asthma in children. *Proc Am Thorac Soc*. 2007;4(2):133–141

14. Association of State and Territorial Dental Directors. State Laws on Dental "Screening" for School-Aged Children. Available at: http://www.astdd.org/docs/final-school-screening-paper-10-14-08.pdf. Accessed April 13, 2015

15. Cunningham CJ, Elton R, Topping GV. A randomised control trial of the effectiveness of personalised letters sent subsequent to school dental inspections in increasing registration in unregistered children. *BMC Oral Health*. 2009:12(9):8

16. Milsom K, Blinkhorn A, Worthington H, et al. The effectiveness of school dental screening: a cluster-randomized control trial. *J Dent Res*. 2006;85(10):924–928

17. Weist MD, Rubin M, Moore E, Adelsheim S, Wrobel G. Mental health screening in schools. *J Sch Health*. 2007;77(2):53–58

18. Kuo E, Vander Stoep A, McCauley E, Kernic MA. Cost-effectiveness of a school-based emotional health screening program. *J Sch Health*. 2009;79(6):277-285

19. Center for Mental Health in Schools at UCLA. Screening Mental Health Problems in Schools. Available at: http://smhp.psych.ucla.edu/pdfdocs/policyissues/mhscreeningissues.pdf. Accessed April 13, 2015

20. US Preventive Services Task Force. Screening for Major Depressive Disorder in Children and Adolescents. March 2009. Available at: http://www.uspreventiveservicestaskforce.org/uspstf/uspschdepr.htm. Accessed April 13, 2015

21. US Preventive Services Task Force. Screening for Suicide Risk. May 2014. Available at: http://www.uspreventiveservicestaskforce.org/uspstf/uspssuic.htm. Accessed April 13, 2015

22. US Preventive Services Task Force. Universal Screening for Hearing Loss in Newborns. July 2008. Available at: http://www.uspreventiveservicestaskforce.org/uspstf/uspsnbhr.htm. Accessed April 13, 2015

23. Centers for Disease Control and Prevention. School health guidelines to promote healthy eating and physical activity. *MMWR Recomm Rep.* 2011;60(RR-5):1–76

24. US Preventive Services Task Force. Screening for Idiopathic Scoliosis in Adolescents. June 2004. Available at: http://www.uspreventiveservicestaskforce.org/uspstf/uspsaisc.htm. Accessed April 13, 2015

25. Washington State Board of Health. Scoliosis screening — school districts, repealing chapter due to passage of HB 1322 (chapter 41, Laws of 2009). Schools will no longer be required to screen students for scoliosis annually in grades five, seven, and nine. WSR 09-24-112 (2010). Available at: http://apps.leg.wa.gov/documents/laws/wsr/2009/24/09-24-112.htm. Accessed April 13, 2015

26. The Center for Health and Healthcare in Schools. The Maryland story: how one state is ending scoliosis screening. Available at: http://www.healthinschools.org/News-Room/EJournals/Volume-7/Number-4/The-Maryland-Story.aspx. Accessed April 13, 2015

27. Chou R, Dana T, Bougatsos C. Screening for visual impairment in children ages 1–5 years: update for the USPSTF. *Pediatrics.* 2011;127(2):e442–e479. Available at: http://www.uspreventiveservicestaskforce.org/uspstf11/vischildren/vischildart.pdf. Accessed April 13, 2015

SECTION 2

School-Based Health Centers

Veda C. Johnson, MD, FAAP
Yuri Okuizumi-Wu, MD

Background

Comprehensive school-based health centers (SBHCs) are primary care medical centers that combine medical care with preventive and psychosocial services as well as organize broader school-based and community-based health promotion efforts. SBHCs serve multiple roles in the health care system for children and youth. For some, SBHCs function as a gateway to the health care system. For others, SBHCs work in conjunction with their medical home to assist with chronic disease management and to address acute care needs that occur during the school day. For many underserved, at-risk children and adolescents, SBHCs may be the sole source of coordinated, comprehensive, and culturally appropriate primary care, emotional and academic support, and professional advocacy.

> SBHCs provide a sense of security to parents, who rest assured in the knowledge that their child's health care is covered at no or low cost; to school leaders, who recognize that prompt attention to student illness means a faster return to the classroom; and to employers, who appreciate that employee productivity is affected when they are unable to attend to their sick children.

This model of health care delivery has been recognized as an effective means of providing quality health care for children that can significantly reduce barriers to health care for those living in poor communities.[1-3] The barriers of accessibility, affordability, fragmentation of care, and lack of transportation along with the lack of knowledge around how to manage one's health and when to access health care are readily addressed through SBHCs. Being located where children are, providing care irrespective of the patient's ability to pay, and providing care in a coordinated, integrated system in which all providers are operating under the same roof and in constant communication with one another makes SBHCs an ideal model for addressing the complex needs of underserved children and adolescents.

The number of comprehensive SBHCs has increased significantly over the past 15 years. Nationally, the number of comprehensive SBHCs has increased by 230% since 1994, with the latest National Census of SBHCs reporting a total of approximately 2000 SBHCs operating throughout the country. These SBHCs are operating in 48 states/territories in the United States, with 57% located in urban communities, 16% in suburban communities, and 27% in rural communities. Thirty-three percent of SBHCs are located in high schools, 24% are located in elementary or middle schools, and 43% are located in alternative schools or schools with a combination of grade levels.[4]

The initial impetus behind the development of SBHCs was to increase access to health care for adolescents, for whom access was often limited by finance, confidentiality issues, and decreased parental involvement.[1,5,6] Therefore, the majority of health clinics were developed for high school and middle school students. Elementary SBHCs have been on the rise, in part because of the perception that the problems identified at the high school and middle school levels could likely be diminished with early detection and intervention at lower grade levels.[7]

In addition to increasing access to quality health care, SBHCs provide a sense of security to parents, who rest assured in the knowledge that their child's health care is covered at no or low cost; to school leaders, who recognize that prompt attention to student illness means a faster return to the classroom; and to employers, who appreciate that employee productivity is affected when they are unable to attend to their sick children. SBHCs also provide a savings to the public by reducing inappropriate emergency department use among children and adolescents.[8-10]

Although SBHCs may vary on the basis of community need and resources, according to the School–Based Health Alliance (formerly known as the National Assembly on School-Based Health Care), the basic tenets of SBHCs are that they:

- are located in schools or on school grounds and work within the school to become a part of the school (some are also mobile programs that rotate a health care team through multiple schools);
- provide a comprehensive range of services that address the physical and behavioral health needs of students;
- employ a multidisciplinary team of providers to care for the students (ie, nurse practitioners, nurses, social workers, physicians, etc);
- provide clinical services through a qualified health provider, such as a hospital, health department, or medical practice;
- require parents to sign written consents for their children to receive services; and
- have an advisory board consisting of community representatives, parents, and youth to provide planning and oversight.

Services Provided by SBHCs

The services provided by the SBHC complement and expand the work of the school nurse. The health center staffed by an advanced medical provider (ie, nurse practitioner, physician assistant, physician, etc), social worker/mental health provider, and medical assistant in conjunction with the school nurse, along with a fully outfitted clinic space (ie, examination rooms, laboratory, etc), can provide services similar to that offered in a typical doctor's office. In addition, the SBHC staff serves as a resource for school-wide health promotion efforts and often provides wellness support for school administrators, teachers, and other school personnel.

SBHCs offer a variety of services that range from basic primary care to primary care-mental health to a primary care-mental health plus model. According to the 2007-2008 National School-Based Health Care census, 25% of SBHCs operate under the primary care model, 40% operate under the primary care-mental health model, and 35% operate under the primary care-mental health plus model.[4]

> SBHC staff serves as a resource for school-wide health promotion efforts and often provides wellness support for school administrators, teachers, and other school personnel.

In the primary care model, the clinics are staffed by a nurse practitioner or physician assistant with physician oversight and offer a scope of services that covers the spectrum of pediatric care, from diagnosis and treatment of acute and chronic illnesses to reproductive health counseling and management (Table 3.2.1). Depending on the resources within the community, radiological services, expanded laboratory services, as well as emergency treatment can be provided through local hospitals and community health centers.

For the primary care-mental health model, in addition to the primary care model the scope of services include comprehensive mental health services (Table 3.2.2). These services are provided on-site by SBHC staff (eg, licensed

---

Table 3.2.1.

Scope of Services for School-Based Health Centers
Primary Care Model

- Diagnosis and treatment of acute and chronic illnesses and minor injuries
- Routine health and sports physicals
- Health check (Early and Periodic Screening, Diagnosis, and Treatment) screenings/immunizations
- Vision, hearing, and dental screenings
- Laboratory testing
- Nutritional counseling
- Prescriptions for medications
- Anticipatory guidance
- Risk assessments (middle childhood through adolescence)
- Sexually transmitted disease education, screenings, treatment, and counseling (where appropriate)

Table 3.2.2.

Scope of Services for School-Based Health Centers
Primary Care-Mental Health Model

- Primary care services
- Mental/behavioral health
  - Screenings/counseling/medical management
- Substance abuse
  - Screenings/counseling/medical management
- Referrals
  - Management of complex disorders
  - Psychoeducational testing
  - Emergency treatment/hospitalization

clinical social worker, psychologist, substance abuse counselor, etc) or through collaborations with local mental health organizations and providers.

The primary care-mental health plus models expands the primary care-mental health services model to include patient case management, health education (ie, personal hygiene, chronic disease management, substance abuse, violence prevention, self-esteem, safety, etc) and expanded nutritional counseling. It is the most comprehensive SBHC model.

Oral health and reproductive health are additional services offered to varying degrees throughout the 3 SBHC models. A majority of SBHCs offer oral health education and screenings (84% and 57%, respectively), but only 12% have a dental provider on staff. Reproductive health services are primarily offered in middle and high school clinics. Approximately 84% of SBHCS offer abstinence counseling, 68% offer treatment and screening for sexually transmitted infections, and 81% provide pregnancy testing.

Finally, the SBHC staff serves as a resource for school-wide health promotion efforts and often provides wellness support for school administrators, teachers, and other school personnel. In effect, this promotes the basic tenets of the Coordinated School Health Program model developed by the Division of Adolescent School Health of the Centers for Disease Control and Prevention. This program is a coordinated approach to school health that creates a system of care that addresses the needs of the whole child by connecting health with education. It also creates a school environment that promotes and supports healthy lifestyles for students, teachers, and staff. The coordinated school health program model has 8 components that include: health education, physical education, health services, staff wellness, nutrition services, family and community involvement, mental health and social services, and healthy school environment.[11] A systematic review of the literature evaluating the impact of coordinated school health programs on academic achievement revealed positive outcomes for children with asthma when health education and parental involvement were incorporated into the management of these students. It was concluded that school health programs "hold promise for improving academic outcomes for children."[12]

> There is significant evidence in the literature to support the role of SBHCs in increasing access to health care, improving health outcomes and reducing health disparities (ie, mental health, asthma), and reducing medical costs for the most needy children and adolescents in our nation.

Effectiveness of School-Based Health Centers in Improving Health Outcomes and Reducing Costs to the Health System

There is significant evidence in the literature to support the role of SBHCs in increasing access to health care, improving health outcomes and reducing health disparities (ie, mental health, asthma), and reducing medical costs for the most needy children and adolescents in our nation. A study conducted by Mathematica Policy Research found a significant increase in health care access by students who used school-based health centers.[13] Studies conducted by Emory University School of Medicine and Public Health, Johns Hopkins University, University of Cincinnati Medical College of Pharmacy, and Montefiore Medical Center demonstrated improved health outcomes for SBHC students with asthma, as reflected in decreased emergency department use and hospitalizations.[8–10,14] Improved use of peak flow meters and inhaled steroids and compliance with asthma action plans resulting in a significant decrease in hospitalizations was noted after the implementation of SBHC asthma detection and intervention program in Minneapolis, Minnesota.[13] In a study conducted by the University of Colorado and published in the Archives for Adolescent Medicine, it was found that adolescents who had access to SBHCs were 10 times more likely to have mental health and substance abuse visits than those who did not have access to SBHCs.[15] In a follow-up study, it was found that inner-city youth were 21 times more likely to make mental health visits at the SBHC than at the community health center.[16]

In regards to the effect of SBHCs on the cost of health care, research conducted by Emory University, Johns Hopkins University, and University of Cincinnati Medical College of Pharmacy demonstrated significant cost savings for SBHCs attributed to decreased emergency department use and hospitalizations.[8–10] Additional studies by University of Kentucky College of Medicine and the Medical Center of South Carolina validated the findings of reduced emergency department use for students enrolled in SBHCs.[17,18] Cost savings attributed to decreased prescription drug use also were noted in studies by Emory University and University of Cincinnati.

School systems and individual schools offer various opportunities for medical providers to become involved in school health programs.

Finally, researchers at the University of Cincinnati Medical College of Pharmacy were able to demonstrate cost savings from SBHCs attributed to reduced parental productivity losses.[19] It was projected that SBHCs in Cincinnati prevented parental productivity losses by an estimated $540,000 to $1,085,000 over a 3-year period.

Research on the impact of SBHCs on school attendance has demonstrated positive outcomes. Reduced absenteeism was noted for SBHCs enrollees as compared with students not enrolled in SBHCs in studies conducted by Harvard Medical School, and a report by the Dallas Youth and Family Centers revealed that SBHCs contributed to a 50% decrease in absences among students who had 3 or more absences in a 6-week period.[20] The same report revealed that students who received mental health services had an 85% decrease in school discipline referrals. Finally, researchers at Montefiore Medical Center found that SBHCs decreased hospitalizations and absenteeism for students with asthma.[14]

How to Work With Schools

School systems and individual schools offer various opportunities for medical providers to become involved in school health programs. From serving on state and district school boards to providing direct services as a "school physician" or through SBHCs to participating in local school health advisory councils, pediatricians can provide expertise and advocacy toward improving student health. In particular, student health services and school wellness programs are charged with developing policies and procedures that address the mental, physical, and emotional health needs of its students. These initiatives could benefit from community physicians' guidance and oversight. Finally, pediatricians can work with schools to support and promote national and state programs (ie, Race to the Top; a contest created by the US Department of Education to spur innovation and reforms in state and local district K-12 education) that support student achievement through community partnerships that improve overall student well-being.[21]

> Pediatricians can become a crucial link between the SBHC and the community.

Recommendations for Pediatricians

Because school is where children spend a large majority of their time daily, SBHCs offer an opportunity for pediatricians to extend themselves beyond the boundaries of their offices and transform their approach to provide care in the context of the children's developmental, psychological, social, intellectual, and physical needs. SBHCs also allow pediatricians and other health care providers the ability to increase patient access to health care, especially for underserved, at-risk children and adolescents. Pediatricians can participate directly in the care of these patients either through on-site services or through the use of telemedicine. Beyond working directly in a SBHC, pediatricians can become involved in school-based health by volunteering their time to work as a consultant to the school, assist with health education of students, provide in-service training of school staff on relevant health topics, directly communicate with schools on a specific student's medical condition, or advocate for patients through activities such as being members of school advisory councils and school boards. Additionally, pediatricians can further promote wellness for students as well as school staff by providing guidance on school nutrition, helping to develop/implement emergency medical plans, and advocating for educational services and an optimal school environment.[22]

Pediatricians can become a crucial link between the SBHC and the community. Health care providers working in SBHCs should integrate and coordinate with other pediatric medical home practices in the community to ensure that care is not fragmented or competes with other providers. Likewise, community pediatricians should also be aware of the SBHC model to collaborate efficiently with SBHC providers to ensure patients have an appropriate medical home and further advocate for SBHC as an effective model of increasing access to quality health care. Community pediatricians with expertise in implementing the medical home model can also assist SBHCs in their efforts to establish themselves as a medical home.[23]

> It has been demonstrated that when residents are exposed to school health during residency, there is an increased likelihood that they will become involved in school health later in their practice.[25]

Recommendations for Program Directors and Trainees

Schools are unique sites that are ideal for resident training.[3] Core concepts, such as health promotion/risk reduction, interdisciplinary collaboration, and cross-cultural competency, can be explored during rotations in an SBHC and can contribute to fulfilling the requirements proposed by the Accreditation Council for Graduate Medical Education (ACGME) for graduate medical education programs.[24] Working first-hand with children in their daily environment will greatly enhance the trainee's understanding of children's growth and development as a significant contributor to their general well-being. Practical information on individualized education programs (IEPs)/Section 504 plans or the logistics of administering medication at school are important concepts that are not routinely covered in a traditional clinic setting. In addition, it has been demonstrated that when residents are exposed to school health during residency, there is an increased likelihood that they will become involved in school health later in their practice.[25]

Given that SBHCs are primarily located in underserved communities, these sites can serve as a valuable training venue to expose residents and other trainees to the value of providing medical care to at-risk patients in the context of the social determinants of health. The SBHC can serve as a site for weekly continuity clinics as well as required rotations in adolescent pediatrics, community pediatrics, developmental pediatrics, sports medicine, mental health, oral health, asthma and allergy, public health, rural health, and patient advocacy.

The SBHC rotation can enhance the residents' interprofessional exposure to other disciplines (the school staff) and other trainees in the context of improving residents' "systems-based practice competency," among others, such as professionalism and communication skills. SBHCs can also serve as a site where residents and fellows in developmental behavioral pediatrics and adolescent medicine can conduct their ACGME-required quality improvement projects. In addition, SBHCs can serve as training site for pediatric fellows whose areas of focus addresses the most prevalent disorders of childhood (ie, asthma and obesity).

If a rotation or elective cannot be solely dedicated to school-based health, integrating experience in a SBHC within another rotation in these other areas may be possible. Another way to integrate school health may be to cover specific school health issues during every rotation, such as communicable diseases in the school setting during an infectious diseases rotation, or reviewing contraindications to sports participation in a cardiology rotation, or evaluating the school's nutrition and physical education programs during an endocrine elective.

Regardless of whether a trainee eventually pursues a career in primary care or a pediatric subspecialty, all providers working with children can benefit by their experience in a SBHC.

Finally, SBHCs can serve as a venue for extracurricular activities for residents and medical students. Through an "adopt-a-school" or after-school program, they can serve as a resource to enhance the overall health and well-being of the student. They can collaborate with the staff of the SBHC to advance student academic achievement through after-hour tutoring and academic support programs, increase student exposure to the medical profession by participating in career day events and conducting field trips to medical schools and health clinics, and enhance student self-worth by participating in mentoring and self-empowerment programs (ie, Cool Girls [**www.thecoolgirls.org**]).

Take-Home Points

- Comprehensive SBHCs are primary care medical centers that combine medical care with preventive and psychosocial services.
- SBHCs increase access to quality health care and decrease health care disparities among minorities and underserved youth.
- The services provided by the SBHC complement and expand the work of the school nurse.
- SBHCs are ideal places to effectively manage chronic conditions such as asthma, diabetes, and obesity.
- The basic tenets of the Coordinated School Health Program are fulfilled through the SBHC model.
- Pediatricians can provide leadership to school health programs and serve as an important liaison between SBHCs and the community.
- SBHCs are ideal settings for resident and medical student training.

Resources
For additional school health related resources, visit www.aap.org/schoolhealthmanual.

References

1. Brindis CD, Sanghvi RV. School-based health clinics: remaining viable in a changing health care delivery system. *Annu Rev Public Health*. 1997;18:567–587
2. Brindis CD, Klein J, Schlitt J, et al. School-based health centers: accessibility and accountability. *J Adol Health*. 2003;32(6 Suppl):98–107
3. Fisher M, Juszczak L, Friedman SB, Schneider M, Chapar G. School-based adolescent health care: review of a clinical service. *Am J Dis Child*. 1992;146(5):615–621
4. National Assembly on School-Based Health Care. School-Based Health Centers: National Census School Year 2007-2008. Available at: http://www.nasbhc.org/atf/cf/%7BB241D183-DA6F-443F-9588-3230D027D8DB%7D/NASBHC%202007-08%20CENSUS%20REPORT%20FINAL.PDF. Accessed April 13, 2015
5. Schlitt JJ, Rickett KD, Montgomery LL, Lear JG. State initiatives to support school-based health centers: a national survey. *J Adolesc Health*. 1995;17(2):68–76
6. Kisker EE, Brown RS. Do school-based health centers improve adolescents' access to health care, health status, and risk-takings behavior? *J Adolesc Health*. 1996;18(5):335–343
7. The Center for Health and Health Care in Schools. 2002 State Survey of School-Based Health Center Initiatives. Available at: http://www.healthinschools.org/en/News-Room/Fact-Sheets/SBHC-Initiatives/Survey%20Narrative.aspx. Accessed April 13, 2015
8. Adams EK, Johnson V. An elementary school-based health clinic: can it reduce Medicaid costs? *Pediatrics*. 2000;105(4 Pt 1):780–788
9. Guo JJ, Wade TJ, Pan W, Keller KN. School-based health centers: cost-benefit analysis and Impact on health care disparities. *Am J Public Health*. 2010;100(9):1617-1623
10. Santelli J, Kouzis A, Newcomer S. School-based health centers and adolescent use of primary care and hospital care. *J Adolesc Health*. 1996;19(4):267–275
11. National Center for Chronic Disease Prevention and Health Promotion, Division of Adolescent and School Health. Coordinated School Health. Available at: www.cdc.gov/HealthyYouth/CSHP/. Accessed April 13, 2015
12. Murray NG, Low BJ, Hollis C, Cross, AW, Davis SM. Coordinated school health programs and academic achievement: a systematic review of the literature. *J Sch Health*. 2007;77(9):589–600
13. Lurie N, Bauer EJ, Brady C. Asthma outcomes in an inner-city school-based health center. *J Sch Health*. 2001;71(9):9–16
14. Webber MP, Carpiniello KE, Oruwariye T, et al. Burden of asthma in inner-city elementary schoolchildren: do school-based health centers make a difference? *Arch Pediatr Adolesc Med*. 2003;157(2):125–129
15. Kaplan DW, Calonge BN, Guernsey BP, Hanrahan MB. Managed care and school-based health centers: use of health services. *Arch Pediatr Adolesc Med*. 1998;152(1):25–33
16. Juszczak L, Melinkovich P, Kaplan D. Use of health and mental health services by adolescents across multiple delivery sites. *J Adolesc Health*. 2003;32(6 Suppl):108–118
17. Key JD, Washington EC, Hulsey TC. Reduced emergency department utilization associated with school-based clinic enrollment. *J Adolesc Health*. 2002;30(4):273–278
18. Young TL, D'Angelo SL, Davis J. Impact of a school-based health center on emergency department use by elementary school student. *J Sch Health*. 2001;71(5):196–198
19. Guo JJ, Wade TJ, Pan W, Keller KN. School-based health centers: cost-benefit analysis and impact on health care disparities. *Am J Public Health*. 2010;100(9):1617–1623
20. Hall LS. Dallas Youth and Family Centers Program. *Final Report-Youth and Family Centers 2000-2001*. Publication No. REIS01-172-2. Dallas, TX: Dallas Independent Schools District; 2001

21. US Department of Education. *Race to the Top Program Executive Summary*. Available at: http://www2.ed.gov/programs/racetothetop/executive-summary.pdf. Accessed April 13, 2015

22. Bravender T. School performance: the pediatrician's role. *Clin Pediatr (Phila)*. 2008;(6): 535–545

23. American Academy of Pediatrics, Council on School Health. School-based health centers and pediatric practice. *Pediatrics*. 2012;129(2):387–393

24. Kalet A, Juszczak L, Pastore D, et al. Medical training in school-based health centers: a collaboration among five medical schools. *Acad Med*. 2007;82(5):458–464

25. Nader PR, Broyles SL, Brennan J, Taras H. Two national surveys on pediatric training and activities in school health: 1991 and 2001. *Pediatrics*. 2003;111(4 Pt 1):730–734

Populations With Unique Needs

Jeffrey K. Okamoto, MD, FAAP

Background

All children require the social, physical fitness, and educational benefits of schooling. Youth with special or unique needs are no exception. Physicians and other health professionals should use the experience and expertise known about health issues as they relate to schools. This will help ensure the best health and development for these youth, because many of their waking hours are usually spent in school.

This chapter covers youth with common medical issues that schools often find challenging. In addition, youth with mental health needs are covered in Chapter 6, Section 2, and Chapter 9 covers children of immigrant families as well as homeless youth.

Medication Issues in General

Many youth need the effects of medication during the school day. Some youth need medication for an acute illness requiring short-term treatment, perhaps for a few days. Youth with chronic conditions, such as asthma, diabetes, and attention-deficit/hyperactivity disorder (ADHD) may require treatment for years. Chronic health conditions affect more than 14 million school-aged youth (almost 20% of the school-aged population), with approximately half of these being moderate or severe,[1] so almost all schools will have a number of children requiring medication (see Table 3.3.1 for the prevalence of chronic medical conditions in children).[2] Emergency medications, such as epinephrine for severe allergic reactions, or rescue medication for asthma, require special considerations in the school environment.

For acute conditions, physicians may need to fill out a school form informing the school of the need for medication and how to administer this during the school day. There is information that the school needs to ensure that the medication is given properly. Minimally, this should include the name of the student, the name of the medication, the dose, approximate time it should be taken, the diagnosis or reason for the medication, and authorization signatures of the prescribing professional and parent/guardian. The medication should also be labeled properly (by the pharmacy if a prescription medication) and stored in a secure area so that theft (especially of medications that have "street value") is discouraged. Furthermore, physical conditions for storage of the medication (eg, refrigeration) should be clearly outlined and expiration dates should be checked periodically. Involvement of a licensed pharmacist in developing policies for the school district regarding medication storage and labeling would be optimal.

There are several considerations for more chronic conditions. For a child requiring daily or frequent medication use, the child may be able to take advantage of a long-acting medication, given once in the morning by his parents or guardians, or doses of short-acting medication given before and after school. This is optimal as to eliminate the disruption of administering the medication during the school day and

Table 3.3.1. Prevalence of Chronic Medical Conditions in Children[2]

Condition	Cases per 1000
Asthma	135
Learning disabilities	90
ADHD	78
Anxiety	64
Depression	60
Developmental delay	32
Intellectual disability	12
Congenital heart disorders	9
Autism	6.6
Epilepsy	6.5
Cerebral palsy	3.1
Diabetes	2.2
Juvenile rheumatic diseases	1.5
Spina bifida	0.4
Cystic fibrosis	0.3
Cancer	0.2
Inflammatory bowel disease	0.07
Chronic renal disease	0.07

reduces any stigma from peers or school staff on seeing that the child is "different," requiring medication that others do not get. An example of successful home administration is the use of a once-daily long-acting oral form of stimulant medication for ADHD. However, if medication needs to be administered during the school day, a form (for the school nurse or designated staff) such as that discussed previously for acute conditions is essential.

However, many children require administration of medication intermittently throughout the school day. Optimally, a full-time registered nurse for the school would be responsible for dispensing and/or administering medications.[3] This would be a highly trained person with experience and knowledge of adverse effects and who uses safeguards to prevent any wrongful administration of the medication. They usually have a better understanding of each student's health conditions compared with other school staff. However, most schools have reduced the number of school nurses on staff, and most states do not require a nurse at every school. Health aides, and in some situations non-health room staff, all of who are not nurses, may be delegated by a nurse to administer medication at school during the school day.

> All children require the social, physical fitness, and educational benefits of schooling. Youth with special or unique needs are no exception.

Delegation is a formal and serious responsibility that is covered by professional nursing organization guidelines and state regulations, including nurse practice acts.[3] Delegation of nursing duties, such as medication administration, to unlicensed assistive personnel (UAP) at the school requires ongoing training and supervision by a licensed school or registered nurse, which cannot be done informally. An American Academy of Pediatrics (AAP) policy statement covers delegation in greater detail.[3] There are medical liabilities involved, which should be worked out by schools to protect the nurse and UAP involved. Also, the nurse and others should follow privacy protections of the Health Insurance Portability and Accountability Act (HIPAA) and Family Educational Rights and Privacy Act (FERPA) concerning how information is kept regarding the health information of the student, including diagnoses and medications, and determine which school staff members should know about the student's health problems.

Schools sometimes get requests to administer medications in a nonstandard way or to administer complementary or alternative medicine or experimental treatments. The school nurse (or if available, a school physician) would have expertise that other school staff may not have to determine whether this request should be honored. Local and state policies, if any, regarding such situations, should be followed.[4] There is an obligation to resolve any disagreement with the parent/guardian and prescriber.[3] Consideration of research medications used in clinical trials being given in the school setting should include (1) any specific requirements to administer the medication including protocol information, (2) a summary of the study from the research organization, (3) signed parental and prescribing physician permissions, (4) requirements of reporting including adverse event reporting, and (5) any nursing actions that are required on follow-up.[5]

Over-the-counter (OTC) medications do not require prescriptions, but diligence is necessary surrounding the administration of these in schools. These medications can have harmful effects if given improperly and may not be useful if given for the wrong indication. Therefore, schools should probably require a written form for OTC medication administration and limit the use of these medications, especially if the student only needs them for a short time. Some schools have developed policies or protocols that support verbal parental permission, taking into account the difficulty in parents getting physician authorization, and the advantages of keeping students with mild illnesses in school with the use of OTC medication. However, long-term use of OTC medication in school by a student should spark physician visits to ensure correct diagnosis, the continued efficacy and need for the medication, and to ensure monitoring of adverse effects or any problems with medication administration.

Health care professionals should know the policies and procedures for the schools of the children they are caring for to ensure that medications are administered appropriately. The goals would be to optimize the effect of medications, and to decrease the risk of unnecessary medication use and of adverse effects. Another goal would be ensuring trained people, and not untrained people, are in the position of administering medication for children at school.

However, emergency situations sometimes require non-health staff members to quickly assess the situation and administer medication to decrease the

> Health care professionals should know the policies and procedures for the schools of the children they are caring for to ensure that medications are administered appropriately.

risk of death. These situations carry liability for the school staff, the school, and school boards and districts if dealt with incorrectly or poorly. For children thought to be at risk of a medical emergency at school, several strategies are critical. These are related in the AAP policy statement on administration of medications in schools.[3] Schools need to:

❶ Train, delegate, and supervise appropriate UAP who have the knowledge and skills to administer or assist in the administration of medication to students when assessed to be appropriate by the supervising and delegating licensed registered school nurse or school physician in compliance with applicable state laws and regulations.

❷ Permit responsible students to carry and self-administer emergency medications for conditions authorized by school policies and regulations, which also describe students'/parents' rights and responsibilities.

❸ Provide and encourage parents to provide spare life-saving medications in the health office for students who carry and self-administer emergency medications in the event that the life-saving medication cannot be located when a student is in need of the medicine.

❹ Make provisions for secured and immediate access to emergency medications at school at all times, including before and after school hours, on school buses, and during students' off-campus school-sponsored activities.

State laws and policies may limit or expand the role of staff and students at schools to accomplish these strategies. Health care professionals, especially pediatricians, should provide expertise and advocate for needed policies and procedures regarding these issues. However, health care professionals do need to understand their existing state and local laws and policies around emergency medication in schools.

The subsequent sections in this chapter further elaborate on emergency medications for certain conditions and situations, but medications used in emergencies that particularly require training in administration include:

- autoinjectable epinephrine for serious allergic reactions;
- rectal diazepam for seizures; and
- nebulized or inhaler albuterol for asthma.

In situations involving these medications, as with all medications at the school, a school nurse can be essential in these critical functions[3]:

❶ Proper storage of medication for security and safety considerations. Controlled substances need to be double locked.

❷ Designation, training, and supervision of first responders.

❸ Easy access by responsible staff at the school when children are present.

❹ Ensuring an adequate supply of medication is always available, including during school lock-downs or evacuations.

❺ Ensuring an supply of medication, whether parent/guardian supplied or school supplied.[5]

❻ Assignment of staff that will carry and know how to administer the medication on field trips.

❼ Review and replacement of outdated medication.

❽ Return of unused medication to parents and legal disposal of medication done properly. Unused medications should not be flushed into the water system.

❾ Updating the individualized health care plan, if used by the school, which includes information on medications, activity levels, dietary needs, equipment, transportation, and other accommodations.[5]

There will be situations in which the school will not know that a child will require emergency medication. This should NEVER be secondary to the parents/guardians/medical professional not notifying the school about an important health issue. But sometimes, a situation is the first time that a health issue manifests. An example is a child who is having his or her first anaphylactic reaction. Schools need to consider having a supply of emergency medication for such instances. Such medication can help children with either known or yet to be discovered health issues that becomes an emergency at the school.

How to Work With Schools

❶ Learn about local school nursing services, medication policies and forms, and self-administration procedures.

❷ Understand the process of possible delegation by school nurses or registered nurses in having UAP at schools administer medication in school for your patient and how you, as a pediatrician, can minimize risks if this needs to be done.

❸ Write specific, clear, and detailed instructions on dated, standardized school medication forms.

❹ Carefully assess and declare in writing your recommendation concerning students' self-carrying/self-administration on the basis of your patient demonstrating the appropriate developmental, physical, and intellectual capacity to self-carry and/or self-administer an emergency medication at school.

5 Work with schools to ensure that student attendance does not stop because of concerns about the need for medication.

6 Schools should NOT be in the dark about any student's important health issues. This is especially true if the problem may affect school functioning or cause an emergency at school. Families and pediatricians should work together to ensure that schools know about these health issues and are prepared for likely situations involving the student and their health. In particular, teachers should be aware of all their students in class who have emergency medication and where the medication is kept when the student is in school, including if the student carries the medication.

7 Advocate for improved communication systems among schools, families, and pediatricians that support medication-administration services for students at school.

8 Advocate for improved school medication data collection and reporting by schools and school nurses.

Recommendations for Pediatricians

1 Prescribe medications for administration at school only when necessary. Many short-term and long-term medications can be given before and after school.

2 Ensure that parents and guardians are always part of the discussion in your work with schools. Be "family-centered," because the family is the constant in a child's life.

3 Work with state departments of health and/or education, state and local school boards, and school districts to ensure the development and funding of adequate school health program staffing and sound school medication policies and procedures.

4 Support state laws, regulations, or standards that establish specific policies for the safe and effective administration of medications in schools that apply to all state school districts.

Recommendations for Program Directors and Trainees

1 Medical students and especially resident physicians need practice in working with schools in ensuring youth obtain medication and other important medical supports in school environments. Trainees need practice in communicating with schools such as by using forms for administration of medication in school.

❷ Rotations with school nurses or in a school health office are important opportunities to see the dynamics of how schools handle health requests and information, and the advantages and pitfalls of medication management in schools.

❸ Schools appreciate the advocacy by pediatric residents and medical students to strengthen their policies and procedures around medication administration.

Take-Home Points

▪ Consideration of school staff expertise and experience should inform your use of medication within the school environment for your patients. Be aware that schools do not have physicians or even nurses on site all of the time. Delegation by nurses to UAP is a commonplace practice.

▪ The administration of medications to youth in schools requires expertise, exemplified by school nurses or registered nurses supervising this practice.

References

1. Bethell CD, Kogan MD, Strickland BB, Schor EL, Roberston J, Newacheck PW. A national and state profile of leading health problems and health care quality for US children: key insurance disparities and across-state variations. *Acad Pediatr*. 2011;11(3 Suppl):S22–S33
2. American Academy of Pediatrics. *Developmental and Behavioral Pediatrics*. Voigt RG, Macias MM, Myers SM, eds. Elk Grove Village, IL: American Academy of Pediatrics; 2011:2
3. American Academy of Pediatrics, Council on School Health. Policy statement: guidance for the administration of medication in school. *Pediatrics*. 2009;124(4):1244-1251. Reaffirmed February 2013
4. National Association of School Nurses. Policy Statement: Medication Administration in the School Setting. Silver Spring, MD: National Association of School Nurses; January 2012
5. American Academy of Pediatrics, Council on School Health. Medical emergencies occurring at school. *Pediatrics*. 2008;122(4):887-894. Reaffirmed September 2011

Allergies and Anaphylaxis

The topic of allergies in schools been widely publicized because of the serious consequences from reactions that can occur in a school setting. Some children have severe allergies that lead to significant anaphylaxis and sometimes to death. Response of school staff to such situations are often sensationalized and editorialized, particularly around the school not using auto-injectable epinephrine or not responding in a timely manner.

This section will concentrate on food allergies, as these are particularly common, now estimated to occur in 1 out of every 25 children in school.[1,2] Other allergies of note include insect stings and bites, latex rubber allergy (seen particularly in children exposed to rubber gloves and catheters, such as children with spina bifida), and antibiotic medications. Any of these allergies may lead to anaphylaxis, a release of allergic mediators causing a severe systemic reaction, which may include widespread hives, wheezing, problems breathing and swallowing, a feeling of impending doom, low blood pressure, and unconsciousness. Anaphylaxis can lead to death. Anaphylaxis can rarely be caused by a nonallergic phenomenon such as cold or exercise.

In children, food is the most common cause of anaphylaxis.[1] Sixteen to 18% of children with food allergies have had a reaction in school.[3,4] The most common food allergies accounting for 90% of reactions are milk, eggs, peanuts, tree nuts, fish, shellfish, soy, and wheat.[1] It should be kept in mind that the majority of food-related allergic reactions are not anaphylactic, and death is rare.[2] Deaths are more common in youth with peanut, tree nut, and milk allergies; in teenagers; and in those with asthma. About one quarter of deaths in preschool and school-aged children in the United States occurred in school and usually were related to a delay in giving epinephrine.

Epinephrine is the treatment of choice in severe anaphylaxis. This can be delivered with self-injectable devices, which have a premeasured dose, and which can be administered by nonmedical personnel quickly.

Schools that receive federal funding (the majority of public schools) or any facility open to the public must accommodate children/teenagers with food allergy, which is considered a disability under these laws.

Food allergies are relevant in several laws affecting schools, including Section 504 of the Rehabilitation Act as well as the Americans with Disabilities Act (ADA). Schools that receive federal funding (the majority of public schools) or any facility open to the public must accommodate children/teenagers with food allergy, which is considered a disability under these laws. Accommodations can be formalized in a Section 504 plan (the law prevents discrimination on the basis of disability). A student with allergies can also have accommodations in an individualized education program (IEP) under the Individuals with Disabilities Education Act (IDEA) if the child is in special education.[2]

Pediatricians should be aware of state and local laws and policies regarding allergy management in schools. If these do not exist, pediatricians and other health care providers should contribute to the development of thoughtful and comprehensive policies and laws. Particularly useful is guidance on whether non-patient–specific epinephrine should be stocked at the school with standing orders for nurses to deliver the medication in life-threatening situations.[1,5] This is especially useful for the 25% of students who have anaphylaxis without a previous life-threatening reaction. Having epinephrine in stock at schools is a policy supported by the AAP, the National Association of School Nurses, the American Academy of Asthma Allergy Immunology, and the Food Allergy Anaphylaxis Network.

The overall goals of management in schools around students with food and other allergies are: (1) providing a safe environment; (2) training school staff on allergies and how to respond to anaphylactic events; and (3) planning on supports, including for any emergency that may occur in the school environment.[1]

Planning around a student with food allergies should include the development of an individualized health care plan (IHCP), otherwise known as an individualized school health plan (ISHP) or individualized health plan (IHP). As in the IEP for special education, one plan should not be used for several or all youth who are in similar situations, and each student should have a separate, individualized plan. A school nurse should help develop and implement this plan. Pediatricians and other health professionals who know the child's health situation should assist in the development of the IHCP, especially because orders are usually needed from a physician for several elements, including medication administration.[1] The IHCP should take care of day-to-day care and considerations for a child with a significant allergy to foods or other exposure.[2] Also, because of the risk of anaphylaxis, an emergency action plan (EAP) should be developed.

Issues to be addressed for a student with a food allergy include the following. School, local, and state policy should be followed in problem solving these issues.

❶ Safeguarding the environment
  a. Banning a certain food from school is not recommended.[1]
    i. This provides a false sense of security, as friends and peers may bring to school the food to which the student is allergic. It is impossible to fully control what others bring to school.
    ii. This does not help the youth with allergies learn how to live in a world containing the food to which he/she is allergic.
    iii. Other children in the classroom may be reliant on the nutritional value of the food staple to which a student is allergic.[2]
  b. Teaching the student to avoid foods or other allergens
    i. Staff may need to remove food the allergic child is in Kindergarten or classrooms with children with developmental disabilities if the chance of transfer of food from child to child is high.
  c. The student with food allergy should not be physically separated from other children.[2]
    i. If there will be a separate table with "safe foods," several friends and classmates should also participate at that table.
  d. Children should not be ostracized because of their allergic condition.
  e. If a school or classroom does use avoidance techniques, this needs to be communicated with all staff in contact with the school or classroom.[2]
    i. "No Sharing of Food" policies
    ii. Use of commercially prepared and labeled, individually wrapped food items
    iii. Education of those providing foods regarding safe and unsafe foods and label-reading
    iv. Education of cafeteria/food service staff
    v. A ready supply of safe alternative snacks
    vi. Policies of no eating on the school bus and having a means of communication on the bus

❷ Emergency action plans[2]
  a. The following information should be included:
    i. Child's name
    ii. Identifying information (picture may be helpful)
    iii. Contact information for family
    iv. Specifics about the food allergy including symptoms
    v. Treatments for particular scenarios

      vi. Instructions to activate emergency medical services (EMS). Contact with a food can cause a biphasic reaction, with a second reaction hours after the initial reaction, or rebound after treatment with epinephrine. 911 and activation of EMS is necessary after use of epinephrine because of these issues. Twenty percent of people who receive epinephrine have such a secondary reaction.[2]

      vii. If a student is supine during treatment for a reaction, both school staff and EMS needs to be careful about not raising the student to the upright position because of the possibility of "empty-ventricle syndrome" which occurs with pooling of blood into the lower extremities in anaphylaxis.[2]

  b. Who will be carrying out this plan? Is there a nurse located at the school versus a nonlicensed medical aide or assistant?[2]

      i. Some school personnel cannot make a medical/nursing assessment and gauge which treatment is appropriate (antihistamine versus epinephrine, for example). In these cases, using epinephrine and calling EMS may be the plan when a child is symptomatic.

      ii. A simple means to instruct when epinephrine should be administered is to suggest that it be injected for significant respiratory (eg, tightness of the throat, hacking cough, hoarseness, shortness of breath, wheezing, etc) or cardiovascular symptoms (eg, paleness, blue skin tone, decreased consciousness/confusion, poor pulses, etc) or if there is progression of symptoms or involvement of more than 1 organ system (eg, more than a few hives).

      iii. Coaches, field trip supervisors, specialty or substitute teachers, after-school advisers, and others involved with the student require training on the emergency action plan.

      iv. Schools need to consider a system to ensure that epinephrine, both for the school in general and for a particular student, does not expire.

❸ Will the student carry epinephrine and self-administer if needed?

  a. This is dependent on the student's developmental level and skills, parental considerations, and the school situation as well as legal issues in the state or locality.

  b. If self-administration will occur, the student needs to be taught how to properly store and administer the medication.

  c. Designated school staff should still be trained to administer medication in case the student is not able to do so with a severe reaction.

    d. Having the epinephrine available in more than the health room or cafeteria is critical for quick response to an allergic reaction; therefore, methods for the student to have this nearby, wherever he or she is, needs to be considered.

4 School staff

    a. School staff need to be trained in

        i. Awareness of food allergy in youth

        ii. Signs and symptoms of allergic reactions

        iii. Prevention of food allergic reactions

        iv. Treatment of allergic reactions

    b. Education on recognition and management of allergic reactions must be routine. This education should include staff members who are involved in both school activities and extra-curricular activities and other activities related to the school, on or off the school grounds. Field trips and sports events outside the school grounds are possible situations where allergic reactions may occur. The National Association of School Nurses suggests this be at least annually.[1]

    c. Communication is paramount. Teachers, physical education teachers/coaches, school bus drivers, and playground supervisors need to be aware of students who have food allergies and have access to EAPs.

    d. Schools should establish overall emergency plans for allergic reaction, to include delineation of personnel responsible to remain with the student, those who are to activate the EMS system (call 911) and those whose job it is to contact the parent(s).

5 Working with parents and guardians

    a. Parents/guardians may fear school attendance because of the risk of contact with the food to which the student is allergic.[6]

    b. Parents should consider having their child with a significant allergy wear medical information jewelry.

School nurses are key to development of the IHCP and EAP for a student with significant food allergies. School nurses are usually the most educated and skilled school staff member, short of having a school-based physician, which most school districts do not have. Also, immediate treatment and the creation of an EAP are more likely when a school nurse is involved.[7]

How to Work With Schools

Please see the guidance in the AAP clinical report "Management of Food Allergy in the School Setting" for many important strategies for supporting children with allergies in schools.[2]

1 Support the creation of evidence-based policies and procedures for schools and school districts around allergy and anaphylaxis management in schools.

2 Help your patients' family and their schools draft and finalize an emergency care plan for a child at risk of a life-threatening allergic reaction in school.

3 Support the creation of an IHCP, otherwise known as an ISHP or individualized IHP for a child with food or other allergies.

4 Supply the school with a list of foods to be avoided and possible safe substitutions that can be used.

Recommendations for Pediatricians

The AAP clinical report "Management of Food Allergy in the School Setting" contains the following guidance:

1 Pediatricians and other health professionals need to evaluate when a child or teenager has an allergy that can lead to anaphylaxis. This may need to be done in conjunction with a pediatric allergist, who may want to perform physician-supervised oral food-challenge testing. Information from the clinical history, laboratory and skin testing, and any examination findings after reaction need to be synthesized to determine whether a child/teenager has a possibly life-threatening food allergy condition. Although any food can elicit a serious reaction, certain foods such as peanuts and other nuts, milk, seafood such as fish and shellfish, egg, soy, wheat, and seeds (such as sesame) particularly are associated with significant reactions. A past history of allergic reactions, and other conditions such as asthma, should be factored into the risk of future anaphylaxis.

2 Prescriptions for self-injectable epinephrine should be written for school (in addition to home). There should be considerations of how many auto-injectors to have for the school and whether to have one for the student to carry and one to be stored in the health room. Also, pediatricians need to recognize self-injectable epinephrine devices have expiration dates and remind parents to obtain new prescriptions regularly.

3 Pediatricians should work with parents who fear school attendance secondary to fears of allergic reactions in school. Pediatricians should help parents work together with schools so that their children will be safe even with their allergies and will also get the benefits of being in school. Pediatricians, other medical professionals, and families need to work together to determine the level of exposure that might be dangerous for a particular student (ingesting, smelling, and/or touching the allergen) to have an appropriate level of vigilance by family members, school personnel, and others.

Recommendations for Program Directors and Trainees

❶ Pediatric residents should have opportunities to assist in the development of IHCPs and EAPs for youth with significant allergic reactions. This can be done in a rotation at the health office at the school or in a school health rotation.

❷ The topic of allergies in school could potentially be a great topic for a resident quality improvement project.

Take-Home Points

❶ Pediatricians and other health care professionals need to ensure that parents and schools work together to have students with significant food and other allergies reap the benefits of school environments while being safe.

❷ Advance planning for children with known allergies to food or other materials enable appropriate support by school personnel. This includes teaching the child to avoid allergens; training appropriate school staff, including those in contact with the child, about allergies and responding to allergic reactions; and having appropriate medications available in all situations in which the student participates.

References

1. National Association of School Nurses. Position Statement: Allergy/Anaphylaxis Management in the School Setting. Silver Spring, MD: National Association of School Nurses; June 2012

2. Sicherer SH, Mahr T; American Academy of Pediatrics, Section on Allergy and Immunology. Clinical report—management of food allergy in the school setting. *Pediatrics*. 2010;126(6):1232-1239

3. Nowak-Wegrzyn A, Conover-Walker MK, Wood RA. Food-allergic reactions in schools and preschools. *Arch Pediatr Adolesc Med*. 2001;155(7):790–795

4. Sicherer SH, Furlong TJ, DeSimone J, Sampson HA. The US Peanut and Tree Nut Allergy Registry: characteristics of reactions in schools and daycare. *J Pediatr*. 2001;138(4):560–565

5. National Association of School Nurses. Board Statement: Non-Patient Specific Epinephrine in the School Setting. Silver Spring, MD: National Association of School Nurses; January 2011

6. Roy KM, Roberts MC. Peanut allergy in children: relationships to health-related quality of life, anxiety and parental stress. *Clin Pediatr*. 2011;50(11):1045-1051

7. Greenhawt M, McMorris MS, Furlong TJ. Self-reported allergic reactions to peanuts and tree nuts occurring in schools and child care facilities. *J Allergy Clin Immunol*. 2008;121(2):S95

Asthma

· · · · · · · ·

Asthma is the leading chronic illness among children and adolescents in the United States. Approximately 10% of all children in school have asthma.[1] Unfortunately, asthma causes much school absenteeism, leading to an average of 10.5 million missed school days each year. There is also a disproportionately higher percentage of asthma in children from low-income, inner-city environments. In comparison to the general population, these children are also more likely to visit the emergency department, be hospitalized, or die from their asthma.

Asthma is a chronic condition in which bronchoconstriction and inflammation of small airways leads to wheezing, cough, and respiratory distress. Children with asthma still die in the United States because of inadequate treatment, the severity of asthma exacerbations, or both. A strong collaboration between parents, schools, and health care professionals can help ensure that each student who suffers with asthma is provided with the healthiest learning environment possible.

A strong partnership between school and health care provider can also help ensure that schools have an adequate understanding of asthma and its many medications. Medication management can include short-term and long-term medication, and there are a variety of routes of administration. Depending on the frequency and severity of a student's asthma and the student's ability to take medication, medications are individualized for each student. Some students require episodic relief medications that are hand held and used only for symptomatic relief. Some students are on longer-term medications taken orally and inhaled, with additional medication used over and above these if the student has more severe symptoms. Although these are individualized, pediatricians and other health care providers have many guidelines to inform appropriate care to decrease morbidity and mortality in this population. Descriptions of the different medications and their use are beyond the scope of this section but can be found in many references and guidelines. One metric of optimal treatment is not having limitations in school or exercise.[2]

Pediatricians should be aware of state and local laws and policies regarding asthma management in schools. Particularly useful is guidance on whether asthma medications can be carried and self-administered by a student. Ways schools can strengthen the support of their students with asthma include:

❶ Establishing strong links with asthma care professionals, including pediatricians, to ensure appropriate and ongoing medical care.

❷ Targeting students who are the most affected by asthma at school to identify and intervene with those in greatest need.

③ Building a team of enthusiastic staff in school, including a full-time school nurse, to support programs for children with asthma.

④ Using a coordinated, multicomponent, and collaborative approach that includes school health services, including the school nurse and school-based physicians if available, asthma education for students, and professional development for school staff.

⑤ Tracking the outcomes of students with asthma using appropriate measures (see goals of supports stated later in this section).

Issues that need to be considered in the school environment include:

① Safeguarding the environment[3,4] which can affect how asthma manifests in youth in schools.

   a. Are the school building, buses and other transportation for students, and school activities, including sport events, tobacco smoke free? Also, buses should be encouraged to turn the engine off, helping to reduce fume exposure, when parked in front of the schools.

   b. Does the school help to reduce or prevent students' contact with allergens or irritants, indoors and outdoors, that can make their asthma worse? Allergens and irritants include mold, dust mites, cockroaches, and strong odors or fumes from things like bug spray, paint, perfumes, and cleaners. Does the school exclude animals with fur or feathers?

② Will the student carry and use his or her own medications?

   a. If not, is there ready access to medications?

   b. Will the child use an inhaler? Some inhalers should be used with spacers (with face mask for younger ages).

③ Emergency action plans (EAPs)

   a. In an emergency, such as fire or extreme weather, or if a student forgets his or her medicine, are there medication and standing orders to use these?[3]

   b. What school personnel will be following the emergency action plan if not a school nurse? Is the plan appropriate for the level of training of these school staff?[3] Teachers and physical education teachers/coaches should be aware of children with asthma in their classrooms. Parents and their children's health care providers should work to make school staff in contact with their child aware that the child has asthma and educate them on what the plan is for any worsening of the asthma.

   c. Are medications available for school use? What is the mechanism for refilling prescriptions and obtaining medications when supplies run low?

d. How will the parent be notified when a student has an asthma attack and who will be responsible for notification? Not every student who has an asthma attack needs to be sent home or to the emergency department. Many times, the child will have a good response to treatment and be able to go back to class. However, the parent (and health care provider, if possible) still needs to be notified.

❹ Sports and physical education

a. Does the student have exercise-induced asthma?

i. Who will supervise the student with asthma during these times?

b. Will the student self-administer medication prior, during, or after these activities?

c. Are there alternate activities if a sports activity is contraindicated that will allow the child to remain involved? Will the student have issues with their grade or teasing/bullying about engaging in alternate activities?

❺ Training in the school

a. Who will train staff and students about asthma, and will a student who is having an asthma attack be supported? Is the school nurse or someone else doing the training?

b. All those who are responsible for students should be trained, and it should not be assumed that there will be a school nurse available.

c. Parents have related being worried about not having a full-time school nurse and having anxiety with nonmedical school personnel supervising care and administering medications for their child one with asthma.[5] A few parents believed their child knew more about administering medications than the school personnel.

❻ Emergency preparedness of a school[6]

a. Determine whether the school has:

i. Nebulizers on campus

ii. Spacer devices, which are helpful for students using hand-held inhaler medications that are more effective with spacer devices.

iii. Peak flow meters

iv. Self-injectable epinephrine

v. Oxygen (rural programs were more likely to have this and self-injectable epinephrine)

vi. An asthma EAP for every child with asthma

vii. A plan for dealing with respiratory emergencies, including delineated roles for personnel: who stays with the student, who activates the emergency medical services (EMS) system (calls 911), who contacts the parent(s)

The goal of supports for students with asthma include students: (1) being free from asthma symptoms without coughing, wheezing, problems breathing, or chest tightness or at most having only minor symptoms; (2) being able to go to school every day; (3) not missing class time; (4) being able to participate fully in school activities, including play and sports activities; (5) having no adverse effects from medications; and (6) having no emergency department visits or hospitalizations.

There are a plethora of model asthma education programs. These vary in the age of the students targeted (elementary through high school), whether all students versus only those identified with asthma are targeted, who the person leading the teaching is (volunteer, school nurse, classroom teacher), and teaching techniques used (structured program, computer program). It is clear that families, students, and school staff need to learn about asthma but also that pediatricians and other health care providers need to prescribe the correct medications and provide solid evidence-based medical care.[7] Implementing evidence-based clinic practice guidelines for asthma has demonstrated effectiveness. There have been multiple programs showing an improvement in asthma skills and knowledge and sometime outcomes, but these are dependent on students and school staff participation in some programs and on physician participation in others.[7]

School-supervised care has been shown to improve asthma control in several studies.[8] Nonadherence to asthma therapy can be improved with school staff routinely observing the child taking medication. This is because there is an average minimum of 180 school days per year. Also, asthma exacerbations occur seasonally and during the school year. Lastly, schools are natural environments for youth to be educated on health and illness.[8]

Be knowledgeable about state laws and school policies concerning asthma care at school, accommodations under Section 504 of the Rehabilitation Act of 1973, and availability of rescue medication, including "self-carry" policies.

How to Work With Schools

There are multiple ways for pediatricians to be involved with schools in support of children with asthma:

1. Share information about the child's asthma with the school with permission from the parents/guardians, especially in high-risk severe cases, but in all cases no matter the frequency and severity.

2. Share written asthma EAPs for your patients with the school nurse. This allows the nurse to provide individual education for your patient by discussing and reinforcing the plan with the student.[7]

3. Support asthma education at schools that your patients attend. Partner with school nurses in teaching asthma classes.

4. Be knowledgeable about state laws and school policies concerning asthma care at school, accommodations under Section 504 of the Rehabilitation Act of 1973, and availability of rescue medication, including "self-carry" policies.

5. Advocate at the state level for full-time school nurses and asthma education in all your schools.

6. Advocate for changes in school policy to allow children to self-carry their own medications. For older children and adolescents, this is an important step to encourage them to progressively manage their own disease.[5]

7. As there are more and more non-medically trained school health staff, they require training, such as in asthma symptoms and responses.[5]

Recommendations for Pediatricians

1. Use community resources, including school-based educational programs, for asthma self-management education of your patients.

2. Pediatricians and parents need to ensure that the school has any medications needed in the care of a student with asthma.

Recommendations for Program Directors and Trainees

1. Medical students and residents can coteach asthma training programs at schools.

2. Pediatric residents should have opportunities to assist in the development of individualized health care plans (IHCPs) and emergency action plans (EAPs) for youth with asthma. This can be done in a rotation at the health office at the school or in a school health rotation.

Take-Home Points

❶ Asthma requires attention for your patients with this chronic condition to attend school regularly.

❷ IHCPs and EAPs are important for your patients to obtain supports at the school to increase school performance and full participation in all activities.

References

1. Centers for Disease Control and Prevention. *Asthma in the US, Growing Every Year. Vital Signs. May 2011.* Available at: http://www.cdc.gov/vitalsigns/Asthma. Accessed April 13, 2015

2. Joint Task Force on Practice Parameters, American Academy of Allergy, Asthma and Immunology; American College of Allergy, Asthma and Immunology; Joint Council of Allergy, Asthma and Immunology. Attaining optimal asthma control: a practice parameter. *J Allergy Clin Immunol.* 2005;116(5):S3-S11

3. National Heart, Lung, and Blood Institute, National Asthma Education and Prevention Program School Asthma Education Subcommittee. How Asthma-Friendly Is Your School? Available at: http://www.nhlbi.nih.gov/health/resources/lung/asthma-friendly-html. Accessed April 13, 2015

4. Lara M, Rosenbaum S, Rachelefsky G, et al. Improving childhood asthma outcomes in the united states: a blueprint for policy action. *Pediatrics.* 2002;109(5):919-930

5. Monsour ME, Lanphear B, DeWitt T. Barriers to asthma care in urban children: parent perspectives. *Pediatrics.* 2000;106(3):512-519

6. Sapien RE. Preparing for asthma-related emergencies in schools. *Pediatrics.* 2007;119(3):651-652

7. Frankowski B. Asthma education: are pediatricians ready and willing to collaborate with schools? *Pediatrics.* 2009;124(2):793-795

8. Gerald LB, McClure LA, Mangan JM, et al. Increasing adherence to inhaled steroid therapy among schoolchildren: randomized, controlled trial of school-based supervised asthma therapy. *Pediatrics.* 2009;123(2):466-474

Diabetes

Diabetes is a common condition, with an increasing incidence because of the rise of obesity seen in all states (see Table 3.3.1, page 60, to compare diabetes with other conditions). In the United States, it is estimated there are approximately 215,000 children and teenagers with diabetes.[1] These children and teenagers with diabetes can participate fully in school activities and succeed but require some attention and planning because of the short-term or long-term problems from hyperglycemia or hypoglycemia. Processes in the school to monitor and manage diabetes help to prevent students from having morbidity from such symptoms, optimize school performance, and promote health and long-term well-being.[1]

Diabetes mellitus is a condition in which glucose is not used properly by the body. The body and brain needs glucose as an energy source. Diabetes may be secondary to poor insulin production or insulin resistance by the body.[1] If not treated or if poorly managed, diabetes usually leads to problems such as hypoglycemia and hyperglycemia. Hypoglycemia (low blood sugar) can occur quickly and can cause problems with impaired cognitive and motor function, which can lead to the student not being able to get help or give help to themselves.[2] Hyperglycemia (high blood sugar) tends to develop more slowly, over hours or days, but can lead to life-threatening diabetic ketoacidosis (DKA). Long-term complications of poorly treated diabetes mellitus include retinopathy, cardiovascular disease, renal disease, and/or poor blood circulation in the extremities that can lead to gangrene and the need for amputation.

Diabetes is relevant in several laws affecting schools, including IDEA, Section 504 of the Rehabilitation Act, and the ADA. Schools that receive federal funding (the majority of public schools) or any facility open to the public must accommodate children/teenagers with diabetes, which is considered a disability under these laws. Accommodations should be formalized in a Section 504 plan (the law prevents discrimination based on disability) or in an individualized education program (IEP) under IDEA law.

Although each child's situation is unique and plans need to be individualized to the school's and family's situation, there are several common themes that need to be considered. Main issues that need to be addressed include:

❶ Provision of diabetes care

    a. Autonomy of the child/teenager versus need for supervision and assistance[1,2]

        i. Increasingly, it is easier to monitor one's own blood sugar, but this requires some technical ability and the ability to analyze results.

        ii. Knowing the carbohydrate content in food intake and other dietary information for a healthy diet, in order to adjust insulin, is a skill.

        iii. Giving the right insulin dose by pen, syringe, or pump is critical for good management.

        iv. Will the student carry supplies, and how should the student reach a parent or the school nurse if he or she needs help?

        v. What permission does the student have to:

            1. Visit the school nurse or other trained school personnel?

            2. Have snacks to prevent hypoglycemia?

            3. Use the restroom and have access to fluids?

        vi. School staff and parents need to make decisions on how much the child or teenager is responsible for, keeping in mind what local and state guidelines and policies allow. This is dependent on the child's developmental level, both cognitively and socioemotionally.

        vii. Learning how to best care for diabetes as a student allows good skills and knowledge as an adult.

        viii. The student's level of sophistication in self-care usually changes with training and maturity, so these considerations need to be revisited regularly.

    b. What are the parents'/guardian's roles in the school process?[1]

        i. Parents are crucial to the discussion about the student's role in care.

        ii. Coordination of school/home regimens. A logbook for the school to record glucose and ketone results that the parents can review as frequently as necessary is useful. Sometimes the glucose meter memory is used for this purpose.

        iii. Supplies and maintenance of devices, materials for proper disposal of materials. This includes daily supplies, such as insulin or testing materials, but also supplies for hypoglycemia treatment, including glucose and/or glucagon.

        iv. Dialogue with medical professionals, the school nurse and other school staff. The school needs to know how to reach the student's parents/guardians for routine questions but also for emergencies. Releases should be signed for open communication between the family members and school personnel involved with planning and implementation of diabetes supports in the school.

    c. Responsibility of school personnel[1]
        i. There should be clarity on who should perform what roles at all times. General guidance to all without specifying who can and who will take what roles can be problematic.
            1. Which staff will be supervising or assisting in blood glucose monitoring, insulin administration, and emergency treatments? Is this the school nurse or a designated staff person?
            2. Who is the backup for all roles?
            3. Who will notify the parents/guardians of any change in the schedule (monitoring, treatments, diet, etc) and determine when to do so?
       ii. Ongoing diabetes education and training for staff, at the level necessary—for example, the school nurse requires a high level of training if he or she has a high level of responsibility at the school. Other staff with routine or emergency tasks will require the requisite level of training.
      iii. Location in the school for privacy may be desired by some students families for diabetic monitoring and treatment. But does the student want to do this in the classroom and not go somewhere else?

2 Student with newly diagnosed diabetes versus someone with an older diagnosis
    a. If a youth has a new diagnosis of diabetes—it is assumed the youth and others who support them (including school personnel) do not know much about the disease, monitoring, and treatments.
    b. Someone with a longer history of diabetes—the youth and their support system (including school personnel) probably know more than a student with a new diagnosis, but the youth and support people may have gaps in knowledge, so this needs to be explored sensitively and on an ongoing basis.

3 Monitoring of blood glucose[2]
    a. How will equipment and supplies be accessed and replenished?
    b. Frequency? Continuous blood glucose monitoring?
    c. Need to avoid low blood sugar levels causing symptoms during school activities
    d. Need to avoid high blood sugar levels that lead to later complications of diabetes

4 Need for food intake monitoring[1]
    a. Do snacks need to be given routinely in school? Snacks may be essential in preventing abnormal blood sugar levels. How is this timed in regard to the typical schedules for all students?

    b. Food content, amounts, and timing—the family, together with the school, needs to coordinate this with the schedules of the other students in the school.

    c. Instruction and direction is necessary, especially when young students are affected, about what to do about food for parties and other nonroutine events.

5 Engagement in physical activity[1]

    a. Essential in maintaining good health

    b. Risk of hypoglycemia, requires rescue strategies in any plan

6 Administration of medication

    a. Oral medication

    b. Insulin injections[1]

        i. Doses and timing depending on blood glucose levels and carbohydrate intake

        ii. Storage

        iii. Physician authorizing parents to make certain adjustments in dosing regimen?

    c. Insulin infusion pump

        i. Lack in insulin in the pump can lead to DKA unexpectedly

7 Response to hypoglycemia[1]

    a. School staff knowledge in identifying symptoms

    b. Staff response

        i. Administration of glucagon?

        ii. Because of possible problems with consciousness and motor ability, the student with hypoglycemia should not be left alone or sent alone elsewhere to seek help.

        iii. Treatment should be given where the child is (such as the classroom), readily available, and given immediately.

8 Response to hyperglycemia

9 Diabulimia—identification and management[3]

    a. Prior to diagnosis, students with type 1 diabetes probably will lose a lot of weight.

    b. If insulin is the treatment, this encourages fat storage.

    c. Female adolescents with type 1 diabetes are at higher risk of eating disorders.

    d. Some teenagers, especially if female, learn that reducing or eliminating insulin treatment leads to weight loss.

    e. Poor regulation of blood sugar if insulin is not used properly leads to complications.

10 Availability of resources including medication for ALL situations in school and related to school

11 Discrimination from students or teachers because of the diabetes

More useful information can be found in the section on seizure disorders in this manual, which relates a Section 504 plan for a child with epilepsy. There are many considerations in that plan (such as location of supplies and equipment and field trips and extracurricular activities) that are important to consider for a child with diabetes, although the symptoms and treatments are different.

The school staff member who has the skills and knowledge to meet the comprehensive health care needs of students with diabetes in schools is the school nurse.[2] School physicians and other professionals also have the expertise but are not as widely available in many schools. Health aides, without training, do not have the experience or background to provide comprehensive care for a student with diabetes in the school environment.

Planning around a student with diabetes should include the development of an individualized health care plan (IHCP), otherwise known as an individualized school health plan (ISHP) or individualized health plan (IHP). As in the individualized education program for special education, one plan should not be used for several or all youth who are in similar situations, and each student should have a separate, individualized plan. A school nurse should develop and implement this plan. Pediatricians and other health care professionals who know the child's health situation should assist in the development of the IHCP, especially because orders are usually needed from a physician for several elements, including medication administration.[1,2]

The goals of a school plan for a student's diabetic care should be: (1) normal or near normal blood glucose, minimizing the episodes of hyperglycemia or hypoglycemia; (2) normal development and growth; (3) emotional and social well-being; and (4) academic success.[2] The plan should consider daily needs but also emergency management for situations that have a risk of occurring. The plan also needs to consider requirements in field trips and other out-of-classroom situations, including athletic events.

Importantly, it has been shown that in children with poorly controlled type 1 diabetes, school nurse supervision over monitoring of blood glucose levels and adjustments in insulin dosage helps control blood glucose better.[5] Good blood glucose regulation is strongly linked to the prevention of later diabetic complications.[5,6]

Families are essential in creating and sanctioning such plans, and school staff members need to be part of the development, because they are key in implementing any IHCP properly. School staff can be trained with several strategies, including a National Diabetes Education Program developed by the National Institutes of Health (NIH).[4] Teachers, administrators, and other school staff members who would respond to or assist in the monitoring and management of a student's diabetes usually do not have an adequate understanding of the condition and issues without such training. The school needs to include bus drivers, sports coaches, and others in diabetes training as they may need to respond to the child's needs at some point.

School nurses and others should monitor the implementation of the IHCP and evaluate the effectiveness of the plan. Development of the IHCP is a function of nursing and should not be delegated to unlicensed personnel.[2] Other than the creation of the IHCP, provision of other nursing tasks, such as insulin administration, can be delegated by the school nurse. State laws and nurse practice acts needs to be followed to delegate properly. Importantly, it has been shown that in children with poorly controlled type 1 diabetes, school nurse supervision over monitoring of blood glucose levels and adjustments in insulin dosage helps control blood glucose better.[5] Good blood glucose regulation is strongly linked to the prevention of later diabetic complications.[5,6]

Early onset of diabetes (younger than 5 years) and poor diabetes control (especially if this causes ketoacidosis, unconsciousness, or seizures) have been shown to be associated with adverse cognitive effects, including poor verbal IQ, problems with nonlanguage-based skills, attention, and memory.[7] Although the age of onset cannot be affected by a student's supports, diabetic control can be.

How to Work With Schools

1. Parents/guardians, physicians, and school staff need to work together to help school nurses create a comprehensive IHCP for a student with diabetes.
2. School staff require training on diabetes to assist or respond in both daily and emergency care situations. Physicians and other medical personnel can support such training.

Recommendations for Pediatricians

❶ Pediatricians should support children and teenagers cared for in the hospital and clinic by being part of the development of plans in the school to manage diabetes properly.

❷ Prescriptions and orders for school use should be clear and straightforward. Supplies will be needed for both home and school environments.

❸ Collaborating with school personnel on IHCPs in the school lessens the risk of emergencies and need for hospitalization.

Recommendations for Program Directors and Trainees

❶ Pediatric residents should have opportunities to assist in the development of IHCPs and emergency action plans for youth with diabetes. This can be done in a rotation at the health office at the school or in a school health rotation.

❷ Rotations in classrooms that have children with special needs help medical students and residents understand the dynamics and issues surrounding children with chronic diseases in the school environment.

Take-Home Points

❶ Support the development of IHCPs for students with diabetes.

❷ Ensure that the care at home and at school is coordinated for a student with diabetes. Ensure that supplies for monitoring and medication are secure for both environments.

❸ Youth with diabetes have many issues that need to be addressed to help them be successful academically, socially, and physically.

References

1. American Diabetes Association. Diabetes care in the school and day care setting. *Diabetes Care*. 2012;35(4):939
2. National Association of School Nurses. Position Statement: Diabetes Management in the School Setting. Silver Spring, MD: National Association of School Nurses; January 2012
3. Hasken J, Kresl L, Nydegger T, Temme M. Diabulimia and the role of school health personnel. *J Sch Health*. 2010;80(10):465-469
4. National Institutes of Health. *Helping the Student with Diabetes Succeed: A Guide for School Personnel*. National Diabetes Education Program. NIH Publication No. 10-5217. Bethesda, MD: National Institutes of Health; September 2010
5. Nguyen T, Mason K, Sanders C, Yazdani P, Heptulla R. Targeting blood glucose management in school improves glycemic control in children with poorly controlled type 1 diabetes mellitus. *J Pediatr*. 2008;153(4):575–578
6. Diabetes Control and Complications Trial Research Group. Effect of intensive diabetes treatment on the development and progression of long-term complications in insulin-dependent diabetes mellitus. *N Engl J Med*. 1993;329(14):977–986
7. Taras H, Potts-Datema W. Chronic health conditions and student performance at school. *J Sch Health*. 2005;75(7):255-266

Children at Risk of Emergencies in School

The American Academy of Pediatrics (AAP) policy statement "Medical Emergencies Occurring in Schools" states that the average school-aged child spends 28% of the day and 14% of his or her total annual hours in school. There are 72.3 million children younger than 18 years living in the United States (according to the 2000 US Census). The Maternal and Child Health Bureau of the US Department of Health and Human Services estimates that of this group, 18 million children and adolescents have special health care needs or a chronic illness. Children with special health care needs or chronic illness account for 25% of the pediatric patients seen in hospital emergency departments each year. Despite its critical importance, school emergency preparedness is frequently inadequate because of barriers such as geographic and physical facility conditions, staffing, staff education and training, and financial resources."[1-3] In a 2004 survey, 68% (391 of 573) of school nurses had managed a life-threatening emergency requiring emergency medical services (EMS) activation during the past school year.[4]

EMS services, such as ambulances, respond to calls from schools. Injuries are the chief complaint listed for two thirds of EMS calls from schools. Injuries are causes of morbidity and mortality, both for children with and without special needs. These injuries are often related to participation in sports.[3]

Children with special health care needs are particularly at risk of medical emergencies in school. These emergencies include status asthmaticus, diabetic crises, and status epilepticus.[1] Problems with breathing and seizures lead to one quarter of calls to EMS from schools.[3] Some episodes of problems with breathing and seizures are incidental, happening for the first time for these children, and are not predictable. But breathing issues and seizures often occur around children who are known to have chronic conditions such as asthma and epilepsy. Parents and their children's health care providers should work with schools to ensure that schools are informed and that planning for each child that has such conditions occurs. Then schools can manage these issues calmly and with expertise. These children may require special equipment; preparation and training of personnel, medications, and supplies; and/or transport decisions and arrangements.[1,3]

How to Work With Schools

Please see the policies in the AAP policy statement "Medical Emergencies Occurring in Schools" (**http://pediatrics.aappublications.org/content/122/4/887**) for many important strategies around preparing for emergencies around all youth in schools.[1]

For children with special needs, the AAP policy statement makes several recommendations:

❶ Students and staff members with chronic medical conditions or other special health care needs are more susceptible to medical emergencies and require schools to have a heightened sense of readiness. Students should have an updated individualized health plan (IHP) prepared by the school nurse with input from the family and the primary care clinician. The IHP contains information on medications, activity levels, dietary needs, equipment, transportation, and other accommodations. Using this information, the school can then plan for accommodations for daily classroom activity, field trips, and the emergency needs of the student. The IHP can assist school teams in developing individualized education programs (IEPs) or Section 504 plans.

❷ Staff who care for students with special needs should have an awareness of the conditions and be trained to respond to emergencies (eg, seizures, asthma, diabetic ketoacidosis, hypoglycemia, sickle crisis) until a health care professional arrives. This capacity is especially important in the event of a community disaster in which the EMS prehospital emergency-response system may not be readily available.

❸ Any equipment or medication required for emergency management of a student or staff member (eg, evacuation chair or self-injectable epinephrine device) should be easily accessible.

❹ Individual emergency action plans (EAPs), developed from information in the IHP, should be copied and made available for transport with the child if he or she requires hospital treatment and/or management in the event of a community-wide disaster. The emergency information form, developed by the AAP and the American College of Emergency Physicians, is useful in developing both an IHP and an EAP.

❺ Some parents may opt not to disclose a child's disability to teachers out of concern about stigmatization. In these cases, basic awareness training to all staff at the beginning of the year is a prudent approach.

Recommendations for Pediatricians

The AAP policy statement "Medical Emergencies Occurring in Schools" has these recommendations:

❶ **Communication:** Maintain a strong, open, and ongoing line of communication with the school nurse and/or the school physician (when available) regarding the individual student's medical condition and current management in coordination with the parent/caregiver. This linkage informs the school nurse of any changes or updates to the student's IHP, EAP, 504 plan, or IEP when applicable. The emergency information form (developed by the American College of Emergency Physicians and the AAP) is one such tool that can be completed by the primary care clinician and may be used to communicate with the school nurse.[5] The school nurse plays an important role in developing and implementing health plans, activating physicians' orders, and interpreting physicians' instructions for staff, students, and families.

② **Familiarity:** Be familiar with the emergency action plan and the disaster plan of the patient's school, the school resources, and staffing and provide advice on issues that might affect the student's disease management and outcome.

③ **Parent engagement:** Advise parents to become familiar with the school's emergency plan and help them evaluate how the plan meets the needs of their children.

④ **Advocacy:** Get involved with the school district's school Health Advisory Council and provide input on health-related policies that will affect individual patient care, including school wellness policies and emergency plans.

⑤ **Drafting health plans:** Participate in the drafting of IEPs and 504 plans as needed. If a student with a particular special health care need or chronic disease has special education needs, an IEP may be developed by using the IHP as a foundation for details on the student's disease-management routine. To qualify for an IEP, a child must have an impairment that substantially affects his or her academic performance.

⑥ **Orders:** Provide a clearly written problem list, daily care instructions, accommodations, and orders for the use of emergency medications (eg, self-injectable epinephrine, albuterol) and the necessary current prescriptions to keep these medications and devices available in school for use in a particular student's emergency. This information is used by the school nurse to create the student's IHP and EAP.

⑦ Be available to assess the individual student after an emergency and assist in a prompt and safe return to school and provide support to parents whose child sustained a medical emergency in school.

⑧ Review the documentation and details of the student's school emergency, provide feedback, and provide instructions that amend the individual EAP as necessary.

⑨ Communicate directly with the school physician (where available) as needed.

> Children with special health care needs are particularly at risk of medical emergencies in school. These emergencies include status asthmaticus, diabetic crises, and status epilepticus.[1] Problems with breathing and seizures lead to one quarter of calls to EMS from schools.[3]

Recommendations for Program Directors and Trainees

1 Medical students and especially resident physicians need practice in working with schools in ensuring youth have IHPs, EAPs and appropriate medical supports in school environments. Trainees need practice in creating practical and appropriate IHPs and EAPs.

2 Rotations with school nurses or with a school health office are important opportunities to see the dynamics of how schools handle health requests and information, and how IHPs and EAPs are created.

3 Schools appreciate the advocacy by pediatric residents and medical students to strengthen their policies and procedures towards children with special care needs around possible medical emergencies in the school setting.

Take-Home Points

1 Children can have various types of medical emergencies in schools. The most common are injuries. Also common are problems with breathing and seizures.

2 Planning between pediatricians, parents and guardians, school nurses, and the school staff can lessen anxiety and stress around medical emergencies in schools, and better equip the school staff in handling these situations, especially in those occurring in children with chronic conditions and other special health care needs.

References

1. American Academy of Pediatrics Council on School Health. Medical emergencies occurring at school. *Pediatrics*. 2008;122(4):887-894
2. Sapien RE, Allen A. Emergency preparation in schools: a snapshot of a rural state. *Pediatr Emerg Care*. 2001;17(5):329–333
3. Loyacono TR. Responding to school emergencies. *Emerg Med Serv*. 2005;34(4):43–44, 46, 48 passim
4. Olympia RP, Wan E, Avner JR. The preparedness of schools to respond to emergencies in children: a national survey of school nurses. *Pediatrics*. 2005;116(6):e738-e745
5. American Academy of Pediatrics, Committee on Pediatric Emergency Medicine and Council on Clinical Information Technology, American College of Emergency Physicians and Pediatric Emergency Medicine Committee. Emergency information forms and emergency preparedness for children with special health care needs. *Pediatrics*. 2010;125(4):829-837

Seizure Disorders

Children with epilepsy should thrive in school environments. However, problems that parents and the school worry about include status epilepticus; harm to the child from seizures, including death; the reaction of classmates and peers to seizures[1]; school staff reaction to seizures; whether the child will be treated unfairly because of epilepsy,[1] and the effects of seizures and anticonvulsants on learning and activities in the school environment. Because epilepsy is fairly common, occurring in 6.5 children of every 1000,[2] chances are that any particular school will have some experience with a child with epilepsy. Even if it is the school's first experience, preparation and discussions with school staff can help alleviate the anxiety around reacting to seizures.

A seizure is excessive electrical activity of the brain. This may cause jerking of parts of the body (what most people think what a seizure looks like), other types of unusual movements, and/or a change or loss of consciousness, such as staring spells.[3] Epilepsy, or a seizure disorder, is diagnosed when seizures are recurrent and not from a reaction from low blood sugar or other chemical imbalance, acute infection, or injury. Status epilepticus is a continuous seizure or recurrent seizures without resumption of consciousness, for 30 or more minutes and is considered a medical emergency. Convulsions lasting more than 20 or 30 minutes can cause brain damage.[4] Children with recurrent seizures, therefore, commonly receive anticonvulsant medication. Some children are on multiple medications, usually because the seizures are intractable and difficult to treat. Child neurologists are particularly expert at helping to manage children with epilepsy and to decrease the risk of status epilepticus.

The Epilepsy Foundation document "Model Section 504 Plan for a Student with Epilepsy" has the following important considerations for a protocol to be followed for any particular child with epilepsy in school[5] (supplemented by other references as indicated):

❶ Provision of epilepsy care
   a. Staff member training about epilepsy and first aid to a child with seizures. This includes staff for extracurricular activities, field trips, or other school events and bus drivers.
   b. Which staff should respond when seizures occur
   c. What students should be educated about epilepsy and what to expect
   d. Recognition of seizures or possible seizures
   e. Responding to seizures calmly, not calling an ambulance, how and when to allow return to classroom activities, and when to call 911[1]

2 Student level of self-care and location of supplies and equipment
   a. What can the child do independently to care for himself or herself
   b. When should staff assist or supervise
   c. Activation of school nurse, or person delegated by the school nurse, to give medication
   d. Where medication and supplies are kept

3 Exercise, physical activity, and rest periods
   a. Participation is permitted, except in what situations
   b. Physical education teachers and coaches should be able to recognize seizures and assist with first aid
   c. Medications should be available at physical education location and sports sites
   d. If the child has to rest after a seizure, where the safe, supervised, comfortable setting will be (this does not have to be with a school nurse at the school health office)

4 Ketogenic diet (this is a special diet that helps some children have less or no seizures)
   a. Access to food and liquid to maintain the diet
   b. Parent/guardian role in providing premeasured quantities of required food for the diet
   c. School staff to be trained to maintain the diet and to prevent violations
   d. Which classmates will be trained as to not share their food with the student on the diet
   e. Alternatives for the student on the ketogenic diet during parties and celebrations, including playing a special role during the occasion

5 Vagus nerve stimulator (VNS)
   a. Which school staff will be trained about the VNS
   b. Which staff member will activate the device if a seizure occurs, as related in a seizure action plan
   c. Log and sharing of this information when the VNS is used with parents/guardians

6 Routine and emergency use of medications
   a. Prescribed doses of medication as related in the seizure action plan
   b. Which staff member and backup staff member to administer diazepam, as related in the seizure action plan, including all school-related activities in which the child might engage

7 Field trips and extracurricular activities

   a. Participation in all activities without restriction and with necessary supports and accommodations, including supervision and assistance by school staff

   b. Nonrequirement that the parent/guardian accompany the student

   c. What trained person will be designated and available for first aid or medication administration

   d. The student's anticonvulsant medication will travel with him or her to any field trip or activity, including those out of school

8 Classroom work and tests

   a. If there is a seizure during a test, retaking the test at another time without penalty

   b. If adverse effects from medication affect ability to concentrate, that extra time be given for assignments or tests without penalty

   c. If waking up late to avoid early morning seizures, that the student not be penalized for missed work and make up time be given

   d. The student should be given make up time for any school time missed because of seizure care, illness, or medical appointments

9 Instructions and communication

   a. Substitute teachers are given written instructions for seizure care and what school staff is involved in the care for that student around seizures

   b. Communication to parents/guardians about any seizures that occur, what aid was given, and any other relevant information

   c. Any unusual response to seizures triggers 911 and a call to the parents/guardians

10 Emergency evacuation and shelter in place

   a. The plan would be in effect with any emergency evacuation or shelter in place.

   b. The school nurse or designee, as related in the 504 plan, would provide seizure care and transport medication. This person would be in touch with the child's parents/guardians regarding their instructions for seizure care.

11 Emergency contacts, including names and contact information about physicians

---

Preparation and discussions with school staff can help alleviate the anxiety around reacting to seizures.

The Epilepsy Foundation has several other tools to support a student with epilepsy in school. This includes a questionnaire for a parent to complete for the school nurse to use. Also, they have a "seizure action plan" helpful for the school to manage seizures in a child with epilepsy. There is a template for the student to give information about their seizures. A "teacher information sheet" informs the teacher of a child about the seizure condition. There is also a form available for the teacher to write a report on seizures that they observe called a "teacher anecdotal record" with a medication adverse effect portion.

Epilepsy is not an intellectual disability or a mental health condition. Some children with epilepsy do have an intellectual disability, mental health issue, or associated medical problem, but many children do not. Unfortunately, misinformation or misunderstanding about epilepsy among teachers and school staff can have a detrimental effect on their attitude toward a student with epilepsy.

Children with epilepsy can be "A" students in their school, but sometimes they have learning problems. Sometimes, the learning difficulty is secondary to a brain disorder that contributes to the epilepsy. Sometimes seizures are occurring often throughout the school day, interfering with learning. Anticonvulsant medication can cause concentration or other difficulties for learning. Some children with epilepsy have depression, causing low energy and a decreased attention span.[1] Learning disabilities are more common in children with epilepsy but may be present unrelated to the epilepsy.[6] The prevalence of learning disabilities in the general population—90 out of 1000 children—is much more than epilepsy.[2] Therefore, several things need to be considered for a child with epilepsy who is not learning well, and any contributing factor should be addressed. The pediatrician has a major role in helping the child and his or her family with any and all of these.

How to Work With Schools

❶ It is the role of parents/guardians and medical professionals, including pediatricians, to inform school staff about children with epilepsy.[1] Information will help dispel myths and unnecessary fears that the school has about a child with seizures. The right information to the right people can make a big difference.

❷ Decreasing misinformation may lessen the stigma associated with epilepsy.

❸ An emergency action plan or seizure action plan for a student with epilepsy will help guide the school on what to do with occurrences of seizures.

❹ Calling an ambulance may not be the right response for a typical seizure in the school environment occurring in a child with epilepsy. This may take a child out of school unnecessarily. However, the school needs to know what to do rather than call 911.

Recommendations for Pediatricians

1 Pediatricians have a major role in determining any medical factors leading to poor learning by a child with epilepsy. This can include effects from the epilepsy itself, anticonvulsant medications, depression, learning disability, and other factors. A pediatrician who is an effective medical home will investigate, or effectively utilize consultants, in evaluating and then managing issues leading to poor school performance.

2 Different types of seizures require different responses from schools. Pediatricians are an excellent resource to help the school understand these issues.

Recommendations for Program Directors and Trainees

1 Assisting community pediatricians or subspecialists such as child neurologists in their work with a school is a terrific role for pediatric residents. This may include drafting seizure action plans, education of school teachers and staff around seizures, and collaborating with the school nurse on individualized health plans for each student with epilepsy.

2 Neurology residents and neurodevelopmental and behavioral fellows should be involved with schools.

Take-Home Points

1 Children with seizures are sometimes stigmatized and wrongly thought to be intellectually disabled or have a mental health disorder. Pediatricians and school personnel should work together to ensure that children are not stigmatized.

2 Children with epilepsy require planning between medical professionals, such as pediatricians, and the school to ensure that barriers to learning are evaluated for and managed, such as possible learning disabilities, medication effects, depression, or absences from school because of medical appointments or hospitalizations.

References

1. American Academy of Pediatrics, Council on School Health. Medical emergencies occurring at school. *Pediatrics*. 2008;122(4):887-894. Reaffirmed September 2011
2. Sapien RE, Allen A. Emergency preparation in schools: a snapshot of a rural state. *Pediatr Emerg Care*. 2001;17(5):329–333
3. Loyacono TR. Responding to school emergencies. *Emerg Med Serv*. 2005;34(4):43–44, 46, 48 passim
4. Margolis LS, Gross G. *Legal Rights of Children with Epilepsy in School and Child Care—An Advocate's Manual*. 2nd ed. Landover, MD: Epilepsy Foundation of America; 2011
5. Epilepsy Foundation. Model Section 504 Plan for a Student with Epilepsy. Available at: http://www.epilepsynorcal.org/docs/Sample_504.pdf. Accessed April 13, 2015
6. Epilepsy and Your Child's School. Available at: http://www.webmd.com/epilepsy/children-school. Accessed April 13, 2015

HIV/AIDS

HIV and AIDS continue to be an important problem for students, especially adolescents and young adults. Five percent of people infected with HIV in the United States were 13 to 24 years of age at the time of diagnosis. The estimated number of cases of HIV/AIDS increased among 15 to 19 year olds and 20 to 24 year olds, and AIDS is one of the top 10 causes of death in the latter group.[1]

School Attendance and Activities for the Student With HIV/AIDS

Students with HIV/AIDS should have every right and opportunity to be successful in school. Attending school and participation in school activities decreases isolation, promotes a sense of belonging, and provides environments promoting normalcy.

Teachers and school administrators may have fears about the transmission of HIV in the school setting. Such transmission has not been documented.[2]

Students with HIV who have no symptoms cannot be identified from their peers. Therefore, teachers and school personnel should understand universal precautions around all students in school. Students with AIDS may be more symptomatic, but they rarely need to be kept from school for their own safety. Symptoms may necessitate home schooling temporarily or, more rarely, for greater spans of time when the disease progresses. Such decisions should be made by the student, his or her family, the student's pediatrician or other trusted medical professional, and the school. HIV/AIDS is relevant in several laws affecting schools, including the Individuals with Disabilities Education Act (IDEA), Section 504 of the Rehabilitation Act, and the Americans with Disabilities Act (ADA). Schools that receive federal funding (the majority of public schools) or any facility open to the public must accommodate children/ teenagers with HIV/AIDS. Accommodations should be formalized in a Section 504 plan (the law prevents discrimination based on special health care needs) or in an individualized education program (IEP) under IDEA law.[2]

The majority of students with HIV have normal cognitive functioning. However, some students may have cognitive effects from HIV and require special education and other supports. Neurodevelopmental and cognitive effects may be ameliorated by antiretroviral treatment.[2]

Some students with HIV/AIDS require multiple medications.[3] Standard procedures around administration of medication in a school should be used. Especially for such students, development of an individualized health care plan (IHCP), otherwise known as an individualized school health plan (ISHP) or individualized health plan (IHP), is important. Occasionally, students may have

> Attending school and participation in school activities decreases isolation, promotes a sense of belonging, and provides environments promoting normalcy.

progression of their disease and become ill enough that they may require special consideration in support by school personnel. As in the IEP for special education, one plan should not be used for several or all youth who are in similar situations, and each student should have a separate, individualized plan. A school nurse should develop and implement this plan. Pediatricians and other health professionals who know the child's health situation should assist in the development of the IHCP, especially since orders are usually needed from a physician for several elements, including medication administration.

Confidentiality must be assured. HIV and AIDS are still stigmatized. However, school personnel administering medication should be informed of the student's diagnosis, and the adverse effects of the medication being used. The student's age-appropriate assent and consent of the family is necessary. However, nondisclosure should not prohibit the student from attending school.[2]

How to Work With Schools

1. Pediatricians should work with school personnel in ensuring that students with HIV/AIDS attend school without discrimination or isolation.
2. Education of school staff about HIV, AIDS, transmission, and safeguards is essential for schools to feel comfortable and competent in supporting all students at their school.

Recommendations for Pediatricians

1. Pediatricians and other health professionals should help students with AIDS transition to special education and home schooling environments if this is necessary.
2. Pediatricians should help students with HIV and their families understand the chronic illness aspects of this infection.

Recommendations for Program Directors and Trainees

1. Pediatric residents should be part of the development of IHCPs for students with HIV/AIDS.
2. They can be helpful in disseminating information about HIV and other associated information in schools for both students and staff.

Take-Home Points

1 Children with HIV/AIDS should receive the education all students deserve.

2 Special supports for students who cannot attend school should be planned and implemented in collaboration between families, schools, and their pediatrician or other health practitioner.

Prevention of HIV/AIDS

Sexually transmitted diseases (STDs) reflect the role of schools in healthy student behaviors. Goals of school-based health education include delay in sexual activity and the use of condoms if a youth does engage in intercourse.[4] Other goals include education about getting HIV from either contaminated blood from the sharing of equipment in the use of illicit drugs or from unprotected sex that may occur while under the influence of drugs.

Rates of HIV/AIDS reflect the usefulness of condoms. The high rates of pregnancy and STDs, including HIV, reflect the low use of condoms and other contraception in American students who are sexually active.[4] The correct use of condoms is a crucial preventive mechanism to prevent HIV transmission. Policies and programs to encourage condom use are, therefore, desirable, including making condoms available in schools.[4] Factors that need to be considered in promoting the use of condoms include cost, access, availability, and confidentiality. Condoms need to be latex, and not natural lamb, as the latter have pores that can allow viruses such as HIV and herpes to be transmitted during intercourse. Condoms have the advantages of minimal side effects and not requiring a prescription. Also, condoms promote the role of male students in taking responsibility in preventing pregnancy and disease in sexual intercourse.

Increased understanding of the usefulness of condoms does not necessarily translate into increased use. There are multiple factors[4] affecting teenagers' use of condoms, including:

1 Peer influences (are peers supportive in using condoms?)

2 "Invulnerability" and the feeling that practicing safe sex is not required

3 Fear of HIV/AIDS or other diseases

4 Self-image

5 Overcoming any embarrassment in buying condoms

6 Believing that spontaneous sex is better compared with "planned" sex

7 Instruction in using condoms
 a. Sexuality education, including the usefulness and instruction on use
 b. Literacy level of the instructions on the packaging may be higher than the student's

8 Belief that condoms can prevent HIV/AIDS and other diseases

9 Feeling that the student can convince their partner in the use of condoms

10 Availability of physician in discussing condom use

11 Ready availability (adolescents carrying a condom are 2.7 times more likely to use them)

Preventing illicit drug use has similar considerations in peer influences, the sense of "invulnerability," and the importance in teaching healthy behaviors in schools. Students should also be aware of HIV transmission with contaminated tattoo needles or reused tattoo ink.[5]

Although improved access to new or sterile needles and syringes may decrease the transmission of HIV, this approach is controversial with many states. There does not seem to be an increase of drug use with better access to new or sterile equipment, or because of syringe-exchange programs. Therefore, such programs should be made more widely available.[5]

How to Work With Schools

1 Schools affect healthy behaviors, including condom use, in 3 main ways[4]:
 a. Information
  i. Comprehensive sexuality education is critical – teaching of responsible decision making is the goal, including
   1. Abstinence – this is the surest way of preventing HIV transmission
   2. Effective contraception for sexually active students
 b. Motivation for healthy behaviors, including communication between partners
  i. Interpersonal skill building
   1. Interactive communication
   2. Assertiveness for healthy behaviors
   3. Negotiation
   4. Conflict avoidance and resolution
   5. Refusal skills for negative peer pressure
  ii. Use of media and activities to teach skills including role playing exercises
  iii. Peer support systems

   c. Availability of condoms barriers and restrictions should be removed

      i. As part of comprehensive health programs versus HIV/AIDS-specific activities

     ii. Condoms freely available versus restrictive dispensing only after parental permission and counseling—these details may be decided by coalitions of parents, medical professionals, teachers, school staff, administrators, and school boards.

    iii. Condoms do not cause greater rates of sexual activity and intercourse; creating barriers to condom use do not decrease sexual activity

    iv. Schools are where adolescents are, so they are important places for condom availability

Pediatricians and other health care professionals can work with schools and other community partners to improve healthy behaviors by being involved in endeavors and initiatives in the above 3 areas. Partners can include families, religious groups, and other community organizations, health departments, and the media.

❷ Schools are part of community efforts in preventing the onset of illicit drug use and decreasing or eliminating drug use once it starts. Pediatricians should be part of the development and implementation of such efforts. Advocate for programs that make sterile/new needles and syringes more readily available and for syringe-exchange programs.

Recommendations for Pediatricians

❶ Engage youth in care. They should be counseled not to start high-risk behaviors. Also, pediatricians and other practitioners should identify risk factors in their patients including illicit drug use. Other risks factors associated with injection drug use may include tobacco, marijuana, and alcohol use. Depression and a history of childhood sexual abuse are also correlated with illicit drug dependence.[5] The use of screening tools, such as the CRAFFT tool or the Guidelines for Adolescent Health Survey, may be helpful in identifying risks.[1] Treatment and counseling of underlying issues that may cause increased risk of HIV exposure should be done in a nonjudgmental and supportive manner.

❷ Testing for HIV infection should be offered to all adolescents at least once by 16 to 18 years of age when the prevalence in the patient population is more than 0.1%. If the prevalence is lower, routine HIV testing is recommended in sexually active adolescents or those with risk factors. High-risk youth should be tested annually. Consent of the adolescent should be enough, although parental involvement is always desirable. Free and community-based testing programs may be used by pediatricians if cost or confidentiality are issues for the youth being tested.[1]

❸ Pediatricians and other health professionals are critical resources for availability and facilitating condom use. Patients who have talked to their health care provider about HIV show 1.7 times more condom use.[4]

Recommendations for Program Directors and Trainees

❶ Medical students and pediatric residents may be excellent resources for schools to provide education regarding STD transmission (including HIV), condom use, and a variety of other topics. This may be within a comprehensive health education curriculum or for special projects.

❷ Fellows in infectious diseases and adolescent medicine can be a great resource for the schools concerning students with HIV/AIDS.

Take-Home Points

❶ Students who are abstinent from sexual intercourse, use condoms if involved in sexual activity, do not engage in injectable illicit drug use, and involve themselves in other healthy behaviors decrease their risk of HIV and AIDS.

❷ Pediatricians and schools have major roles in education of students in healthy behaviors that will prevent HIV transmission.

References

1. American Academy of Pediatrics, Committee on Pediatric AIDS. Adolescents and HIV infection: the pediatrician's role in promoting routine testing. *Pediatrics*. 2011;128(5): 1023-1029

2. American Academy of Pediatrics, Committee on Pediatric AIDS. Education of children with human immunodeficiency virus infection. *Pediatrics*. 2000;105(6):1358:-1360. Reaffirmed March 2013

3. American Academy of Pediatrics, Council on School Health. Policy statement: guidance for the administration of medication in school. *Pediatrics*. 2009;124(4):1244-1251. Reaffirmed March 2013

4. American Academy of Pediatrics, Committee on Adolescence. Condom availability for youth. *Pediatrics*. 1995;95(2):281-285

5. American Academy of Pediatrics, Committee on Pediatric AIDS. Reducing the risk of HIV infection associated with illicit drug use. *Pediatrics*. 2006;117(2):566-571. Reaffirmed May 2012

Children With Terminal Illness

Some children attending school have a terminal illness. It is thought that on any given day, approximately 4000 children in the United States are within 6 months of dying from some type of known serious medical condition.[1] Also, some children are medically fragile and are at risk of having significant medical issues at school. However, school is a vital social environment for youth, and a student with a terminal illness or who is medically fragile may greatly desire to be with friends and peers in school. Participation in school activities may greatly increase the quality of life for a student with significant medical issues. The support of parents/guardians, medical professionals, and school staff can enable the child with terminal illness to participate in school.

Federal legislation such as the Individuals with Disabilities Education Act (IDEA) and Section 504 of the Rehabilitation Act supports all youth, no matter the medical condition or disability, to have access to school.[2]

What should happen when these children become more ill or critical while in school? School administrators, teachers, and health staff at the school can be uncomfortable with the responsibilities over the child with a terminal illness or who is medically fragile at their school. Clarity of roles and responsibilities and clear directions for the care of these children can be accomplished with good planning and collaboration between families, school staff, pediatricians, and other professionals.

Part of this planning should be the development of an individualized health care plan (IHCP), otherwise known as an individualized school health plan (ISHP) or individualized health plan (IHP). As in the individualized education program (IEP) for special education, one plan should not be used for several or all youth who are in similar situations, and each student should have a separate individualized plan. A school nurse should develop and implement this plan.[3,4] Important elements for each IHCP include[1,3]:

1. Clarification of care necessary in acute situations versus end-of-life situations. Discussion should include what should happen if a youth is in distress, rather than in a life-threatening situation.

2. Elaboration on comfort measures such as oxygen, suctioning, pain measures, control of bleeding, holding, and positioning

3. If there are situations for comfort measures only (see discussion below regarding do-not-attempt-to-resuscitate [DNAR] orders), an area for this to happen should be designated.

4. Which school staff needs to know about the particular youth's situation and receive education about procedures

5 Whether skilled nursing will be based at the youth's school (rather than as an external support)

6 Whom to contact in case of an emergency

7 When emergency medical services (EMS, such as an ambulance) should be involved

8 Is there a DNAR order (see below)?

9 If the youth should die at school, what is the plan?

   a. Where will the student be moved to within the school and when?

   b. Who will pronounce the death?

   c. Transportation and mortuary arrangements

10 How field trips are handled

11 Enabling self-care, depending on the child's developmental and social capabilities

12 How a child gets to school—what transportation method is necessary

13 How spiritual, psychological, emotional, and social needs should be addressed

Creation of the IHCP may be supported by the use of a school physician consultant.[2] The consultant can help schools communicate directly with the youth's physicians. The consultant can recommend what intensity of services would be appropriate when there are disagreements between family, school staff or medical professionals. One area of possible disagreement is the use of DNAR orders.

In 1974, the American Heart Association articulated that cardiopulmonary resuscitation (CPR) is not indicated for all patients. In 1994, the American Academy of Pediatrics and National Education Association (NEA) produced guidelines regarding do not resuscitate (DNR) orders.[3] DNR orders evolved into DNAR orders, highlighting that resuscitation is not always successful. In some places, this is called allow natural death (AND). DNAR orders allow some supports to be used (such as oxygen or bag-mask ventilation) while not allowing measures such as chest compressions or cardiac defibrillation.[5] Having a DNAR does not mean medical care is abandoned or is of lower quality but is part of the deliberate and planned management of a child's particular situation.[1]

Although others such as medical professionals or school staff can advise parents and guardians, family members have the authority to make decisions for their children, unless it is a case of abuse or neglect. Parents should determine where the child is in the progression of the illness and whether cardiopulmonary resuscitation (CPR) and other similar life-sustaining measures would merely prolong the inevitable. They can weigh whether CPR would or would not be in the child's best interest[5] and determine whether a DNAR order should

> The support of parents/guardians, medical professionals, and school staff
> can enable the child with terminal illness to participate in school.

be implemented in their child's school. However, it is important to understand
that parents usually have limited input into school curriculum, discipline, and
most school activities. Implementing a DNAR order in a school setting rubs
parental authority against school autonomy.[6]

School administrators may be emotional about students having DNAR
status, worry about student response to a death on the campus, have major
ethical issues with DNAR orders, and believe that their staff is unprepared
to carry out such orders.[7] DNAR orders reflect the difficulties of our society
"striking a comfortable balance between protecting the sanctity of life and
honoring the wishes of individuals with terminal conditions."[8] This is particularly difficult with youth, who are seen as having so much potential, and who
require family members to make decisions for them.

Eighty percent of school districts did not have a policy, protocol, or regulation to support DNAR orders in a survey of the 50 largest cities, and all state
capitals.[5] Most districts surveyed would not support DNAR, or did not know
whether they could. Acceptance of DNAR orders varies according to state.
Therefore, knowledge of state and local laws and regulations is essential.

However, a white paper produced by a national hospice and palliative organization recommends "orders to forgo resuscitative efforts (DNR) outside of
hospitals must be honored in school and other public and non-hospital settings,
including the emergency medical system." In a court decision in Massachusetts—
ABC Schools v Mr and Mrs. M—the court related that the school could not shield
the staff from liability if they did not follow the DNAR order.[3]

Qualities that DNAR orders for schools should have include[1,3]:

❶ Parents and guardians should create the DNAR order in conjunction with
their pediatrician or trusted health care professional.

❷ The DNAR order should provide clear, explicit directives for the staff to
follow in case of a cardiac or respiratory arrest.

❸ The DNAR order is a family decision. Also, students who are 18 years or
older, if competent, need to approve the DNAR order.

❹ DNAR orders should be dated—these should be time-limited with renewal
every few weeks as necessary.

❺ A DNAR order may be revoked at any time, but this needs to be
communicated to all involved.

❻ The DNAR order should be for an individual youth.

❼ The DNAR order should be reviewed by the district legal counsel to ensure that state and local laws are followed.

These are not orders to "do nothing" and should not decrease the quality of care the child receives. What school staff SHOULD do should be clearly stated in the IHCP.

Some mention should be made of fragile or terminal children who would not benefit from a school setting. Children "who are unable to interact with their environments, recognize usual caregivers, or benefit from an educational program" may be better served by respite or medical day care outside of a school environment.[9]

How to Work With Schools

❶ Pediatricians and other health care professionals should work together with school staff to ensure appropriate care of children who are medically fragile and/or with a terminal condition in school.

❷ Health care professionals are critical in development of DNAR orders. But this needs to be done within the rules, regulations, and laws locally and for the state in which the child attends school, if the DNAR is to be used at school. Parents and their pediatricians should work together with nursing personnel, teachers, administrators, legal counsel, and EMS personnel when a DNAR order is considered and/or implemented.

❸ The DNAR order should be part of a comprehensive IHCP, with careful planning and discussion, including solving disagreements.

❹ Pediatricians can be important resources to schools, including special educators, in understanding youth who have chronic conditions, especially those who are medically fragile or terminal. Parents and school personnel particularly had trouble with the following areas for their youth with chronic conditions[10]:
   a. How to inform the school about the youth's condition
   b. How to have the youth reintegrate back into school
   c. Monitoring of health status
   d. Teaching school personnel about unexpected health problems
   e. School staff expectations

❺ Pediatricians should work with local and state authorities responsible for laws regarding end-of-life care, and the EMS policies affecting out-of-hospital DNAR orders. Rational procedures and legal protections need to be well developed, to protect the school, school staff, and EMS members who follow DNAR orders and other elements of the IHCP. These laws and policies should respect the rights and interests of dying children.

Recommendations for Program Directors and Trainees

❶ Program directors should collaborate with schools to provide physician training within schools around youth with special needs. Pediatric and family practice residents can better understand school issues in supporting these youth, be involved in IHCP and DNAR order planning (with supervision from community or school pediatricians and other professionals), and become skilled in school/physician interactions.

❷ Trainees and their mentors may be excellent resources for age-appropriate educational programs about death and dying in certain situations for local school systems and parent-teacher organizations.

Take-Home Points

❶ Children who are terminal and medically fragile can greatly benefit from being in school, and pediatricians should work with parents and school staff to ensure such children are able to participate in school.

❷ IHCPs and DNAR orders require planning and consideration of multiple factors, but these permit the integration of children who are terminal or medically fragile into school.

References

1. American Academy of Pediatrics, Council on School Health, Committee on Bioethics. Honoring do-not-attempt-resuscitation requests in schools. *Pediatrics*. 2010;125(5):1073-1077. Reaffirmed July 2013
2. Taras H, Brennan JJ. Students with chronic diseases: nature of school physician support. *J Sch Health*. 2008;78(7):389-396
3. National Association of School Nurses. Do Not Attempt Resuscitation (DNAR) Issue Brief. Silver Spring, MD: National Association of School Nurses; June 2012
4. White G. Nurses at the helm: implementing DNAR orders in the public school setting. *Am J Bioethics*. 2005;5(1):83-85
5. Kimberly MB, Forte AL, Carroll JM, Feudtner C. Pediatric do-not-attempt-resuscitation orders and public schools: a national assessment of policies and laws. *Am J Bioethics*. 2005;5(1):59–65
6. Diekema D. Pediatric DNAR orders and public schools. The American Journal of Bioethics. 2005;5(1):76-77
7. Hone-Warren M. Exploration of school administrator attitudes regarding do not resuscitate policies in the school setting. J Sch Nurs. 2007;23(2):98-103
8. Collier J, Sandborg C. The first step: DNAR outside the hospital and the role of pediatric medical care providers. *Am J Bioethics*. 2005;5(1):85-86
9. Children's International Project on Palliative/Hospice Services (ChIPPS) Administrative/Policy Workgroup of the National Hospice and Palliative Care Organization. A Call for Change: Recommendations to Improve the Care of Children Living with Life-Threatening Conditions. Alexandria, VA: Children's International Project on Palliative/Hospice Services; October 2001
10. Kliebenstein MA, Broome ME. School re-entry for the child with chronic illness: parent and school personnel perceptions. *Pediatr Nurs*. 2000;26(6):579-582

Technology-Dependent Students

Technology-dependent students are a subset of youth who are medically fragile. Technology keeps more children alive. Although often impaired in some areas of daily living, technology also allows youth previously cared for in institutions, hospitals, or at home to be able to explore the world and their community. Equipment has become portable, with batteries replacing power cords. Power wheelchairs and other assistive devices allow greater mobility. Augmentative communication devices and other technologies allow communication by youth previously silent. These children are now able to attend school and also reap the benefits of the social and academic environments schools provide.

Parents and other family members caring for these youth also have needed respite when these technology-dependent youth are in school. But these youth pose significant challenges for school staff, administrators, and peers in addition to being challenging to parents and guardians, medical professionals, and others working to integrate these children into daily school routines.[1]

Examples of youth who are technology-dependent include those on ventilators, those requiring tube feeding, those receiving intravenous nutritional support, and those who have medical devices that support vital functions of the body.

The last survey through a Congressional Office in Technology Assessment in 1987 estimated that between 11,000 and 68,000 children were dependent on technology. This is probably an underestimate now, with the longer survival of youth with chronic previously terminal conditions, increased survival rates of preterm infants, and the greater availability of technology.[1]

A youth who is technology dependent requires an individualized health care plan (IHCP), otherwise known as an individualized school health plan (ISHP) or individualized health plan (IHP). This will promote school attendance, which is often a problem with children who have medical needs requiring complex support and many physician visits. The IHCP also helps integrate a youth who is technology dependent into school environments. Understanding the child's potentials in addition to limitations enable school staff to have realistic expectations for the youth's growth and development. The school nurse is instrumental in this process. Parents and guardians are also key, both in decision making for their child and in orienting their youth's medical situation to school staff.[1] The school nurse may not be with the child for the entire school day, so school staff need to be trained. Nurses may have to delegate nursing duties to nonmedical school staff, such as teachers, much less to health aides (see explanation on delegation elsewhere in this chapter).

Parents of technology-dependent children, of course, worry about the capabilities of school staff and want to ensure the health and safety of their child in school. They worry about the infection risks from peers and school staff. They worry about their child being isolated when peers are engaged in an activity of which their child cannot be part. Their children may worry about the stigma of treatments or procedures that make them different from peers.[1] These issues should be discussed in preparing the IHCP, and solutions should be pursued. Important IHCP elements are discussed elsewhere in this chapter.

> Examples of youth who are technology-dependent include those on ventilators, those requiring tube feeding, those receiving intravenous nutritional support, and those who have medical devices that support vital functions of the body.

How to Work With Schools

❶ Pediatricians and other medical professionals need to provide information to appropriate school staff on the technology used by their patients who are entering the school environment.

Recommendations for Pediatricians

❶ Pediatricians and other medical professionals are important members of any school team developing an individualized health care plan (IHCP) for a student who is technology dependent.

Recommendations for Program Directors and Trainees

1 Program directors should collaborate with schools to provide physician training within schools around youth with special needs. Pediatric and family practice residents can better understand school issues in supporting these youth, be involved in IHCP planning (with supervision from community or school pediatricians and other professionals), and become skilled in school/physician interactions.

Take-Home Points

1 Although pediatricians and other health care providers may be comfortable with the technology that their patients use in the hospital or home settings, school staff and administrators need support in incorporating these children in a school environment. Planning prior to attendance in school ensures the safety of the youth who is technology dependent and allows the youth to take advantage of the academic and social stimulation of the school environment.

Reference

1. Rehm RS, Rohr JA. Parents', nurses', and educators' perceptions of risks and benefits of school attendance by children who are medically fragile/technology-dependent. *J Pediatr Nurs*. 2002;17(5):345-353

Lesbian, Gay, Bisexual, Transgendered, and Questioning Youth

Students who are lesbian, gay, bisexual, transgender, or questioning (LGBT) often have trouble with peers in the school environment. This can range from teasing and bullying to significant violence against these students. Although the medical community in the past used to classify homosexuality and other "sexual minority" youth as pathological, this has changed. An example of this is the reclassification of homosexuality in 1973 from a mental disorder to a form of sexual orientation/expression in the *Diagnostic and Statistical Manual* published by the American Psychiatric Association. Major health professional organizations now do not classify homosexuality as a mental health condition.[1]

Sexual orientation is a person's pattern of physical and emotional arousal toward others, whether male or female. Homosexual individuals are attracted to others of the same sex, as contrasted with heterosexuals, who are attracted to others of the opposite sex. Homosexual males are gay and homosexual females are lesbian. Bisexual individuals are attracted to both sexes. Transgender individuals want to be a gender (male or female) other than what they are biologically. Transvestites dress in the clothing of the other gender and derive pleasure from doing so. Some adolescents are still questioning their sexual orientation, with more than 25% uncertain about their sexual orientation at 12 years old but decreasing with age to around 5% of 18-year-olds.[2]

LGBT students report being harassed at high rates—about 9 out of 10 in the year prior to one survey.[2] Many of these students also reported lower grades because of the harassment. Two thirds of LGBT students related that they felt unsafe and almost one third skipped at least 1 day of school because of this.[3] Other consequences of being LGBT include sexually transmitted diseases (STDs), unintended pregnancies, violence, being victims of bullying, alcohol and other drug use, tobacco use, depression, problems with weight management, and suicide.[4] A higher risk for suicide has been replicated in different community and national studies and across other countries as well.[5]

School environments can affect the risk of suicide in LGBT youth.[5] A study based on the Oregon Healthy Teens Survey looked at the responses of more than 30,000 students, with 4.4% identified as gay, lesbian, or bisexual. Among students who identified as gay, lesbian, or bisexual, 21.5% were more likely to attempt suicide in the previous 12 months, compared with 4.2% of heterosexual students. A social environment that was more supportive towards lesbian, gay, and bisexual youth showed significantly fewer suicide attempts. Supports studied included gay-straight alliances in schools, antibullying policies particularly including LGBT students, and antidiscrimination policies including sexual orientation.[5]

Unfortunately, school environments that are critical of sexual minorities can cause these students to feel isolated and subject them to harassment and violence. Nonheterosexual students are punished disproportionately by schools.[2] They are at risk of dropping out of school in addition to being kicked out of their homes.[2] Transgendered students are discriminated against and victimized in school and criminal justice systems in qualitative studies.[6]

A comment about gay or lesbian parents is also warranted in this section. Same-sex parents may face discrimination by the school in volunteer or leadership work at the school.[7] The research indicates that parents who are in the sexual minority do not cause cognitive, social, or emotional problems in their children. A prospective, longitudinal study of lesbian parents examining adolescent children not only showed that their children are well adjusted, they were more competent and had fewer behavioral problems than peers with heterosexual parents.[8] Gay and lesbian parents raise children whose sexual orientations are not different from the general population.

How to Work With Schools

The following guidance is from the American Academy of Pediatrics clinical report "Sexual Orientation and Adolescents"[2]:

❶ Pediatricians and other health care professionals can help create awareness of LGBT issues in their communities and schools.

❷ Pediatricians can advise when and how factual sexual orientation materials should be available to students in school and other community environments.

❸ Pediatricians can support the development and maintenance of support groups for sexual minority youth in schools.

❹ Pediatricians can create a supportive social environment for LGBT youth in their schools, including establishing or strengthening gay-straight alliances in schools, creating antibullying policies particularly involving lesbian, gay, or bisexual students, and developing and establishing antidiscrimination policies, including those dealing with sexual orientation.

Recommendations for Pediatricians

❶ All youths, including those who know or wonder whether they are not heterosexual, may seek information from physicians about sexual orientation,
STDs, substance abuse, or various psychosocial difficulties. The pediatrician should be attentive to various potential psychosocial difficulties, offer
counseling or refer for counseling when necessary, and ensure that every
sexually active youth receives a thorough medical history, physical examination, immunizations, appropriate laboratory tests, and counseling about
STDs (including HIV infection) and appropriate treatment if necessary. Not
all pediatricians may feel able to provide this type of care. Any pediatrician
who is unable to care for and counsel nonheterosexual youth should refer
these patients to an appropriate colleague.[2]

❷ Pediatricians and other health care professionals should ask a youth who is
LGBT about the school environment—whether it is supportive or hostile,
and support the youth while keeping in mind the attitudes and practices of
the school. Also, pediatricians and other providers should not assume that
the school, friends, and peers know of their patient's sexual orientation.
Medical professionals should be cognizant of the student's status at home
and in school.[9]

❸ Pediatricians should support gay and lesbian parents in their clinical work.[10]
This should include any desired discussions by families on how to explain
their family constellation to their preschool and school-aged children (for
instance, how to explain the absence of a father when meeting with lesbian
parents).[11] Another important time is during the middle school and high
school years. Sexuality and conformity are important issues during these
years. Teenagers may find it hard to discuss their family situations with
friends and classmates. This can be an important discussion moderated
by the pediatrician in the office.

Recommendations for Program Directors and Trainees

❶ Medical students and residents can be advocates for LGBT youth by supporting school efforts in education around sexual orientation, strengthening
support group efforts, and bringing factual LGBT medical information
to school staff. This may be done during adolescent medicine rotations or
developmental-behavioral pediatrics rotations (both of which are mandatory in US pediatric residency curricula).

Take-Home Points

❶ LGBT youth are at great risk of harassment and violence because of their sexual orientation or beliefs. They, like all adolescents, deserve educational opportunities and social interactions without creating a milieu that encourages suicide, drug use, school dropout, and many other deleterious effects.

❷ Schools can be critical in supporting LGBT and questioning youth.

References

1. American Psychological Association. Just the Facts About Sexual Orientation and Youth: A Primer for Principals, Educators, and School Personnel. Washington, DC: American 2008. Available at: www.apa.org/pi/lgbc/publications/justthefacts.html. Accessed April 13, 2015

2. Frankowski B; Committee on Adolescence. Sexual orientation and adolescents. *Pediatrics.* 2004;113(6):1827–1832

3. Kosciw JG, et al. *The 2009 National School Climate Survey: The Experiences of Lesbian, Gay, Bisexual and Transgender Youth in Our Nation's Schools.* New York, NY: Gay Lesbian and Straight Education Network; 2012

4. National Association of School Nurses. Policy Statement: School Health Education about Human Sexuality. Silver Spring, MD: National Association of School Nurses; June 2012

5. Hatzenbuehler ML. The social environment and suicide attempts in lesbian, gay and bisexual youth. *Pediatrics.* 2011;127(5):896–903

6. Himmelstein KEW, Brückner H. Criminal-justice and school sanctions against nonheterosexual youth: a national longitudinal study. *Pediatrics.* 2011;127(1):49-57

7. National Association of School Nurses. Policy Statement: Sexual Orientation and Gender Identity/Expression (Sexual Minority Students): School Nurse Practice. Silver Spring, MD: National Association of School Nurses; January 2012

8. Gartrell N, Bos H. US national longitudinal lesbian family study: psychological adjustment of 17-year-old adolescents. *Pediatrics.* 2010;126(1):28–36

9. American Academy of Child and Adolescent Psychiatry. Practice parameter on gay, lesbian, or bisexual sexual orientation, gender nonconformity, and gender discordance in children and adolescents. *J Am Acad Child Adolesc Psychiatry.* 2012;51(9):957–974

10. Perrin, EC and Kulkin H. Pediatric care for children whose parents are gay or lesbian. *Pediatrics.* 1996;97:629

11. Stein M. A Difficult adjustment to school: the importance of family constellation. *J Dev Behav Pediatr.* 2002;23(3):171–174

Resources

For additional school health related resources, visit www.aap.org/schoolhealthmanual.

SECTION 4

Role of the School Physician[a]

Cynthia DiLaura Devore, MD, MS, FAAP
Lani S. M. Wheeler, MD, FAAP

Background

Overview

Physicians play an important role in promoting the optimal biopsychosocial well-being of children in the school setting. Although the practice of medicine in the pediatric medical home or pediatric medical subspecialist's office might be managed in one way, an extension of medical home goals, objectives, or orders into the educational setting creates a different set of issues and concerns that might require adjustment of traditional medical care for a child. Schools have certain resources and limitations that affect the way they are able or, sometimes, willing to intervene in the medical management of a child. The school physician can be a valuable liaison between the medical home, the school, and the family. The school physician can also be a mediator, focusing less on what is right for a parent or the school and more on what is essential to the well-being of a child, especially when there are disputes over care. By understanding the roles and contributions physicians can make to schools, pediatricians can support and promote school physicians in their communities and improve the health and safety of children.

---

[a] Chapter excerpted/adapted from policy statement American Academy of Pediatrics, Council on School Health. Role of the school physician. *Pediatrics.* 2013;131(1):178-182

> Millions of children spend roughly 7 hours per day, 180 days per year in school[10] and may only visit their medical home once annually.

History of Physicians in the School Setting

Physicians associated with schools have held a variety of titles over the years. For the purpose of this chapter, a school physician is any physician who serves in any capacity for a school district, such as, but not limited to, an advisor, consultant, medical director, volunteer, team physician, medical inspector, or district physician.[1] This chapter does not address the role of physicians in school-based health centers[2] or the role of community pediatricians as private providers to school-aged children. Information on these topics is available on the American Academy of Pediatrics (AAP) Council on School Health (COSH) Web site (**http://www.aap.org/sections/schoolhealth/**).

The tradition of a school physician dates back to the late 1800s, as parents and public officials recognized that public school facilities needed national systematic medical inspection for hygiene and building safety concerns.[3] Over time, and during the polio epidemic of the 1950s, the role of the school medical inspector expanded to include containment of prevalent infectious diseases of childhood[3,4] and eventually as an important vehicle to manage universal immunization.[5] Modern school physicians focus on the needs of individual children as well as public health of the school community.[3,6,7] They often assist schools to accommodate students with special health care needs, manage acute and chronic illness, and oversee emergency response, environmental health and safety, and health promotion and education.[8,9]

Millions of children spend roughly 7 hours per day, 180 days per year in school[10] and may only visit their medical home once annually.

In 1999, Dr. Jocelyn Elders, former US Surgeon General, acknowledged the interdependence of health and education when she said, "You cannot educate a child who is not healthy, and you cannot keep a child healthy who is not educated."[11] Additionally, *Bright Futures: Guidelines for Health Supervision of Infants, Children, and Adolescents* encourages public schools and public health communities to become partners in prevention efforts.[12] Despite the value of coordinating health and education, physicians are not effectively and consistently involved in schools across the nation. As a result, American children have varying levels of medical support and safety, depending on the community in which they live. Well-placed school physician expertise can contribute to the creation of policies and practices that provide sound evidence-based structure to coordinated school health teams.

Current Laws Pertaining to the Physician in Schools

Currently, there is no single national set of school health laws. School health services are primarily regulated by state or local governments or individual school districts and vary.[13–15] Some states mandate school physicians; most do not.[16,17] However, "no one has systematically identified the full range of relevant legal authorities pertinent to schools that may help shape the health of children and adolescents."[15]

Federal law guarantees antidiscrimination and equal protection to individuals with disabilities.[18–20] These laws, such as the Individuals with Disabilities Education Act (IDEA) and Section 504 of the Rehabilitation Act, require states receiving federal funding for education to provide "related services," such as school nursing, as part of a child's individualized education program (IEP). However, the US Supreme Court ruled that school districts are not required to provide physician services for individual students, except for diagnostic or evaluative purposes for special education services.[13–15] This ruling's broad interpretation has limited funding to schools for physician services, despite the fact that many states, and the AAP, established basic minimal health services schools should provide, even though they might not have established guidance for pediatrician involvement.[21]

The AAP recommends that all schools have a registered professional school nurse, hereafter referred to as school nurse, to provide health services in schools.[22] The AAP also recommends that every school district have a school physician.[23] The American Medical Association not only recommends that school health be provided by "a professionally prepared school nurse" but also that "health services in schools must be supervised by a physician, preferably one who is experienced in the care of children and adolescents. Additionally a physician should be accessible to administer care on a regular basis."[24]

Despite a scarcity of laws addressing school physicians, pediatricians remain leaders in child health care and are integral members of the school health team.[22,25–29] Certainly, pediatricians need to know the laws that apply to their patients and themselves. All pediatricians will benefit from collaboration with their AAP chapter, state and local health departments, and school district to

Key to this discussion, and worthy of reiteration and emphasis, is that the AAP recommends a school nurse for every school and a school physician for every school district.

understand the laws specific to their roles in the schools. However, the lack of uniformity of laws or standards of best practice for school physicians complicates the role physicians have in schools and results in a difference of health care for children depending on the schools they attend and the communities in which they reside.

Key to this discussion, and worthy of reiteration and emphasis, is that the AAP recommends a school nurse for every school and a school physician for every school district.

How to Work With Schools

Current Roles and Relationships for School Physicians

The roles and types of relationships for physicians working in schools are broad. Involvement can range from fulfilling mandated services, serving as a **provider** of direct services, such as mandated physical examinations, or simply being an **advisor** to a school health advisory group. The role can be one of **consultant** when called on by the superintendent of the district or the Board of Education, or it can be of **leader** of a coordinated school health program. School physicians function on the basis of the medical and social needs or demands of the community, the school district's priorities, and state laws. School physicians not only bring value to the quality of health services but also may provide a cost savings to districts, with decreased liability from physician oversight of sound school health programs. School physician-coordinated concussion-management programs, established climate standards for outdoor activity, or guided anaphylaxis management protocols can potentially save lives, reduce morbidity, improve outcomes, and prevent potential costly litigation against school districts.[30-33]

States fund schools on the basis of student attendance, so a school physician can potentially save schools money by decreasing absenteeism through advocacy and education, such as in improved asthma or diabetes management.[34-37] The COSH Web site (**http://www.aap.org/sections/schoolhealth/**) provides guidance on these activities and how pediatricians can work with schools. Table 3.4.1 offers a summary of the various roles and responsibilities of a school physician. A model for the clinician on working with schools to improve asthma outcome is available,[38] as is a primer for the pediatrician on school health activities.[39]

Establishing a working relationship with a school district can be challenging, because physicians can have a professional relationship with schools in many

Table 3.4.1. Roles for School Physicians

Mandated services	Programmatic leadership

• Physical examinations (grade mandated, special education, work permits, sports participation)
• Oversight of return to sports (eg, concussion management programs)
• Active member on teams/committees (eg, special education, wellness, health education).
 	
Consultation
 	
• Write standing nursing orders/protocols
• Athletic advisor/team physician
  – Oversee health aspects of athletic programs and best practice standards
    ▪ Infectious diseases especially for close contact sports
    ▪ Participation of athletes with serious medical conditions
  – Adaptive physical education for acutely injured or chronically disabled youth
  – Mixed-gender competition
• Develop policies
  – Contagious diseases/pandemics
  – Bullying
  – Restraint, suspension, expulsion
  – Chronic school absenteeism
• Develop protocols
  – Delivery of medications
  – Anaphylaxis management
  – Seizure management
  – Asthma education and management
  – Diabetes care
• Assist in the management of specific medical emergencies or immediacies
• Participate at the building level in comprehensive, multidisciplinary teams and wellness councils
	• Health program evaluation and quality improvement
	  – Health education
	  – Physical activity and education
	  – Mental health promotion
	  – Staff wellness programs
	  – Family and community education
	  – Nutrition and food services
	• Liaison with primary care physicians regarding specific concerns
	• Professional performance development
	• Evaluation and collaborative oversight of nursing staff and other health service providers, including one-on-one nurses and door-to-door transportation
	• Review emergency care plans for children with life-threatening conditions
	• Classroom observation of children with special needs
	• Health education curriculum development
	
	Direct consultation with principals or the superintendent
	
	• Medical-legal issues
	• Parent attorneys or advocates in accommodation disputes and hearings
	• Building and playground health and safety
	• Bloodborne pathogen incidents
	• School closure related to illness or weather extremes or infections that affect public health

ways, such as a full- or part-time employee, an independent contractor, or a volunteer on a school health advisory group. Clearly, it is important for a pediatrician contemplating involvement with a school district to determine how much time is needed and how the he or she can be adequately reimbursed for his or her expertise. An hourly rate, billed monthly, consistent with community standards payable on an agreeable arrangement is probably one of the easier ways for a physician to be reimbursed for services. Some pediatricians prefer to estimate a total amount over a school year and divide that figure into twelve equal parts. Others choose to bill by the patient seen, if the primary service is performing mandated physicals. The problem with such an arrangement, though, is that the reimbursement is dependent on the reliability of children showing up for scheduled physicals, which means a physician could block out hours to be at school only to find virtually no patients present. Whatever the arrangement, it is reasonable for a school physician to bill a school district for their time at a rate that is fair and reasonable for all.

Where feasible, a school physician does not serve as a private physician for a child in that school district, however, because doing so can create a potential conflict of interest between the private physician, as representative/advocate for a patient versus the school physician as a representative of the school district. Maintaining some degree of objectivity allows the school physician to function as a mediator among all parties without suggestion of bias when advocating for what is best for the child.

Whatever the relationship, once a school district asks a physician to participate in hands-on medical practice for compensation in exchange for services, a clear definition of district expectations of the physician is essential. An agreement, accounting for laws governing the relationship of the physician to the public school district, should define indemnification and liability. It is critical that physicians understand the specifics of the relationship and that the legal implications are articulated clearly in a written agreement renewed periodically, often annually.

Although community volunteerism is attractive, physicians should take some precautions before volunteering to serve as a school or team physician, especially if the state's law requires medical oversight in the school. It is essential that the pediatrician know and understand state laws that address whether a district has an obligation to hire a medical director. It is also important for school physicians to remember that school districts pay for consultants in architecture, education, law, and accounting, for example, and often at premium rates. Those salaries are public record, which allows the school physician to compare his or her salary as reimbursement for medical expertise with other nonmedical professionals.

Regardless of the type of relationship, the physician should notify his or her professional liability insurance company of involvement in school health activities and determine whether the insurance covers such activities. If covered, the school physician should have this decision in writing. If a district has a legal obligation to provide compensation for physician services, this will allow the physician to schedule adequate time for the school district and to improve the quality and consistency of service.

Recommendations for Pediatricians

Given the contribution a school physician can make to the overall well-being of a child within the context of the school setting, the AAP recommends the following as a policy basis for school health:

1. Pediatricians should advocate that all school districts have a school physician to oversee health services. The school physician's roles and responsibilities should be well defined, fairly compensated, and outlined within a written contract.
2. Pediatricians should support their patients and local school health programs by working closely with the school health services team. In districts without school physicians, pediatricians should educate districts about the benefits of having a school physician and work to foster private-public partnerships for school physicians.
3. School physicians should be experts in key school health topics and be educated about the medical-legal environment in which they practice. They need to provide proper notification of their role and responsibility to their medical liability insurer and should collaborate with their AAP chapter, state and local health departments, and school district to understand the laws specific to their role in the schools.
4. Community pediatricians should be knowledgeable about key school health topics and how to work effectively with schools their patients attend.
5. Pediatricians should consider becoming a school physician or serving on school boards or school health advisory groups to develop sound school health policies and community programs.
6. All physicians who work with school-aged children should recognize the value to the child when there is a comprehensive, coordinated team effort among the child's medical home, the school, and family.

❼ Pediatric medical investigators should consider further research to determine how comprehensive coordinated school health programs under the direction of a school physician can improve health care in schools and enhance the goals of the medical home without attempting to replace it.

❽ AAP districts and chapters should support school health and school physicians and use the school physician's expertise to advocate for important changes to state and local school health policy. Additionally, AAP districts and chapters should advocate to develop and promote school health policies that benefit children by advocating for additional research on the benefits of school physicians in school health services.

Recommendations for Program Directors

Schools are complex systems that are able to offer students and residents a unique perspective on how pediatricians seek to optimize child health through policies, programs, practices, education, and measures. Reviewing local school district physician roles and responsibilities, compared with national "best practices," can be enlightening for trainees. Examining the pros and cons of the many controversial issues surrounding schools is an exercise that sharpens a student's sensitivity to the nuances of public health issues and policy making for schools. Program directors can arrange for training opportunities to ensure that pediatric residents learn the critical school health knowledge base and work directly with school physicians, school nurses, and school districts. Group discussions of on-site observations can expand learning for a group of trainees. Experiences such as attending a school health advisory council or a school board meeting are valuable learning tools. School health activities are excellent ways to solidify the trainees' competencies in systems-based practice, interpersonal and communication skills, and professionalism as the trainee has to work with various professionals in a system of care.

Critical School Health Knowledge Base for Physicians

Ideally, school physicians should be board-certified pediatricians or physicians with expertise in pediatrics.[24] In addition to basic training in child growth and development, disease processes, and well-child care, including adolescent and reproductive health and sports medicine, physicians who work with schools need additional expertise in key school health topics.[38-40] The degree of mastery required depends on the extent of the physician's role with schools. Overall, a school physician can become a positive liaison between the medical home, the family, and the school.[8]

Although all pediatricians need to understand infectious diseases, school physicians need a well-honed understanding of infections in a public setting. This might include outbreak control, cluster investigation, or public health tasks, including risk assessment (public health risk) and risk management (public relations control). It also necessitates that the school physician has a good set of resources to assist in complicated or unusual situations, such as pandemics.

School physicians need a strong understanding of immunization requirements, particularly for exemptions, such as the difference between medical contraindications versus medical precautions, with a focus on the importance of community safety in addition to individual protection.

Medical-legal issues arise often in school health, and because of their leadership role, school physicians are often asked for what amounts to legal opinions perhaps better referred to attorneys. Yet, because of the trust and respect physicians hold in many school situations, school physicians might be asked to offer an opinion, necessitating that the school physician understand the difference in his or her state among laws or statutes, regulations for various state departments, (eg, health and education), and local community standards of care. For example, a community standard might become the legal barometer used in courts of law, even taking precedence over existing laws and regulations. State and district school and public health laws, regulations, and policies are all an important critical knowledge base for the school physician.

The Individuals with Disabilities Act, Section 504 of the Rehabilitation Act, and the Americans with Disabilities Act (ADA) have established standards for mandatory accommodations and supports for children in the school setting. School physicians, as mandated members exploring school programming for children with special health care needs, such as a committee on special education, must have an understanding of these various standards to provide fair and balanced guidance to the school district to provide reasonable accommodations, advocacy for the child, and support for the parents.

Although pediatricians are familiar with the Health Information Portability and Accountability Act (HIPAA), many are not aware of the Federal Educational Rights and Privacy Act of 1974 (FERPA, also known as the Buckley Amendment). Physicians are obligated to follow HIPAA, not FERPA. Schools are mandated to follow FERPA, not HIPAA. How they intersect in the school setting, therefore, is truly critical in the knowledge base of a school physician, particularly because caution is needed not to allow excessive concern over confidentiality to overshadow legitimate concern over patient safety, care, or management. The medical home, the school physician, and the family need to work cooperatively within the context of these important laws to ensure that everyone who needs to know important health information has it.

Adolescent health (eg, brain development and reproductive health) brings a unique perspective to the work of a school physician. Although pediatricians working in a private setting might be fully aware of the needs of adolescents, such ensuring they are knowledgeable about reproductive health and safety, each community and every school district has a different population. How a board of education wishes to have its population of adolescents educated about matters such as these, among others, therefore, can be sensitive and requires careful attention and sometimes education of the community by the school physician to ensure that adolescents are given the tools they need to navigate their teenage journey.

Sports medicine, unless otherwise managed by a sports medicine physician or clinic, will fall to the school physician, who, by default, will become the team physician and the advisor to the physical education program. Therefore, a school physician will need to understand matters such as injury prevention, the value of regular conditioning, the risks of exercise in weather extremes, both hot and cold, or what constitutes temporary or permanent disqualifying conditions for sport activities. Other issues also affect physical activity programs in the school setting and require consultation by a school physician, such as hydration and sanitation on the field, mixed-gender competition, advanced athletic placement, return to play following injury, or postconcussion management. Determination of the level of physical activity participation based on school resources and limitations for the child with special health care needs is important. These needs might range from severe, permanent physical impairment to more common medical conditions, such as asthma, seizures, or diabetes. School physicians might provide education to coaches and physical education staff or school nurses about caring for the injured athlete, providing adaptive physical education for the child with special health care needs, or scheduling or cancelling outdoor activities to accommodate climate stress.

The value of physical education, proper nutrition, and physical activity at school are inherent to the prevention efforts of pediatricians in combating childhood obesity. School physicians have an excellent opportunity to instill the concept among educators that physical activity and sensible nutrition can enhance mental and academic performance.

Emergency preparedness is another area of expertise required of a school physician. For example, in dealing with children with special health care needs, the school physician might help develop emergency evacuation plans for non-ambulatory children. During the H1N1 influenza epidemic, school physicians were critical in assisting schools on issues of social distancing, isolation, quarantine, all of which affected children's ability to attend senior prom, final examinations, or even graduation events. Extended lock-downs, sheltering, or evacuation planning for potentially widespread catastrophic community events, from natural to manmade disasters, might be required of a school physician.

Some school physicians become involved in environmental and occupational health, such as indoor air quality concerns, cancer cluster investigations, or sick building syndrome claims. A school physician needs to understand these issues at least enough to find appropriate community resources to assist in areas outside his or her expertise.

The interplay between health and learning are part of the critical knowledge base of a school physician. Medical, emotional, attention, and learning problems can affect learning, and the school physician who views the total child might be able to put together a puzzle by finding a critical missing piece that will assist all concerned. To do this, school physicians sometimes require ready access to social services resources, including ways to assist families in finding access to health insurance and other community assistance programs, even if only referring them to the proper resources within the school or larger community.

Importantly, all school physicians need to become familiar with the 8 components of a coordinated school health model. These include (1) a strong interplay among health services, (2) health education, (3) healthy and safe environment, (4) physical education and activity, (5) nutrition services, (6) counseling/psychology/social services, (7) staff health promotion, and (8) family/community involvement. Ideally, all of these components warrant close team work and alliances or partnerships among the medical home, the educational home, and the family home to afford the child the best possible outcomes physically, intellectually, emotionally, educationally, and spiritually.

Table 3.4.2 contains a nonexclusive summary list of essential areas of expertise required of a school physician. The list of areas of expertise might be considered essential competencies/milestones/entrustable professional activities for a school health rotation/experience.

Table 3.4.2. Critical Knowledge Base for School Physicians

- Infectious diseases (eg, outbreak control)
- Public health (eg, risk assessment and management, resources)
- Immunizations (eg, school requirements and medical contraindications)
- Medical-legal issues
    - State and district school and public health laws, regulations and policies
    - IDEA, Section 504, and ADA
    - FERPA and HIPAA and how they intersect in the school setting
- Adolescent health (eg, brain development and reproductive health)
- Sports medicine*
    - The value of physical education and physical activity at school
    - Injury prevention
    - Conditioning
    - Disqualifying conditions
    - Hydration
    - The effects of climate extremes on athletes
    - Concussion management
    - Adaptive physical education
- Emergency preparedness (eg, children with special health care needs)
- Environmental and occupational health (eg, indoor air quality)
- Health and learning (eg, medical, emotional, attentional, and learning problems that affect learning)
- Social services resources (eg, access to health insurance and assistance programs)
- A coordinated school health model (eg, health services, health education, healthy and safe environment, physical education and activity, nutrition services, counseling/psychology/social services, staff health promotion and family/community involvement)

*Unless there is a separate team physician.

Recommendations for Trainees

Regardless of their future plans for primary or specialty care, trainees should become well versed in the basic school health knowledge base. They should become familiar with the laws and regulations that govern school health in their states, particularly how their state department of health and state department of education intersect. They should learn the difference between laws, regulations, or guidance and determine how they affect the practice of medicine, such as learning the timing of mandated vaccines for school entry versus the medical model for vaccines, which sometimes differ. They should become comfortable with the rights of children with special health care needs or hand-icapping conditions and facile with a comprehension of laws such as IDEA, ADA, Section 504, FERPA, and HIPAA. The 10 components of the Centers for Disease Control and Prevention coordinated school health model are also an important tool new pediatricians can use when talking to schools. They can consider their current and future collaboration with school physicians, school nurses, and schools to improve the biopsychosocial health and well-being of their patients. They should recognize the value and necessity of coordinating the goals of the medical home within the school setting and the family home. New community pediatricians might find it helpful to make time to visit local school districts when they initially establish their careers after training to become familiar with the administration, meet the school nurses, and inquire about school district policies relevant to the health and safety of children. Young pediatricians with an interest in school health should also consider joining the AAP Council on School Health for ongoing education and updates on school health.

Take-Home Points

* Advocate with your local school districts for a school nurse in every building and a school physician in every district.
* Learn your state and local school health laws and regulations.
* Collaborate with your state and local school physicians and school nurses and learn about the philosophies, priorities of health services, resources, and limitations within the school district.
* Help your patients and their families with school health issues, especially the management of chronic conditions and special health care needs at school.
* Consider expanding your role with local schools to include school physician activities.
* Join the AAP Council on School Health.

Resources

For additional school health related resources, visit www.aap.org/schoolhealthmanual.

References

1. Massachusetts Office of Health and Human Services. Template for Massachusetts School Physician/Medical Consultant Role. Commonwealth of Massachusetts; 2014. Available at: http://www.mass.gov/eohhs/gov/departments/dph/programs/community-health/primarycare-healthaccess/school-health/publications/. Accessed December 1, 2015

2. American Academy of Pediatrics, Committee on School Health. School health centers and other integrated school health services. *Pediatrics.* 2001;107(1):198–201

3. Markel H, Golden J. Children's public health policy in the United States: how the past can inform the future. *Health Aff (Millwood).* 2004;23(5):147–152

4. Minna Stern A, Reilly M, Cetron M, Markel H. "Better off in school": school medical inspection as a public health strategy during the 1918-1919 influenza pandemic in the United States. *Public Health Rep.* 2010;125(Suppl 3):63-70

5. Apr 26, 1954: Polio vaccine trials begin. This Day in History. Available at: http://www.history.com/this-day-in-history/polio-vaccine-trials-begin. Accessed April 13, 2015

6. Wilson KD, Moonie S, Sterling DA, Gillespie KN, Kurz RS. Examining the consulting physician model to enhance the school nurse role for children with asthma. *J Sch Health.* 2009;79(1):1–7

7. Schetzina KE, Dalton WT, Lowe EF, et al. Developing a coordinated school health approach to child obesity prevention in rural Appalachia: results of focus groups with teachers, parents, and students. *Rural Remote Health.* 2009;9(4):1157

8. Taras H, Brennan JJ. Students with chronic diseases: nature of school physician support. *J Sch Health.* 2008;78(7):389–396

9. Yaffe JM. Developing and supporting school health programs. Role for family physicians. *Can Fam Physician.* 1998;44(Apr):821-824

10. US Census Bureau. School Enrollment 2000. US Census 2000 Brief. Available at: http://www.census.gov/prod/2003pubs/c2kbr-26.pdf. Accessed April 13, 2015

11. Morse C. Joycelyn Elders says U.S. must transform its sick care system. *Cornell Chronicle.* February 18, 1999:A1

12. Hagan JF, Shaw JS, Duncan PM, eds. *Bright Futures: Guidelines for Health Supervision of Infants, Children, and Adolescents.* 3rd ed. Elk Grove Village, IL: American Academy of Pediatrics; 2008

13. Brener ND, Wheeler L, Wolfe LC, Vernon-Smiley M, Caldart-Olson L. Health services: results from the School Health Policies and Programs Study 2006. *J Sch Health.* 2007;77(8):464–485

14. Centers for Disease Control and Prevention. The Centers for Law and the Public's Health: a collaborative at Johns Hopkins and Georgetown Universities. A CDC Review of School Laws and Policies Concerning Child and Adolescent Health. *J Sch Health.* 2008;78(2): 69–128

15. Jones SE. A CDC Review of School Laws and Policies Concerning Child and Adolescent Health: executive summary. *J Sch Health.* 2008;78(2):69-72

16. Pennsylvania Code. School Health. Available at: http://www.pacode.com/secure/data/028/chapter23/chap23toc.html. Accessed April 13, 2015

17. New York State Education Department. School health services to be provided. Available at: http://www.p12.nysed.gov/sss/schoolhealth/schoolhealthservices/Article19Sections.html#902. Accessed April 13, 2015

18. US Department of Education. Building the legacy: IDEA 2004. Available at: http://idea.ed.gov/. Accessed April 13, 2015

19. US Department of Justice. Americans with Disabilities Act: ADA home page. Available at: http://www.ada.gov/. Accessed April 13, 2015

20. US Department of Education. Protecting Students with Disabilities: Frequently Asked Questions about Section 504 and the Education of Children with Disabilities. Available at: http://www2.ed.gov/about/offices/list/ocr/504faq.html. Accessed April 13, 2015

21. Taras H, Duncan P, Luckenbill D, Robinson J, Wheeler L, Wooley S, eds. *Health, Mental Health and Safety Guidelines for Schools.* Elk Grove Village, IL; American Academy of Pediatrics; 2004. Available at: http://www.nationalguidelines.org/. Accessed April 13, 2015

22. American Academy of Pediatrics, Council on School Health, Magalnick H, Mazyck D. Role of the school nurse in providing school health services. *Pediatrics.* 2008;121(5):1052–1056

23. Devore CD, Wheeler LS, American Academy of Pediatrics, Council on School Health. Role of the school physician. *Pediatrics.* 2012;131(1):178–182

24. American Medical Association. Policy Statement H-60.991: Providing Medical Services through School-Based Health Programs. Chicago, IL: American Medical Association; 2012. Available at: https://www.ama-assn.org/ssl3/ecomm/PolicyFinderForm.pl?site= www.ama-assn.org&uri=/resources/html/PolicyFinder/policyfiles/HnE/H-60.991.HTM. Accessed April 13, 2015

25. American School Health Association. Physicians in Schools, Preschools, and Child Care Centers. Kent, OH: American School Health Association; 2004

26. General Laws of Massachusetts. Chapter 71: Public Schools. Section 1: Public schools. Section 53: The school committee shall appoint one or more school physicians. Available at: http://law.onecle.com/massachusetts/71/53.html. Accessed April 13, 2015

27. Laws of New York. Employment of health professionals. Available at: http://public.leginfo. state.ny.us/LAWSSEAF.cgi?QUERYTYPE=LAWS+&QUERYDATA=$$EDN902$$@ TXEDN0902+&LIST=LAW+&BROWSER=EXPLORER+&TOKEN=54954571+ &TARGET=VIEW. Accessed April 13, 2015

28. Ohio Revised Code. Title [33] XXXIII EDUCATION Chapter 3313: BOARDS OF EDUCATION. 3313.71 Examinations and diagnoses by school physician. Available at: http://statutes.laws.com/ohio/title33/chapter3313/3313_71. Accessed April 13, 2015

29. Rhode Island Rules and Regulations for School Health Programs. Section 8.2: School Physician. Available at: http://sos.ri.gov/documents/archives/regdocs/released/pdf/ DOH/5471.pdf. Accessed April 13, 2015

30. Associated Press. La Salle settles injured player's lawsuit. ESPN College Football Web site. Available at: http://sports.espn.go.com/ncf/news/story?id=4700355. Accessed April 13, 2015

31. Seattle/Local Health Guide. Zack's Story: CDC highlights Washington sports concussion law. Available at: http://mylocalhealthguide.com/zacks-story-cdc-highlights-washington-sports-concussion-law/. Accessed April 13, 2015

32. Hood J. Family sues restaurant over seventh-grader's fatal food allergy. *Chicago Tribune.* March 18, 2011. Available at: http://articles.chicagotribune.com/2011-03-18/news/ct-met-peanut-allergy-lawsuit-20110318_1_food-allergy-peanut-products-katelyn-carlson. Accessed April 13, 2015

33. Fox News. Two Georgia Teens Die During Football Training Camp, August 3, 2011. Available at:

34. http://www.foxnews.com/sports/2011/08/03/teen-dies-during-football-training-camp/. Accessed April 13, 2015

35. Richmond CM, Sterling D, et al. Asthma 411: addition of a consulting physician to enhance school health. *J Sch Health.* 2006;76(6):333–335

36. Centers for Disease Control and Prevention. Coordinated School Health. Available at: http://www.cdc.gov/healthyyouth/cshp/. Accessed April 13, 2015

37. Young MA, Phillips PH. Changing the role of the school physician: the Newton Study. *J Sch Health.* 1966;36(9):424–432

38. Wheeler L, Buckley R, Gerald LB, Merkle S, Morrison TA. Working with schools to improve pediatric asthma management. *Pediatr Asthma Allergy Immunol.* 2009;22(4): 197-206

39. Nader P. A pediatrician's primer for school health activities. *Pediatr Rev.* 1982;(4):82-92

40. Kleinschmidt EE. Special educational qualifications for the school physician. *J Sch Health.* 1939;9(1):13-19

41. Neilson EA. Health education and the school physician. *J Sch Health.* 1969;39(6):377–384

SECTION 5

The School Nurse

Erin D. Maughan, PhD, MS, RN, APHN-BC
Shirley Schantz, EdD, ARNP

Background
. . . .

School nurses are the health care representatives in the school setting.[1] They perform a pivotal role in the health and well-being of children and staff, especially with the significant increase in the number of children with chronic disease and special health care needs over the last few decades.[2] School nurses make a difference in the school setting: they decrease the number of students who experience asthma exacerbations[3]; help manage diabetes care[4]; and keep students in their seats in their classrooms at a higher rate than non-licensed school personnel.[5] A school nurse in the building frees up 1 hour per day of principal time.[6]

School nurses address social determinants and disparities (such as poverty, minority populations) that affect the health and learning readiness of children in the school setting.[7] It is essential for pediatricians to appreciate the demographics and roles of school nurses, the variety of school nursing models that exist, the culture of education, and laws that affect school health services.

Demographics

School nurses have served a critical role in improving public health and in ensuring students' academic success for more than 100 years. Currently, there are more than 75,000 school nurses in the United States, and approximately 75% of schools have a full- or part-time school nurse assigned to their building.[8]

> The American Academy of Pediatrics (AAP) identifies 7 key roles of the school nurse[1]: clinicians, leaders, advocates, health promoters, educators, policy makers, and community liaisons.

The National Association of School Nurses (NASN) recommends that school nurses are registered nurses (RNs) with a baccalaureate degree in nursing.[2] Approximately 72% of school nurses have a bachelor's degree or higher,[9] and There are approximately 3500 nationally board-certified school nurses (written communication with Nadine Schwab MPH, BSN, RN, NCSN, FNASN, executive director of the National Board for Certification of School Nurses, 2013). Many states also offer state certification for school nurses. The majority of school nurses have been nurses for 10 or more years and are 50 years or older, with 40% of these nurses expecting to retire in the next 5 years.[9]

School nurses are responsible for the care of all the children in the school, taking special care to provide case management for children with chronic conditions. It is estimated that 13% to 18% of all children have chronic conditions such as asthma, diabetes, seizures, and severe, life-threatening allergies.[10] The number of children with these conditions has increased steadily over the past decade. In addition, between 2002 and 2008, there has been a 60% increase in the number of children in special education with health impairments attributable to an acute or chronic condition.[11] School nurses are responsible for the care and case management of all these students as well as all the care of other students and school staff in the building.

Role of the School Nurse

The American Academy of Pediatrics (AAP) identifies 7 key roles of the school nurse[1]: clinicians, leaders, advocates, health promoters, educators, policy makers, and community liaisons.

In addition to providing care and case management for students with chronic illnesses while they are in school, school nurses provide acute care for illnesses and injuries on a daily basis, use their assessment skills to identify need and develop health care plans to address students' health needs, and facilitate the provision of accommodations for children with special health care needs to attend school.

School nurses are the health experts in the school. They provide leadership, direction, and advocacy related to the health needs of the entire organizational school system.

School nurses are health advocates. School nurses perform screenings that help identify students with specific individual health care needs that have the potential to affect learning. School nurses use the information to make appropriate referrals. Screenings may include vision, hearing, height/weight, blood pressure, dental, or other screenings. School nurses also advocate for policy changes that provide for healthier environments that benefit the entire school community.

School nurses are health promoters. They promote a physical and mental health environment that is safe and secure. They monitor for infectious disease outbreaks and support full and adequate immunization for all children. School nurses address the safety of playground equipment (especially when playground injuries occur) and monitor outdoor air quality for all outdoor play and activities. School nurses advocate for programs to reduce bullying and violence. They address and assess for mental health issues, drug use, and abuse. They are in the ideal position to address and intervene for health risks that potentially lead to absenteeism, depression, sexual activity, and much more. The result is a child/adolescent that has a healthy and safe learning environment.

School nurses are educators. They provide education and support to students with chronic and acute illnesses and teach students about personal health and healthy behaviors, how to manage asthma triggers and avoid allergens, hygiene, prevention of infectious disease, first aid, pregnancy prevention, substance use prevention, and numerous other health concerns that arise in today's society. In some states, school nurses are also certified health teachers and serve as the health educator in the school community.[9]

Schools nurses are collaborators. They provide the bridge between students/families and health care providers, ensuring that each child is connected to a medical home. Their expertise ensures that schools provide the appropriate accommodations for students with special needs. School nurses use data to demonstrate the continuing need for health services in schools and communities. They collaborate with pediatricians and other community partners to address social determinants and health disparities (such as poverty, ethnicity, culture, language, environment, etc), each of which can have a significant effect on health care and a student's ability to learn.[12] School nurses are also well positioned to serve as coordinators in the Whole School, Whole Community, Whole Child (WSCC) model of the ASCD (formerly the Association for Supervision and Curriculum Development) and the Centers for Disease Control and Prevention (CDC).[13]

School health services are one concern facing schools. The ASCD and CDC recommend schools choose a collaborative approach of health within the school and with the community. The WSCC model builds on the coordinated school health model and includes community involvement; family engagement; health education; physical education and physical activity; nutrition environment and services; health services; counseling, psychological, and social services; employee wellness; social and emotional climate; and physical environment. The new WSCC model includes 10 components necessary for a healthy environment that promotes academic success.

Each component of the WSCC model is significant, and the components often overlap. For example, many mental health concerns mask themselves as physical symptoms, necessitating consultation between the school nurse and counselor; a child with diabetes must know the carbohydrate content of foods to accurately calculate how much insulin is needed, necessitating consultation between the school nurse and nutrition services; and a student with asthma may need accommodations in physical education class, necessitating consultation between the school nurse and physical education teacher. For a collaborative school health approach to be successful, it is critical to have someone coordinate all the components. This is a logical responsibility for the school nurse, who has the knowledge and case management skills necessary and already works with each of the areas as he or she ensures the best health outcomes for all children. Pediatricians are encouraged to be members of the WSCC model through community involvement or serve as a medical director/advisor for a school or school district.

In the past, school health was seen as a separate "silo" from primary health care and even public health. The Affordable Care Act (ACA), which has placed increased emphasis on coordinated care organizations,[14] will enable school nurses to enhance bridges and collaborations with community partners and health care providers.

ROLE OF THE SCHOOL NURSE

School nurses:

- Facilitate normal development and positive student response to interventions.
- Provide leadership in promoting health and safety, including a healthy environment.
- Provide quality health care and intervene with actual and potential health problems.
- Use clinical judgment in providing case management, self-advocacy, and learning.
- Actively collaborate with others to build student and family capacity for adaptation, self- services.[2]

> When deciding what to delegate, nurses consider the 5 rights of delegation
> (the right person, the right task, the right circumstance, the right supervision,
> and the right direction).[16]

Models of Care and Delegation

The roles of school nurses differ depending on the needs of the students, schools, and also workload. Only 50% of school nurses serve 1 building, the rest cover more than 1 school building.[9] School nurses who work in 1 or 2 buildings tend to provide direct care to children and staff. School nurses who are in large buildings, or who oversee multiple buildings, often work with licensed practical nurses (LPNs), health aides, or unlicensed assistive personnel. In the last assessment of staffing, there was no difference in the staffing of school nurses in Title I (lower socioeconomic schools) compared with non-Title I schools.[8]

States also require different nursing licenses, although many states now belong to a nurse licensure compact. Each state has a separate Nurse Practice Act that outlines the scope and responsibility of the registered nurse. This document also directs what tasks may be delegated. Delegation is the transferring of responsibility for a specific nursing activity or task to another person (Table 3.5.1). The decision regarding delegation should be made by the nurse delegating the task. Many educators and some health care providers need to understand this very important concept. In addition, nurses cannot delegate nursing assessment, only health care tasks.

When deciding what to delegate, nurses consider the 5 rights of delegation (the right person, the right task, the right circumstance, the right supervision, and the right direction).[16] *The right person* means that the nurse determines that the person to whom they are delegating the task has the skill set necessary to perform that task. *The right task* means it is something that is appropriate to delegate to another. *The right circumstance* means the task is routine. *The right supervision* and *right direction* refer to proper training, guidance, and observation of the task by the nurse to the person being trained.

Delegating is not a simple decision and must only be done after careful consideration.[15] Many districts have algorithms or flow sheets to determine whether delegation is appropriate. Because each state has different rules regarding what can be delegated, practices differ greatly from state to state. It is critical that pediatricians know the laws in their states. It is also critical that pediatricians, when determining what nursing or medical care should take place in the school setting, know the circumstances in that school: the RN provides direct care or tasks are delegated.[16,17] The safety of the child must be the first consideration. Nurse Practice Acts and licensure issues become even more of a concern when a school nurse accompanies a student on a field trip that crosses state lines.

Table 3.5.1. Overarching Principles of Delegation

- The nursing profession determines the scope of nursing practice.
- The nursing profession defines and supervises the education, training, and utilization for any assistant roles involved in providing direct patient care.
- The registered nurse (RN) takes responsibility and accountability for the provision of nursing practice.
- The RN directs care and determines the appropriate utilization of any assistant involved in providing direct patient care.
- The RN accepts aid from nursing assistive personnel in providing direct patient care.[16]

Culture of Education

The majority of school nurses are employed by school districts. The goals of education and schools are very different than the goals of health. Schools focus on test scores, accountability, and state standards; health focuses on the physical, emotional, and social well-being of children. In recent years, education has suffered funding cuts with the added responsibilities of educating increasingly diverse populations.[18] The worlds of education and health complement each other, as the student must be healthy to learn. The 2 worlds collide when one world does not recognize the importance and priority of the other. Educators' focus and expertise is related to learning and test scores, and they may not always understand the complexity of children's health and effect their health has on their ability to learn. This issue can be especially complicated when budgets are perceived to be tight, necessitating delegation of health tasks to nonmedical staff. Such an approach brings with it potential risks and may not be in the best interest of the students.

School nurses address this issue every day. Pediatricians must keep this in mind when prescribing medical procedures, including medication, to be given during the school day. This is important in understanding why school administrators may not appreciate the consequences of changing the lunch and physical education schedule of a child who has diabetes and the potential health risks. School administrators may not understand why a child should be excluded from school or when it is appropriate for the student to return.

School Nurses and School-Based Health Clinics

There is a need to better understand the distinction between school nurses and school-based health clinics (SBHCs). SBHCs complement school nursing by using a shared case-management structure.[19] SBHCs started in the 1970s in elementary schools as a way of addressing the need for better access to care; they have since expanded into middle and high schools. The clinics are located in or close to the school, provide primary care, and usually employ doctors, advanced practice nurses (nurse practitioners), or physician assistants. Each clinic is different but often provides a range of medical, mental health, and/or dental services. There are only 1930 SBHCs in the country but more than 75,000 school nurses.[20] School nurses are predominantly RNs with bachelor's degrees who oversee all children in the school, perform population-based screenings, and provide triage to children's specific needs if there is an SBHC. Some schools have both a school nurse and a SBHC. An SBHC does not replace the need for a school nurse. Although there is a clear distinction between the 2, collaboration between the school nurse and the SBHC can have a significant effect on the students' and school community's overall health.

The funding streams of SBHCs and school nurses are usually different,[19] with the majority of school nurses being salaried by the education system and SBHC funding coming from state departments of health.

Laws Affecting School Health Services

Education is overseen mostly at the state level. This means each state and local district has governance related to what happens in schools. However, several significant federal laws have passed that greatly affect school health services. These laws include the Individuals with Disabilities Education Improvement Act of 2004 (IDEA, which grew out of the Education of All Handicapped Children Act of 1975),[21] Section 504 of the Rehabilitation Act of 1973,[22] the Americans with Disabilities Act (ADA),[23] and the Health Insurance Portability and Accountability Act (HIPAA).[24] IDEA[21] mandates that all children have the right to an education. Before the law was passed, children with autism or Down syndrome were not afforded a public education. There are different sections to IDEA. Part B outlines the rights of children to ensure that the needs of the students are met and their rights are protected and what schools must comply with to obtain funding for these students. Part C refers to early intervention programs (birth to 3 years). The purpose of the program is to find children with developmental delay and provide appropriate services for them. These services may include, but are not limited to, physical therapy or speech therapy.

The ADA mandates equal education opportunities for all students, including children with complex medical conditions. In the past, children with disabilities were not allowed or able to attend public school. The ADA dramatically changed this and schools, by law, opened their doors to all children under the age of 21. Many of these children require medical treatments or other nursing care during the school day.[23]

Section 504 of the Rehabilitation Act further clarifies that schools have to provide appropriate nursing care during the school day.[22] It indicates that reasonable accommodations must be made for children with "physical or mental impairment that substantially limits one or more major life activities." For example, a child with diabetes must be allowed to test his or her blood sugar when needed. It is important to note, however, that the law did not mandate any funding to support the necessary accommodations schools must provide.

HIPAA was passed to protect patients' privacy of their health care records.[24] It allows for the sharing of medical information needed for patient care. The law only applies to health plans and health care providers who transmit specific types of information electronically (such as financial/administrative). HIPAA law has caused much confusion, especially in the school setting. Many health care providers in the community believe they cannot share health information with the schools, even when treatment is needed in the school setting, but this is not accurate. HIPAA allows for sharing of medical treatment information to the school nurse for treatment occurring in school, even without parent consent.[24] Of course, it is always better to have written consent from the parent. Part of the confusion is because education has its own confidentiality law, the Family Educational Rights and Privacy Act (FERPA).[24] FERPA only applies to schools that receive federal funding and is meant to protect student education records in the very broadest sense. In many schools, student health records (including children with special health care needs) are included in a section of their education chart. The chart or health information should only be available to those who need to see it. However, this is also interpreted broadly at times. The US Department of Education and US Department of Health and Human Services published a joint paper explaining how the 2 laws can work together in the school setting.[24]

> Health care providers develop medical care plans for the treatment plan and care of the child; school nurses develop individualized health care plans to assist in the treatment plan and health care goals of the child while in school.

As mentioned earlier, education is under local (district or state) control, and each state has a variety of laws related to school health services. Laws related to mandated routine screenings (such as vision and hearing) and assessments required (immunizations or physical examinations for school entrance) are common in many states and may even be district level policy. Because each state and district is different, it is important for the pediatrician to contact school nurses directly for correct information. Another reliable resource for information related to school health is the state school nurse consultant, who may be employed by the State Office of Education or the State Department of Health (or both). The state school nurse consultant provides leadership and oversight related to school health services and school nursing practice for the state and has the knowledge and resources related to state laws and practices.

How to Work With Schools and School Nurses

There are many ways for pediatricians and health care providers to work with school nurses for the benefit of the students and their health. In fact, it is critical they work collaboratively for individual children and the entire school population. Collaboration and clear communication between the school and provider is vitally important in the development of care plans, medication administration, immunizations, screening results and referrals, health promotion efforts, and emergency preparedness.

Care Plans

Communication among the provider, family, and school (nurse/teacher) is critical for successful management of children with chronic conditions during school activities. One of the key ways providers, families, and school nurses can work together is in the development of a care plan. This should be a collaborative effort and supported by the school, health care team, parents, and students.

It is important that terms such as care plan and emergency medical plan are used correctly by providers. Health care providers develop medical care plans for the treatment plan and care of the child; school nurses develop individualized health care plans to assist in the treatment plan and health care goals of the child while in school. Health care providers often establish emergency care plans with information for emergency department doctors, when needed; school nurses develop emergency care plans for teachers and staff to educate them about how to respond to a child's emergency in the school. The audiences and settings are different and must be considered in developing school health care plans. For example, health care providers and school nurses must take into account the model of health care in the school and if treatments can be appropriately and legally delegated. Health care providers and school nurses must also consider school policies and procedures that may affect the situation and identify what equipment is available and appropriate in the school. Emergency care plans that may be used by nonmedical school staff should avoid medical jargon and be the quick resource for the unlicensed or lay person in an emergency.[25]

Although the school nurse is the person who oversees health care plans in the school setting, it is critical that the school nurse (RN), family, and health care provider work together on the development of the care plan for the benefit of the student.[25] School nurses develop individualized health care plans; however, health care providers may assist in the development of portions of the plan. For example, the National Asthma Education and Prevention Program recommends every child with medically diagnosed asthma have a current asthma action plan on file with the school nurse.[26,27] Several asthma action plan templates have been developed and kept at the health care provider's office. Whether the child has newly diagnosed asthma, has an exacerbation, or needs a change in treatment plan, the pediatrician can assist the family with completing the asthma action plan and greatly encourage the family to provide it to the school for the nurse to have on file. The asthma action plan is vital for consistent care for the child during the school day. Students spend half of their waking hours at school, and there is a good possibility that a student with asthma will need care during this time. Asthma action plans facilitate that the treatment plan continues while the student is in school. The HIPAA and FERPA laws *allow* for school nurses to communicate directly with health care providers and their office staff to obtain the information needed to complete a school care plan. A sample asthma action plan and other school medical forms for common chronic conditions such as diabetes or seizure disorders that are needed by school nurses to develop the necessary care plans are available on the AAP Council on School Health Web site.

Health care plans prepared by the school nurse benefit students. They provide an intentional framework for the care of the whole student and assist that student to fully access his or her educational program which promotes academic success. The health care plan is a valuable tool that increases communication between nurses and school staff, which ultimately supports student achievement. Health care plans also clearly delineate issues surrounding the delegation of nursing tasks and provide an evidenced-based plan for both chronic and acute care situations. Initiating and implementing effective health care plans to attain expected outcomes is considered a standard of school nursing practice.[28]

There are a variety of health care plans seen in the school setting (Table 3.5.2):

Table 3.5.2. Care Plan Comparison[29]

Care Plan	Author	Purpose
Individualized health care plan	School nurse in collaboration with health care provider, parent, and student	A nursing document based on nursing diagnosis, interventions and expected outcomes Written in nursing language Written in response to medical orders
Emergency care/action plan	School nurse in collaboration with health care provider, parent, and student	Outlines the appropriate response in an emergency situation (at school, on field trips, etc) Written in lay language with easy-to-follow steps for school staff Written for students with potentially life-threatening health concerns
Section 504 plan	Section 504 plan coordinator for school district in collaboration with parent, school nurse, and specialized instructional support personnel	Legal document that protects individuals with disabilities Written in lay language Addresses disabilities that limit one or more major life activities

Individualized Health Care Plan

The individualized health care plan (IHCP) is the document that provides a comprehensive assessment of a student's health care needs and outlines a management plan to care for a student's health in the school setting.[30] The need for an IHCP is determined by the school nurse and based on required nursing care rather than the educational entitlements that include special education or the accommodations of a Section 504 plan.[31] Priority for IHCP development must be given to those students who are at risk of a life-threatening emergency health crisis.[29] The components of a quality care plan include:

- nursing assessment;
- nursing diagnosis;
- outcome identification;
- planning;
- implementation; and
- evaluation.

The school nurse has the unique nursing and physical assessment skills in the school setting to provide a strong foundation for writing the IHCP. Factors that are included in this assessment include a review of medical records and orders, interviews with key stakeholders (including the student and parent), consultation with health care providers, and physical assessment. This information is used to develop nursing diagnoses and a plan of care for the student while in school.[30] These assessments lead to the identification of appropriate nursing diagnoses, development of strong student-centered goals, and implementation of meaningful nursing interventions. This process supports identified student outcomes. The plan also includes contact information, medications to be given at school, any known allergies, diet modifications, activity modifications, environment modifications, environmental triggers to avoid, symptoms and behavior changes to observe for, and personnel needing training and education. Provisions for field trips and other school activities should be included, as well as a self-management plan appropriate for the child's age and developmental ability. In addition, the plan should include provisions in case of an emergency. This may include additional medications to be included in an emergency kit for the child.

The plan may also include do-not-attempt-to-resuscitate (DNAR) orders. Historically, DNAR orders have been discouraged in the school setting because of the trauma to the bystanders and lack of appropriately trained personnel. However, the number of DNAR orders in the school has increased over the past decade.[32] Few states have allowed for advanced directives for minors out of the hospital. Pediatricians must review the situation carefully before initiating a DNAR order. In particular, they must review district and state policy/law related to DNAR orders; review the liability protection for those who might be involved in a DNAR order, determine whether there is an appropriate process to ensure privacy for the child, speak to emergency medical services regarding their involvement, and most importantly, discuss this issue with the family, child, school nurse, and other school administrators.[24]

Ideally, the school nurse will complete the IHCP and send it to the health care provider and family to review and sign, although not a necessity. A speedy turnaround time by all is important to ensure the highest level of health and safety for the child. The school nurse will continually evaluate the IHCP for effectiveness and renew the plan at least annually, with revisions made as needed.[31] It is imperative that this process be supported by the primary care provider.

The increase in technology, potential for information sharing, and emphasis of care coordination outlined in the ACA promotes the collaboration and coordination between school nurses and health care providers.[14] Several pilot projects have shown that increased communication by sharing health care records improves the management of chronic conditions. One system, in which school nurses were employed by the hospital, was able to alert the school nurse each morning of a student's the emergency department visit after school hours and the outcome. This led to increased school nurse case management and a decrease in asthma exacerbations in school (personal oral communication with conference attendees, 2013). In another model, school nurses were able to access provider health care records (after obtaining parent permission) to the benefit of care for the student in school.[33] Health care providers, school nurses, and families found the increased communication helpful in managing the child's health in school—for example, school health teams and health care providers shared actual laboratory values for daily blood glucose recordings as well as hemoglobin A1c levels. There is also faster communication regarding new treatments or changes in medication.

As the ACA and meaningful use continue to expand the use of electronic health care records, it is important for pediatricians to work with school districts to ensure interoperability of systems. There is currently no standardized system of tracking data (ie, injuries, illness related absences, or other critical indicators) that could inform school and community policies. Health care providers should collaborate with school nurses to advocate for a system that would benefit students, families, school health teams, and health care providers.

Emergency Care Plans/Emergency Action Plans

Many students in school populations are at risk of a life-threatening health crisis. In these situations, the school nurse needs to provide a plan, written in clear, understandable lay language, to guide school staff to make appropriate responses. The format can be a simple statement such as: "If you see this: _____, do this: _____."[30p296]

The components of an emergency care plan (ECP)/emergency action plan (EAP) may include but are not limited to[30]:

- demographic/identifying information (including student picture with parent permission);
- signs and symptoms;
- staff members instructed;
- treatment;
- transportation plan;
- signatures; and
- time frame.

It is recommended that the ECP/EAP be distributed to principals, teachers, field trip staff, cafeteria workers, and transportation staff on a need-to-know basis.[29] A list of all individuals who have a copy of the ECP/EAP should be noted on the bottom of the plan.[29] The school nurse communicates with all parties to ensure understanding of the plan.

Medication Administration

Administering medications in school is necessary for some children. There has been an increase in the numbers, range, and complexity of medications used in schools.[16] As mentioned previously, laws vary from state to state regarding the role of the school nurse in medication administration in schools. School nurses must adhere to the state nurse practice acts that govern their practice. The National Association of State Boards of Education provides a state-by-state guideline for administration of medications in schools.[35]

Each school district should have written policies, procedures, and/or protocols regarding medication administration in the school setting. These procedures should focus on efficiency and safety and ideally should be administered and/or supervised by a school nurse (RN).[16] Medication policies/procedures/protocols should include provisions related to prescription and nonprescription medications; alternative, emergency, and research medication; controlled substances; and medication doses that exceed manufacturer's guidelines.[16,17] The policies/procedures/protocols should also require parental/guardian consent for the school nurse to communicate with the prescribing health care provider to clarify the order, discuss any adverse effects of the medication, or to resolve any other issue associated with the administration of medication in school. In most districts, the policies include forms that must be signed by the provider. It may be helpful, if only working with a few districts, to maintain copies of the appropriate forms at the health care provider's office so that they can be completed as quickly as possible for the benefit of the student. Medication administration in school must always consider the safety of the student first.

When providers are considering and prescribing medications to be given during the school day, they must also be aware that the state has guidelines determining whether nursing activities and/or medications can be delegated to LPNs, vocational nurses, or unlicensed personnel. For example, some district policies do not allow invasive procedures to be delegated to aides or unlicensed personnel. It is critical for the prescribing physician to recognize that if the written policies are not adhered to, the student may not receive the medication as ordered.[36] Health care providers and the school health team strive to provide the best possible care to students to promote health and academic success. If the health care provider has concerns about state, district, or school policies, it is important to speak directly to the school nurse to ensure the safety of the student. Health care providers may also be called on or volunteer to provide training to school staff regarding new medications. These trainings should include reading the medication labels correctly to decrease medication errors, proper techniques of administration, expected effect, adverse effects, proper storage of the medication, standard precautions, and the 5 medication rights (right child, right medication, right time, right dose, right route). It is recommended after these educational trainings to include time for a return demonstration and possibly a test of knowledge. This is critical, especially for unlicensed personnel administering medications. Researchers have found an increase in medication errors when people other than a school nurse administer medications,[37] which should be taken into consideration when determining who administers medications.

When prescribing medication for children to be given at school, it is important for health care providers to include in the prescription additional medication and equipment that may be needed in the school—for example, an inhaler/spacer or epinephrine self-injector for the child at home and another one that can be left at school. Best practice indicates that all medications administered in the school must be in the original container. The prescribing physician can ask the pharmacy to dispense the medication in 2 containers. A waiver may be needed by the insurance company to allow double medications to obtained, but clearly this is a necessity. A health care provider must also indicate whether the child can administer the medication himself/herself while at school. This is especially critical as the child matures. This determination needs to be made in collaboration with the family and the school nurse. All the policies, procedures, and protocols must be determined with the health and safety of the child as the first priority.

Physicians prescribing medications to be administered in schools should adhere to written district policies including (but not limited to)[16,17]:

- Written consent should be given by the parents/guardians for the medication to be administered in school.
- Prescriptions for medication must be dated, written clearly and with detailed instructions by the prescribing physician or primary care provider.
- Medications must be in their original containers.
- Medications should be administered at home when possible.

- Parents should be discouraged from allowing their children to self-administer medications unless specified by policy. Some states allow for students to self-administer select medications for the treatment of asthma or diabetes. There must be written policies to cover this.
- Parents should be encouraged to supply spare life-saving medications for the health office.
- Physicians should collaborate with the school health team (physicians and school nurses) to encourage parent support and participation in their child's health care.

Immunizations, Screening, and Referrals

Each state has different laws and mandates regarding school screenings. The most common mandates are related to immunization entrance requirements and vision and hearing screenings. Although each state may have slightly different immunization requirements, it is important that primary care providers understand that school nurses must abide by and reinforce the laws. (To learn your state requirements, go to: **http://www.cdc.gov/vaccines/imz-managers/laws/state-reqs.html**.) Immunizations given earlier or on a different schedule than the requirement are not considered compliant to state rules. If health care providers administer immunizations at their office, this may mean rescheduling another visit for the vaccine to be given at the right time. Many states are developing immunization databases or registries that allow providers to enter the dates vaccines are given. Registries have been proven successful in tracking immunization compliance.[38] Collaboration between the school health team and primary care providers regarding immunization compliance allows for students to attend school as required.[39] In addition, school nurses serve an important role in promoting immunizations, especially those that may not be required for school, such as human papillomavirus (HPV) and influenza.

School nurses also routinely perform various health screenings in the school, such as vision, hearing, height/weight, and dental screenings. After a screening is conducted, school nurses often provide results of the screenings to parents. Some provide results only when a referral to a health care provider is needed, although some school nurses will provide the results to all parents/guardians.[9] Families are instructed to bring the referral form with them when they see the health care provider. HIPAA and FERPA laws support the sharing of this data if done appropriately and with parent permission.[24]

AAP's *Bright Futures* program[40] provides a comprehensive resource related to standards of care for children, emphasizing prevention in a family-focused approach that empowers families to be more involved in their children's health and development.

The referral process is another example of collaborative team efforts. Referrals to primary care providers by the school nurse and responses and outcomes reported back to the school nurse reinforce the collaborative association between the school nurse, parents, and primary care providers for the health benefit of the child. Some states also have tracking requirements in which school nurses must report the outcomes of referrals. Health care providers giving written feedback to the school nurse facilitates best care for the student.

Prevention and Promotion

School nurses and pediatricians should work together in their efforts to improve the health of children, the health of the community, and all of society. Access to care is a continuing issue, with increasing rates of obesity, chronic illnesses, students with allergies, and other health concerns, and the school setting provides an ideal venue to promote health, wellness, and education promoting disease prevention. Pediatricians often see trends of acute illness or consequences of poor health choices and use these opportunities to discuss these concerns with children and families in the office or quite possibly in the community (using the AAP's *Bright Futures: Guidelines for Health Supervision of Infants, Children, and Adolescents*[40]). The primary care provider must use these opportunities to promote health and disease prevention and educational opportunities that the school provides.

The AAP's *Bright Futures* program[40] provides a comprehensive resource related to standards of care for children, emphasizing prevention in a family-focused approach that empowers families to be more involved in their children's health and development. Pediatricians provide a steady impact on children and families by specifically collaborating with the school nurse, who could accomplish follow-up care and consistent health teaching in the school setting as well.[40] School nurses, in return, contact pediatricians with various concerns and to share resources. This collaborative partnership is successful in benefiting the health care of children. This benefit was identified from the inception of school nursing, when nurses were hired by school districts because children who had been seen by school physicians were not returning to school in a timely fashion.[2] School nurses provided additional training and individual outreach to families and the children who had been treated and could return to school.

Many school districts have medical providers who oversee and assist in evidence-based care and treatment of students and provide expertise related to health policies in schools.[41] Their expertise is valuable when writing medication administration policies (including provisions for over-the-counter and herbal remedies), policies related to foods and drinks sold in the school, various safety guidelines, and emergency preparedness guidelines. Medical providers can also assist in writing appropriate, best practice, exclusion policies related to illness in the school. From a population-level perspective, it could also include expertise and consultation related to written policies or procedures for the treatment of children in the event of an infectious disease outbreak.[25]

Many schools or communities also have wellness committees or health councils that would welcome the participation and insight of pediatricians. Laws and policies may vary, but many districts also may employ a school medical director/doctor[40] who can assist in writing policy, overseeing school health issues, providing referral information, or directly treating children or in many other ways. Pediatricians interested in working with schools should approach the school nurse or school principal to determine appropriate ways their expertise can be used.

Emergencies and Disaster Preparedness

School nurses are often the first responder to an emergency in a school and provide triage and care until other health care providers arrive. Pediatricians should be part of this emergency response planning/disaster team.[42] School disaster plans should have a plan that involves the community responders, primary care providers, and hospital staff that identifies when to access these team members. It is critical to have a pediatrician in the community to provide this assistance when necessary. School nurses work with the community to develop a plan in compliance with plans and terminology of first responders and the disaster/emergency plan within the state.

Recommendations for Pediatricians

The school nurse is a valued partner to the pediatrician. School nurses are the eyes and ears of what children are doing each day to manage chronic conditions, prevent illness, and promote the general health of children and their families. School nurses regularly monitor the progress of children's health in the school and provide additional training to children and their families that pediatricians may not have the time to do. School nurses are the natural extension of the health care team. Building a relationship of trust and partnering with local school nurses can make a pediatrician's life easier and the health of the student better. School nurses often seek community providers who can be collaborators and resources or support for the health concerns they see every day. Partnering is a win-win situation, especially for the child and family.

To strengthen the partnership, pediatricians are encouraged to introduce themselves to the school nurses in their geographic area. Become knowledgeable about what the school nurse sees and faces on a day-to-day basis. Determine, with the school nurse, how communication between the 2 of you can be enhanced. Investigate the possibility of improved communication via electronic health records. For example, the Nemours Student Health Collaboration project has developed a partnership with Delaware public school districts so that school nurses can have access, with parent permission, to providers in Nemours system. This has improved communication and improved continuity of care.[34] Remember to include school nurses on the coordinated care organization teams (outlined in the ACA[14]).

Encourage cross-training so that you can better understand the roles and combined and different educational needs of the school nurse and physician and then resolve to understand and demonstrate the most efficient and collaborative way to work together. For example, the Barbara Davis Center in Colorado provides diabetes education to school nurses, who, in turn, use their knowledge to improve the diabetes management of their students while at school (Sarah Butler, MS, RN, CDE, NCSN, oral communication 2013). Offer support in writing policy or participating on a school health or wellness council. Parents are often overwhelmed when their child is diagnosed with a medical condition. The school nurse can help ease anxiety, answer questions, and reinforce the training and education the families received from health care providers to provide consistent, competent care. Because school nurses see individual children more often, they can also identify gaps of knowledge or concerns that will assist in managing conditions. Support collaboration between the families and the school nurse. This triad of the family, pediatrician, and school nurse will facilitate the treatment plan and education for children and families with health care issues.

As asthma action plans and IHCPs are developed, it is critical that pediatricians and school nurses support efforts to decrease confusion and uncertainty of parents and ensure the best outcomes for their children. Health care providers can assist in opening up lines of communication regarding individual children by encouraging parents to sign release forms in their offices, which allows the providers and school nurse to share appropriate health information. The sharing of information ensures that treatment is not delayed in the school.

Recommendations for Program Directors and Trainees

It is important for pediatric residents to understand the atmosphere in which their children/clients spend each day, which for most is the school setting. Pediatric residents should familiarize themselves with the School Nursing: Scope and Standards,[28] the State Nurse Practice Act, local school policies, and national best practice guidelines for the care of children in a school setting. It would also behoove the pediatric resident to review the AAP's *Bright Futures: Guidelines for Health Supervision of Infants, Children, and Adolescents* for guidance and recommendations about the care of children of all ages and their families.[40] This resource provides specific training to assist residents to understand how to care for children outside of the hospital setting, including focusing on prevention. Program directors may consider including these materials in their pediatric curriculum.

The culture of K-12 education is quite different than medicine, and experience in this setting would be beneficial for the resident to learn the priorities of the school and the issues the school health team and the nurse face in providing health care on a daily basis to many children. These considerations can be reviewed when planning treatment or services that will take place when the child is in school. Interviewing a school nurse and working in an SBHC would also provide valuable learning and experience.

Program directors can use the school nurse and the school team as an extension of the training curriculum by designing rotations that allow the trainees to become familiar with and support the school nurse role. Residents and fellows can provide input about the IHCP, the Section 504 plan, ECPs/EAPs, policies, and several diagnosis-specific action plans. This activity can be a valuable learning tool to pediatric residents, developmental and behavioral pediatric and emergency medicine fellows, and other subspecialty fellows.

Collaborating with the school nurse and the school health team or even adopting a school during the first year of resident training would be invaluable. During this time, residents can partner with the school nurses and school health teams to design and implement quality improvement projects based in schools.

This would allow the trainee and the program director to meet the Accreditation Council for Graduate Medical Education requirements for the practice-based learning and improvement, systems-based practice, communication skills, and professionalism competencies and their milestones. Collaborating with the school nurse may be as simple as an initial phone call.

Take-Home Points

- School nurses are clinicians, leaders, advocates, health promoters, educators, policy makers, and community liaisons.
- Education has rules and policies related to the inclusion of health, but its main focus is academic achievement, and educators do not have training in health care.
- HIPAA protects the rights and confidentiality of patients, and FERPA protects the rights and confidentiality of students. These 2 laws can work together if understood correctly.
- The Nurse Practice Act in every state indicates the scope of the nurse's practice and the extent to which delegation is allowed. It is important to know this information in your state and critical to take this into account when prescribing treatments or medications to be administered in the school setting.
- Schools are the perfect partner to focus on prevention and health promotion. Pediatricians can serve on wellness/health policy committees or partner with the school nurse in health education classes.
- School nurses should/must be included as members of coordinated care teams (ACA).
- Pediatricians should advocate for one nurse per every school building (or 750 well students).
- Pediatricians should encourage all districts to have an assigned school physician who works closely with the school nurses and can serve as a reference if the child does not have a physician.
- School nurses and pediatricians should promote access to health care through the state health insurance programs.
- School nurses and health care providers should promote regular communication as key to ensuring the best outcomes for children with chronic conditions.
- Collaboration, communication, consistent messaging to students and parents, and a mutual respect recognizing that the pediatrician and the school nurse both have a significant role to ensure the primary objective—the health, well-being, safety, and academic success of all children.

> **Resources**
>
> For additional school health related resources, visit www.aap.org/
> schoolhealthmanual.

References

1. American Academy of Pediatrics, Council on School Health. Role of the school nurse in providing school health services. *Pediatrics.* 2008;121(5):1052-1056. Doi: 10.1542/PEDS.2008-0382

2. National Association of School Nurses. Position Statement: Role of the School Nurse. Silver Spring, MD: National Association of School Nurses; Revised 2011. Available at: https://www.nasn.org/PolicyAdvocacy/PositionPapersandReports/NASNPositionStatementsFullView/tabid/462/ArticleId/87/Role-of-the-School-Nurse-Revised-2011. Accessed April 13, 2015

3. Erickson CD, Splett PL, Mullett SS, Jensen C, Belseth SB. The healthy learner model for student chronic condition management—part II: the asthma initiative. *J Sch Nurs.* 2006;22(6):319–329

4. Nguyen TM, Mason KJ, Sanders CG, Yazdani P, Heptulla RA. Targeting blood glucose management in school improves glycemic control in children with poorly controlled type 1 diabetes. *J Pediatr.* 2008;153(4):575–578

5. Pennington N, Delaney E. The number of students sent home by school nurses compared to unlicensed personnel. *J Sch Nurs. 2008;24(5):290-297*

6. Baisch MJ, Lundeen SP, Murphy MK. Evidence-based research on the value of school nurses in an urban school system. *J Sch Health.* 2011;81(2):74–80

7. Fleming R. Use of the school nurse services among poor ethnic minority students in the urban Pacific Northwest. *Public Health Nurs.* 2011;28(4):308–316

8. National Association of School Nurses. *School Nursing in the United States: A Quantitative Study 2007.* Silver Spring, MD: National Association of School Nurses; 2007

9. Maughan ED, Mangena AS. The 2013 NASN School Nurse Survey: advancing school nursing practice. *NASN School Nurse.* 2014;29(2):76-83. Doi: 10.1177/1942602X14523135

10. Bergren M. The case for school nursing: review of the literature. NASN Sch Nurse. 2013;28(1):48–51

11. National Center for Education Statistics. Elementary and secondary education. In: *Digest of Education Statistics, 2011.* Available at: http://nces.ed.gov/programs/digest/d11/ch_2.asp. Accessed April 13, 2015

12. Gorski PA, Kuo AA; American Academy of Pediatrics, Council on Community Pediatrics. Community pediatrics: navigating the intersection of medicine, public health, and social determinants of children's health. *Pediatrics.* 2013;131(3):623–628

13. ASCD. Whole School, Whole Community, Whole Child. 2014. Available at: http://www.ascd.org/programs/learning-and-health/wscc-model.aspx. Accessed April 13, 2015

14. Healthcare.gov. Read the Affordable Care Act. 2012. Available at: https://www.healthcare.gov/where-can-i-read-the-affordable-care-act/. Accessed April 13, 2015

15. National Association of School Nurses. *Position Statement: Nursing Delegation to Unlicensed Assistive Personnel in the School Setting.* Silver Spring, MD: National Association of School Nurses; 2014. Available at: https://www.nasn.org/PolicyAdvocacy/PositionPapersandReports/NASNPositionStatementsFullView/tabid/462/ArticleId/21/Delegation-Revised-2010. Accessed April 13, 2015

16. National Association of School Nurses. *Position Statement: Medication Administration in the School Setting.* Silver Spring, MD: National Association of School Nurses; January 2012. Available at: http://www.nasn.org/PolicyAdvocacy/PositionPapersandReports/ NASNPositionStatementsFullView/tabid/462/ArticleId/86/Medication-Administration-in-the-School-Setting-Amended-January-2012. Accessed April 13, 2015

17. American Academy of Pediatrics, Council on School Health. Policy statement: guidance for the administration of medication in school. *Pediatrics.* 2009;124(4):1244–1249. Reaffirmed February 2013

18. Rhodes JH. *An Education in Politics: The Origins and Evolution of No Child Left Behind.* Ithaca, NY: Cornell University Press; 2012

19. National Association of School Nurses. *The Complementary Roles of the School Nurse and School Based Health Centers.* Silver Spring, MD: National Association of School Nurses; January 2011. Available at: https://www.nasn.org/PolicyAdvocacyPositionPapersandReports/ NASNPositionStatementsFullView/tabid/462/ArticleId/46/School-Based-Health-Centers-The-Role-of-the-School-Nurse-and-Revised-2011. April 13, 2015

20. Lofink, H., Kuebler, J., Juszcak, L., Schlitt, J., Even, M., Rosenberg, J & White, I. *2010-2011 National School-based Health Care Census.* Washington, DC: School-based Health Alliance; 2013. Available at: http://www.sbh4all.org/wp-content/uploads/2015/02/ CensusReport_2010-11CensusReport_7.13.pdf. Accessed April 13, 2015

21. Individuals with Disabilities Education Improvement Act of 2004. 20 USC §§1400 et seq, Pub L No. 108-446, as amended and incorporating the Education of All Handicapped Children Act of 1975, Pub L No. 94-142, and subsequent amendments; regulations at 34 CFR §§300-303 [Special education and related services for students, preschool children, and infants and toddlers]

22. Rehabilitation Act of 1973, Section 504. 29 USC §794 et seq, Regulations at 34 CFR §104

23. Americans with Disabilities Act of 1990, as Amended. Pub L No. 110-325 (2008)

24. US Department of Education, US Department of Health and Human Services. Joint Guidance on the Application of the Family Educational Rights and Privacy Act (FERPA) and the Health Insurance Portability and Accountability Act of 1996 (HIPAA) To Student Health Records. 2008. Available at: http://www.hhs.gov/ocr/privacy/hipaa/understanding/ coveredentities/hipaaferpajointguide.pdf. Accessed April 13, 2015

25. American Academy of Pediatrics. *Managing Chronic Health Needs in Child Care and Schools: A Quick Reference Guide.* Donoghue EA, Kraft CA, eds. Elk Grove Village, IL: American Academy of Pediatrics; 2009

26. National Asthma Education and Prevention Program. *Managing Asthma: A Guide for Schools.* 2003. Available at: http://www.nhlbi.nih.gov/health/prof/lung/asthma/asth_sch. pdf. Revised 2003. Accessed April 13, 2015

27. National Asthma Education and Prevention Program. *Guidelines for the Diagnosis and Management of Asthma.* 2007. Available at: http://www.nhlbi.nih.gov/files/docs/guidelines/ asthgdln.pdf. Accessed April 13, 2015

28. American Nurses Association, National Association of School Nurses. *Nursing: Scope and Standards of School Practice.* Silver Spring, MD: Nursebooks.org; 2011

29. New York State Department of Health, New York State Education Department, New York Statewide School Health Services Center. *Caring for Students with Life-Threatening Allergies.* 2008. Available at: http://www.schoolhealthservicesny.com/uploads/ Anaphylaxis%20Final%206-25-08.pdf. Accessed April 13, 2015

30. Zimmerman B. Student health and education plans. In: Selekman J, ed. *School Nursing: A Comprehensive Text.* 2nd ed. Philadelphia, PA: FA Davis Company; 2012:284-314

31. National Association of School Nurses. Position Statement: Individualized Healthcare Plans. Silver Spring, MD: National Association of School Nurses; 2015. Available at: http://www.nasn.org/PolicyAdvocacy/PositionPapersandReports/NASNPositionStatements. Accessed April 13, 2015

32. American Academy of Pediatrics, Committee on School Health, Committee on Bioethics. Honoring do-not-attempt-resuscitation requests in schools. *Pediatrics.* 2013;125(5):1073–1077

33. Andrews M. School nurses' role expands with access to students' online health records. Kaiser Health News. June 10, 2014. Available at: http://www.kaiserhealthnews.org/Stories/2014/June/10/Andrews-school-nurse-access-to-health-records.aspx. Accessed April 13, 2015

34. National Association of School Nurses. *Position Statement: Standardized Nursing Languages.* Silver Spring, MD: National Association of School Nurses; 2012. Available at: https://www.nasn.org/PolicyAdvocacy/PositionPapersandReports/NASNPositionStatementsFullView/tabid/462/ArticleId/48/Standardized-Nursing-Languages-Revised-June-2012. Accessed April 13, 2015

35. National Association of State Boards of Education. *State School Health Policy Database.* 2009. Available at: http://www.nasbe.org/healthy_schools/hs/bytopics.php?topicid=4110. Accessed April 13, 2015

36. Foley M. Health services management. In: Selekman J, ed. *School Nursing: A Comprehensive Text.* 2nd ed. Philadelphia, PA: FA Davis Company; 2012:1190-1215

37. McCarthy AM, Kelly MW, Reed D. Medication administration practices of school nurses. *J Sch Health.* 2009;70(9):371-376

38. National Association of School Nurses. *Position Statement: Immunizations.* Silver Spring, MD: National Association of School Nurses; 2010. Available at: https://www.nasn.org/PolicyAdvocacy/PositionPapersandReports/NASNPositionStatementsFullView/tabid/462/ArticleId/8/Immunizations-Revised-2010. Accessed April 13, 2015

39. American Academy of Pediatrics, Committee on Infectious Diseases. Recommended childhood and adolescent immunization schedule—United States 2013. *Pediatrics.* 2013;131(2):397–398

40. Hagan JF, Shaw JS, Duncan PM, eds. *Bright Futures: Guidelines for Health Supervision of Infants, Children, and Adolescents.* 3rd ed. Elk Grove Village, IL: American Academy of Pediatrics; 2008

41. Devore CD, Wheeler LS; American Academy of Pediatrics, Council on School Health. Role of the school physician. *Pediatrics.* 2013;131(1):178–182

42. Markenson D, Reynolds S; American Academy of Pediatrics, Committee on Pediatric Emergency Medicine, Task Force on Terrorism. The pediatrician and disaster preparedness. *Pediatrics.* 2006;117(2):e340–e362. Reaffirmed September 2013

CHAPTER

4

Comprehensive Health Education

David K. Lohrmann, PhD, MA, MCHES

Background—High Quality Health Instruction

Health education in schools works! That is, research conducted over more than 20 years has consistently shown that middle and high school students who participated in high quality health instruction are more likely to engage in health-enhancing behaviors—not smoke, avoid alcohol and other drug abuse, abstain from sexual intercourse and/or use protection, eschew violent behavior, and consume a healthier diet.[1] Elementary school students who receive high quality health instruction are more likely to possess effective interpersonal communication and other social and emotional learning skills along with drug refusal skills.[2] They also engaged in lower levels of alcohol and tobacco use and aggressive behaviors.[2]

The curricula on which high quality health instruction is founded share common characteristics:

- research-based and theory-driven;
- focus on specific behaviors;
- include accurate, basic, developmentally and culturally appropriate content;
- use learning activities that engage students in interactive and experiential ways;
- give students opportunities to model and practice skills;
- address social and media influences on behavior;
- strengthen and support individual values and group norms associated with health-enhancing behaviors; and
- provide instruction of sufficient duration to allow students time to master essential knowledge and acquire health skills.[3]

Although all 8 characteristics are important, 2 (inclusion of accurate, basic information and use of interactive learning strategies) deserve special attention because they likely do not epitomize much of the health instruction occurring in schools today. With the current emphasis on teaching "academic" material to help students score better on standardized tests, all teachers, including teachers of health education, are encouraged to build students' vocabularies. Teachers may use this as a rationale for focusing on memorization of lists of terms and key words that are bolded in textbooks. An emphasis on memorization facilitates use of passive learning strategies (eg, lecture, drill, worksheets, etc) that lead to only short-term acquisition of factual knowledge.[4] This approach to teaching and learning is less effective because it does not facilitate adoption of healthy behaviors.[4]

Types of Health Knowledge—Factual and Procedural

Health education has its foundation in the biological science but is not the same as biology; overly-detailed knowledge of anatomy and physiology is not required in order to practice healthy behaviors. For example, a teenager does not need to know extensive cellular level information about disease organisms that are sexually transmitted in order to avoid contracting a sexually-transmitted infection (STI). Factually, they need to know that these types of diseases exist and can have severe consequences. Teens also need to know exactly how these diseases are transmitted along with the limited list of signs and symptoms of STI infection that, if present, require immediate medical attention. More importantly, they need to know that transmission can be prevented by abstaining from risky behaviors and/or effectively using proper protection.

Most importantly, however, teens have to practice and, thus, acquire the procedural knowledge (ie, skills) needed to sustain healthy behavior.[4] Regarding STI prevention, procedural knowledge includes communication skills for discussing behavioral risks and limits with a partner, refusing to engage in risky behavior, and/or negotiating to reduce risk plus consumer skills for purchasing or otherwise acquiring condoms and dental dams and, when needed, for accessing health care. None of these types of skills are covered in a typical science class. They are covered in a high-quality health education class.

Five broad types of teaching strategies have been identified as common to effective health education—role play, group cooperation, interactive technology, team games, and small group discussion.[1]

Appropriate Teaching-Learning Strategies

This is where effective teaching strategies come in—strategies that introduce and explain skills to students, demonstrate use of skills, and, then, provide students the opportunity and time to practice skills in a safe and supportive classroom environment. Acquiring skills this way imbeds both the factual and procedural knowledge in students' long term memories that they can call upon, when needed, to activate healthy behaviors and/or reduce risks when confronted in the real world.[4] To be truly preventive, students need to learn skills in health education before the age when they are likely to encounter real-life risky situations.[4] For example, refusal skills should be learned in late elementary grades before the age at which early-teens are subjected in middle school to peer-pressure to use alcohol. Hence, health education is defined as:

> "Any combination of planned learning experiences using evidence-based practices and/or sound theories that provide the opportunity to acquire knowledge, attitudes, and *skills* needed to adopt and maintain healthy behaviors."[5]

Five broad types of teaching strategies have been identified as common to effective health education—role play, group cooperation, interactive technology, team games, and small group discussion.[1] Learning events based on these types of strategies both promote the practice and acquisition of new skills and require students to employ the effective interpersonal and social skills that form the basis for positive, fulfilling relationships and on-the-job success throughout life. Ideally, students are expected to utilize effective interpersonal and social skills learned in health throughout school beginning in pre-K or kindergarten.[6]

Typically, a classroom observer can determine or sense when effective health education is being provided. In these classrooms, students are actively engaged in learning. They are expected to apply essential health knowledge to their lives by learning specific ways (ie, procedures) for doing things such as managing stress, estimating serving sizes, planning a fitness project, analyzing health-related advertising, choosing appropriate health products, solving real-life problems, setting health goals, and advocating for a healthy environment. They can be observed interacting with classmates in discussions of important issues, making healthy choices and, then, practicing skills that will help them sustain their choices in the real world. They are learning factual information about health in meaningful ways so that they retain what they learn for a lifetime rather than just long enough to bubble in the right answer on a Friday afternoon quiz.

Health Education Standards and Content

Contemporary health education is driven by the US National Health Education Standards[7] (NHESs) that were initially developed to ensure that health education could be included in the national education reform movement if resources became available.[3] Today, almost every state education department has formally adopted and recommended to schools some version of the NHESs. Many states have adopted the NHESs verbatim, whereas others have adapted them in order to conform to existing state statutes or curriculum frameworks. The second edition, published in 2007, includes 8 NHESs with multiple pre-K through grade 2, grades 3 through 5, grades 6 through 8, and grades 9 through 12 indicators for each standard. Indicators describe with greater specificity what students should know and be able to do by the end of the last grade in each sequence. The NHESs[7] are:

1. Students will comprehend concepts related to health promotion and disease prevention to enhance health.
2. Students will analyze the influence of family, peers, culture, media, technology and other factors on health behaviors.
3. Students will demonstrate the ability to access valid information and products and services to enhance health.
4. Students will demonstrate the ability to use interpersonal communication skills to enhance health and avoid and reduce health risks.
5. Students will demonstrate the ability to use decision-making skills to enhance health.
6. Students will demonstrate the ability to use goal-setting skills to enhance health.
7. Students will demonstrate the ability to practice health-enhancing behaviors and avoid or reduce health risks.
8. Students will demonstrate the ability to advocate for personal, family, and community health.

Note that the NHESs do not have specific health topics listed within them for the simple reason that the NHESs are meant to be applied to any and all health topics. Traditionally, pre-K through grade 12 health curricula addressed 10 specified topics, whereas the Centers for Disease Control and Prevention (CDC) has recommended a focus on 6 priority health risk behaviors.[7] The CDC has included a list of 14 topics, based on national health priorities, in nationwide evaluations of health education[8]:

• Alcohol and other drug-use prevention*	• Nutrition and dietary behavior*
• Asthma	• Physical activity and fitness*
• Emotional and mental health*	• Pregnancy prevention
• Foodborne illness prevention	• STD prevention*
• HIV prevention*	• Suicide prevention*
• Human sexuality	• Tobacco-use prevention*
• Injury prevention and safety*	• Violence prevention (eg, bullying, fighting, homicide)*

* Directly relate to prevention of six priority health risk behaviors.

To better illustrate, following is a list of some ways that the NHESs can be applied to instruction about nutrition and dietary behaviors[9]:

- address essential health promotion and disease prevention concepts about nutrition;
- analyze ways in which food preferences and eating patterns are influenced by family, peers, culture, media, technology and other factors;
- practice skills for accessing valid nutrition information and products;
- use communication strategies for resisting pressures to consume unhealthy foods;
- demonstrate skills for making and sustaining healthy food-consumption decisions;
- apply skills for setting and achieving a healthy weight goal via good nutrition;
- practice choosing a variety of healthy food portions at meals, including meals at fast-food restaurants; and
- design a campaign to advocate for the availability of healthy foods at school.

By this point, the congruence between the characteristics of effective health instruction initially discussed and the NHESs may be apparent. Good reason for this congruence exists; the NHESs were developed after much of the research on effectiveness was concluded and were strongly informed by the findings of this research.[3] In essence, the NHESs are purposefully research-based and, therefore, any health curriculum that incorporates the NHESs along with *scientifically accurate health information* should be consistent with well know best practices.[7]

Support for Health Education in Schools

School health education is recognized as an important public health priority. Four health education objectives are included in the US Department of Health and Human Services' Healthy People 2020 document[10] and the US Department of Agriculture Wellness Policy required of schools through the federal child nutrition/school lunch program stipulates that such policies "include, at a minimum, goals for nutrition education, physical activity and other school-based activities to promote student wellness."[11] A 2006 CDC study of the status of school health in the US concluded that "Most states and districts had adopted a policy stating that schools will teach at least 1 of the 14 health topics, and nearly all schools required students to receive instruction on at least 1 of these topics. However, only 6.4% of elementary schools, 20.6% of middle schools, and 35.8% of high schools required instruction on all 14 topics."[9] In other words, although health education is seen as a public health priority, this support is not strongly reflected in the curriculums of US schools. One reason for this lack of attention to health instruction could be that, consistently since at least 1990, health education has not been identified as a school subject by the US Department of Education[12]; federal education policy only stipulates that schools must provide a safe and healthy environment.

Health Education Within Coordinated School Health

Much of what is covered in schools today is taught as a prerequisite to the next level (Algebra I before Algebra II), as something useful later in life (US Government) and/or just because it is believed to be part of a well-rounded education (English Literature). With the exception of reading, few school subjects are intended to be implemented immediately and practiced continually thereafter. Health education is another exception—once learned, students should be expected to apply health knowledge and skills in school immediately and throughout schooling. For example, once learned in health education, students should be expected to practice sound coping, anger management, negotiation, and communication skills in the classroom and throughout the school.[6] This expectation both helps students establish and maintain the positive relationships that are essential to mental health and reduces disruptive classroom behavior, thereby allowing a greater focus on learning. The synergy between healthy behaviors and educational achievement is evident; hence a typical principal's admonition to "get good sleep" and "have a healthy breakfast" the night before and day of that all-important standardized test. Healthy kids learn better and health education helps assure that kids engage in the behaviors that promote their good health.

The corollary to this point is that the school culture and environment must form an ecology which provides cues and supports for healthy behavior.[13] And, as discussed in other chapters, this health culture should extend beyond the school to the family and community. For example, health instruction can be reinforced in other school subjects such as Language Arts when students complete an essay after reading a book with a health theme.[14] To engage families, students can be given homework assignments that they must complete with family members, such as conducting a safety-related inventory of common poisonous products in the home. Regarding the community, students can be involved in service-learning projects through agencies and organizations such as the American Cancer Society, American Red Cross, Habitat for Humanity, a local food bank, a local hospital, or a local parks and recreation department.

Additionally, lessons learned in health education must be supported throughout the school.[13] For example, to support healthy food choices learned in health, nutrition information, including total calories, should accompany foods offered in the cafeteria and foods labeled with symbols such as a green dot (high nutrition, eat as much as you want), a yellow dot (moderate nutrition, eat in limited amounts) or a red dot (minimal nutrition, a "sometimes" food). Lessons learned about preventing the spread of communicable diseases such as HIV and hepatitis are reinforced when students observe a playground aide using universal precautions to attend to a skinned knee or a custodian employing proper procedures for cleaning up a body fluid spill in the hallway, or a school nurse disposing of a used needle in a sharps container.

How to Work With Schools

Because of real pressures to improve reading and mathematics test scores, convincing administrators and teachers to devote sufficient instructional time and attention to health education may prove difficult. They are more likely to teach health if convinced that providing health education can contribute to better test scores or that health education can be delivered in conjunction with reading or math instruction. Examples of both have been provided above; the learning and use of personal and social skills in health education can reduce classroom disruptions, thus leaving more time for direct instruction.[6] Reading and analyzing health-related stories can address both health education and reading/writing standards.[14] Illustrating these connections is most important when working with elementary schools principals where health is supposed to be taught by regular classroom teachers. (In middle and high schools, health is more likely to be provided in specifically designated courses taught by teachers certified in health education.)

Recommendations for Pediatricians

Collectively, pediatricians can help fund and deliver social marketing campaigns in support of school health education. Unlike other subjects such as art and music, no major organized group in the US systematically advocates for school health education. Seeing billboards and hearing public service announcements in support of art or music education is relatively common but totally unseen and unheard are advocacy messages in support of health education such as "Has your child learned about health today?" Organizations of health professionals, perhaps in collaboration with health insurers, pharmaceutical manufacturers, and others, could develop sustained national and/or statewide social marketing campaigns in support of health education. All of these entities have numerous vested interests, both altruistic and pragmatic, for having healthy children and youth so this approach should be a "natural" for them.

A local physician, especially a pediatrician, often has the credibility within the community to act as a health education champion by publically advocating for health instruction and convincing school board members, administrators, and other interested parties to implement high quality, pre-K through grade 12 health instruction. A ready-made avenue for such involvement is leadership of the wellness council that every school or school district involved in the USDA school lunch program must maintain.[12] Wellness councils are charged with advocating for education about nutrition, physical fitness, and other health issues and have the challenge to both expand the amount of health education that is taught and enhance the quality of instruction. A sound starting point is to insist on a thorough review of the current program by using the CDC's Health Education Curriculum Assessment Tool (HECAT), a free, easily-available publication that provides a rational, detailed process and specific criteria for assessing program quality relative to desired content and the NHESs.[8] Once an assessment is completed, wellness council leaders are empowered to develop and monitor implementation of a wellness improvement plan and assure that school officials provide mandated progress reports to the community.[11] Ideally, wellness councils will also assist school officials in securing the additional resources from the community that may be required to fully implement comprehensive health education.

Recommendations for Program Directors and Trainees

During their clinical experience, pediatricians routinely treat numerous diseases and conditions that could be prevented through appropriate health behaviors as basic as proper hand washing or as complex as entrenched eating patterns. Rather than simply treating patients, program directors can motivate trainees to ask questions such as: What health behaviors could this patient have practiced to prevent this? What could schools do through effective health education to assure that this patient has command of the essential knowledge and requisite skills needed to behave in healthy ways? How can I serve my future patients by working with school decision makers and stakeholders, including parents, to assure that they achieve the NHESs? Additionally, program directors (eg, Pediatric and Family Medicine Residency Directors, Adolescent Medicine Fellowship Directors, Pediatric Infectious Disease Fellowship Directors, etc) can use health education in schools as a way to enhance their trainees' experience. Program Directors may consider connecting their trainees with local school administrators and parent-teacher association (PTA) leaders who can, then, work with them to assure that health education is systematically included as a valued subject in the overall school curriculum. They may also offer the services of their trainees to teachers for the purpose of selecting and/or developing and delivering high quality health lessons.

Trainees can use their health education experiences in schools to improve their disease prevention and health promotion competencies and skills, which they can then apply beyond the walls of the clinic to serve a much larger number of individuals. These activities also strengthen their competency in delivering age-appropriate and developmentally-appropriate messages along with their ability to work with school staff on a common goal. Helping trainees understand their role in advocating for health education in schools will further develop their competencies in Systems-Based Practice, as well as Interpersonal and Communication Skills and Professionalism.

Take-Home Points

- Health education "works"—students who experience high-quality health instruction are more likely to behave in healthy ways.
- Health education contributes directly to the mission of schools by ensuring that students are healthy and ready to learn every day.
- The characteristics of high quality health education are well known and are embedded in the National Health Education Standards.
- To be truly effective, health education must be taught consistently across all grades, pre-K through 12.
- The USDA wellness policy mandates for schools to provide a clear opportunity for pediatricians to become involved as leaders of local wellness councils.
- Curriculum improvement can be initiated through use of the CDC's HECAT, followed by implementation and evaluation of a wellness plan that encompasses health education.
- Although clearly a public health priority in the United States, health education is much less of a priority for public education agencies at the national, state, and local levels.
- School officials understand the connection between health and learning but are under tremendous pressure to maintain and/or improve test scores.
- For health education to take its rightful place in the school curriculum, it needs highly-influential advocates such as pediatricians at the national, state, and local levels.
- School officials need strong input from influential community champions, such as pediatricians, in support of education for the whole child, including education for mental, emotional, social, and physical health.

Resources

For additional school health related resources, visit www.aap.org/schoolhealthmanual.

References

1. Herbert P, Lohrmann DK. It's all in the delivery: an analysis of instructional strategies from effective health education curricula. *J Sch Health.* 2011;81(5):258-264

2. O'Neill JM, Clark JK, Jones JA. Promoting mental health and preventing substance abuse and violence in elementary students: a randomized control study of the Michigan Model for Health. *J Sch Health.* 2011;81(6):320-330

3. Lohrmann DK, Wooley S. Comprehensive school health education. In: Marx E, Wooley S, eds. *Health is Academic.* New York, NY: Teachers College Press; 1988:4366

4. Lohrmann DK. Thinking of a change: health education for the 2020 generation. *Am J Health Educ.* 2011;45(5):258-269

5. Brown KM, Torabi MR, Anglin TM, et al; Joint Committee on Health Education and Promotion Terminology. Report of the 2011 Joint Committee on Health Education and Promotion Terminology. *Am J Health Educ.* March-April 2012;43(2). Available at: https://www.questia.com/read/1G1-284015297/report-of-the-2011-joint-committee-on-health-education. Accessed April 13, 2015

6. Learning First Alliance. *Every Child Learning: Safe and Supportive Schools.* Alexandria, VA: Association for Supervision and Curriculum Development; 2001

7. Joint Committee on National Health Education Standards. *National Health Education Standards Achieving Excellence.* 2nd ed. Atlanta, GA: American Cancer Society; 2007

8. Centers for Disease Control and Prevention. *Health Education Curriculum Analysis Tool.* Atlanta, GA: Centers for Disease Control and Prevention; 2007

9. Kann L, Telljohann SK, Wooley SF. Health education: results from the School Health Policies and Programs Study 2006. *J Sch Health.* 2007;77(8):408-434

10. Brenner ND, Demissie Z, Foti K, et al. *School Health Profiles: 2010 Characteristics of Health Programs Among Secondary Schools in Selected US Sites.* Atlanta, GA: Centers for Disease Control and Prevention; 2011

11. US Department of Agriculture. *Local School Wellness Policies: Overview and Action Steps.* Available at: http://www.fns.usda.gov/sites/default/files/lwpoverview.pdf. Accessed April 13, 2015

12. US Department of Education, Office of Planning, Evaluation and Policy Development. *A Blueprint for Reform: The Reauthorization of the Elementary and Secondary Education Act.* Washington, DC: US Department of Education, Office of Planning, Evaluation and Policy Development; 2010

13. Lohrmann DK. A complimentary ecological model of coordinated school health promotion. *J Sch Health.* 2010;80(1):1-9

14. Council of Chief State School Officers. HEAP's Health and Reading Initiative: Improving Reading and Health Literacy through a HEAP of Books. Available at: http://www.heaphealthliteracy.com/reading.html. Accessed April 13, 2015

CHAPTER

5

Physical Education, Physical Activity, and School Sports

Claire MA LeBlanc, MD, FAAP, FRCPC
Blaise A. Nemeth, MD, MS, FAAP

Background

Approximately one third of school-aged children and youth are overweight or obese in the United States.[1] Obese children are predisposed to a number of chronic diseases, including high blood pressure, insulin resistance, type 2 diabetes mellitus, dyslipidemia, obstructive sleep apnea, nonalcoholic steatohepatitis, and lower health-related quality of life.[2] The etiology of obesity is multifactorial, but major contributors include excessive caloric intake and sedentary behaviors and inadequate physical activity and exercise.[2]

The US Department of Health and Human Services recommends 6- through 16-year-old Americans partake in at least 60 minutes/day of moderate to vigorous aerobic physical activity, with vigorous exercise at least 3 days/week. This should include muscle- and bone-strengthening exercise at least 3 days a week. Activities should be diverse, enjoyable, developmentally appropriate, and include energetic behaviors that can be incorporated into the youth's lifestyle at home, in the community, and at school.[3] Healthy People 2020 expands on these guidelines with several active living objectives to reduce screen time to less than 2 hours per day in children older than 2 years and to increase the proportion of children and youth who meet the federal physical activity guidelines in multiple settings. This includes childcare facilities and schools, through daily physical education (PE), regularly scheduled elementary school recess, and active transportation using new legislation to improve the built environment.[4]

Unfortunately, only 3.8% of elementary schools, 7.9% of middle schools, and 2.1% of high schools in the United States provide daily PE or its equivalent for the entire school year.[6]

HEALTHY PEOPLE 2020 PHYSICAL ACTIVITY (PA) OBJECTIVES
PA-3 Increase the proportion of adolescents who meet current federal physical activity guidelines for aerobic physical activity and for muscle-strengthening activity
PA-4 Increase the proportion of the nation's public and private schools that require daily physical education for all students
PA-5 Increase the proportion of adolescents who participate in daily school physical education
PA-6 Increase regularly scheduled elementary school recess in the United States

According to national survey data on students in grades 9 through 12, 32% watched television 3 or more hours per day and 31% played video or computer games at least 3 hours/day on an average school day. Only 28.7% had been sufficiently physically active at least 60 minutes daily for 7 days. Approximately 56% of these students participated in muscle-strengthening activities on 3 or more days per week, and only 31.5% attended PE class daily.[5] Unfortunately, only 3.8% of elementary schools, 7.9% of middle schools, and 2.1% of high schools in the United States provide daily PE or its equivalent for the entire school year.[6] This is in part because of pressures on educators to focus on academic programming; however, research suggests school-based physical activity does not interfere with and may improve student grades.[7] For school officials to successfully develop and implement school health policy promoting physical activity and PE, evidence demonstrating better educational outcomes is key.

Promoting Physical Activity Programs to Educators and Administrators

Physical activity has been demonstrated to reduce adiposity and comorbidities of obesity.[8] High-impact physical activity promotes improved bone health.[9] Other benefits, such as the promotion of psychological well-being, reduction of anxiety and depression, and an improvement in self-esteem and self-concept

cannot be understated.[10] School-based physical activity and healthy eating programs promoting older-to-younger student buddying demonstrate improved
social skills, social responsibility, and less bullying.[11] Sports participation also
provides an opportunity for students to understand and implement concepts
such as respect, responsibility, discipline, fairness, and teamwork.[12] Despite
these benefits, it is the positive effect on academic performance that is central
to influencing education decision makers.[13]

> To meet these standards, students require a minimum of 150 minutes/
> week (elementary school) and 225 minutes/week (middle and secondary
> school) of high-quality classes taught by PE specialists using adequate
> equipment and facilities.

National Standards for School Physical Education

The National Standards for Physical Education provide the framework for
high-quality classes.[14] Specialists in PE need to use appropriate instruction
focusing on movement concepts and the motor skill development required to
perform a variety of physical activities while promoting regular participation by
all students regardless of skill, gender, race, or ethnic group. The program needs
to incorporate the means for students to achieve individual health-enhancing
physical fitness, self-discipline, improved self-judgment, and goal setting.
Additional student goals include learning stress reduction and strengthening
peer relations, including respect for others. There must be ongoing, meaningful
assessments of the PE curriculum and all students participating to determine
total program effectiveness. Monitoring height, weight, and body mass index
provides surrogate measurements of health, but assessing changes in strength,
endurance, and flexibility is of additional value, and these have been standardized through multiple resources. To meet these standards, students require a
minimum of 150 minutes/week (elementary school) and 225 minutes/week
(middle and secondary school) of high-quality classes taught by PE specialists
using adequate equipment and facilities. Physical education class time should
be 30 minutes for grades K through 2 and 45 minutes in grades 3 through 5.[14]
The teacher-student ratio should be no greater than 1:25 (elementary school)
and 1:30 (middle/high school) for optimal instruction. The use of physical
activity as punishment is not acceptable.[15]

Physical Education Programs

The American Academy of Pediatrics (AAP) and the World Health Organization recommend that schools adopt a healthy school-community model in which physical activity is promoted in multiple settings, including physical education.[16,17]

Recommendations for PE Programs in Schools (Modified and Adapted From the AAP Statement[16])

- Promote enjoyable, lifelong physical activity.
  - Develop students' knowledge, attitudes, motor skills, behavioral skills, and confidence.
- Require compulsory quality daily PE programs from kindergarten through grade 12.
- Coordinate PE with health education at each grade.
  - Employ qualified, trained specialists to teach PE classes.
  - Educate all members of the school community about the benefits of physical activity and encourage them to participate.
  - Offer a variety of physical activities for students and staff.
  - Provide opportunities for students and families to participate in physical activities together.
  - Accommodate the needs and interests of all students, including those with illness, injury, disability, obesity, sedentary lifestyles, and disinterest in team or competitive sports.
- Provide a safe, supportive environment for a variety of physical activities. Offer staff development on injury prevention, first aid, and equipment as well as facilities maintenance. Require appropriate use of protective equipment.
- Commit to adequate resources, including program funding, personnel, safe equipment, and facilities.
- Regularly evaluate the district's physical activity programs, including classroom instruction, the nature and level of student activity, and the adequacy and safety of athletic facilities.
- Establish complementary relationships with community recreation agencies and youth sports programs. Encourage student and family participation in these extracurricular programs.

Goal and Structure of Physical Education Programs

The goal of the PE curriculum is to expose students to all components necessary for a lifetime of continued physical activity. Such programs build and strengthen psychomotor, cognitive, affective, safety, and motor skills. Motor skills include muscle strength and endurance, flexibility, coordination, and cardiac strength and endurance. Teaching or expecting physical skills to develop before students are developmentally ready is more likely to cause frustration than long-term success.[12,18,19]

> By 15 years of age, it is estimated that 75% of youth who were previously engaged in organized sports have already dropped out.

Most preschool students have short attention spans and are easily distracted; therefore, pediatric experts recommend free play, teaching motor skills in age-appropriate spaces with emphasis on show-and-tell format, fun, exploration, experimentation, and safety.[2,18,19] Activities might include walking, running, tumbling, throwing, and catching. As motor skills, balance, and visual tracking improve, 6- to 9-year-old students should be encouraged to play using more sophisticated movement patterns with emphasis on fundamental skill development. Organized sports (coed not contraindicated) with short instruction times, flexible rules, and a focus on fun can be initiated.[2,18,19] By late childhood, fully developed visual tracking, motor skills, and balance allow more advanced skill development and better participation in team sports as well as solitary sports. The focus should remain on enjoyment with full participation by all students. Because puberty begins at different times and progresses at different rates, consideration should be given to basing placement in contact sports on physical maturity rather than chronologic age to reduce injury rates.[2,18,19] Supervised strength training may begin in this age group, provided the student uses small free weights with high repetition and demonstrates proper technique.[20]

As children enter into high school, physical activity declines significantly. Students' daily PE class attendance from grades 9 to 12 dropped approximately 50% in 2011.[5] By 15 years of age, it is estimated that 75% of youth who were previously engaged in organized sports have already dropped out. There are many reasons for this disturbing trend. The focus on early specialization through time-intensive travel teams forces children to choose between sports at too early an age and encourages those who are less skillful or less willing to sacrifice their other interests to drop out of sports altogether. Providing more opportunities for children to continue to participate in sports throughout high school on a "less intense" level would be helpful. In addition, the benefits of continued participation in multiple sports throughout high school should be emphasized. There is a lower risk of overuse injuries and athletic burnout with more diverse sports participation. Providing adolescents with a variety of exercises that focus on the individual interest of the student and include friends is crucial for long-term participation in physical activity and healthy lifestyles.[2,18,19]

Episodic Exclusion From Physical Education for Health Reasons

Children periodically experience illness or injury that may interfere with or present a contraindication to physical activity. Many children complain of a variety of ailments sometimes used as reasons to not participate in PE class. As such, teachers and schools rely on medical personnel to confirm the diagnosis and provide recommendations for activity restriction and guidance on safe return to PE. Specific medical ailments precluding participation in sport, such as infections (respiratory, gastrointestinal and dermatologic), head injury, and exacerbations of chronic disease (eg, asthma, seizures and diabetes), have been well outlined in a statement by the AAP Council on Sports Medicine and Fitness and the AAP publication *Preparticipation Physical Evaluation (PPE)*.[21,22] In most cases, decisions require individual assessments by medical personnel to determine the severity of the illness and a return to baseline health before initiating return to play under supervised conditions. In many cases, input from specialists may be required.

Injury and surgery usually require a personalized approach to assessment, with ongoing monitoring of recovery, to determine activity modifications and when it is safe to return to sports participation. Injuries require a twofold determination of limitations: risk of reexacerbation of the original injury as well as the effect on mobility predisposing to subsequent injury. Mild sprains and strains often result in minor limitations, and most students achieve full resumption of activity within weeks. More significant injuries require longer healing times with advancement of activity based on clinical and/or radiographic improvement (in the case of fractures). Rehabilitation to regain range of motion, strength, proprioception, and overall conditioning assists in recovery and return-to-play for athletes. Specific limitations, such as no body contact in football or restricted weight-bearing upper-extremity activities in gymnastics, may allow earlier participation to at least some degree.[23,24] Some physical educators allow such students to perform required rehabilitation exercises in class for credit until they can fully participate. Physical therapy should not be considered a long-term replacement for PE; instead, the goal should be a return to participation, utilizing adaptive programs when necessary.

Other common complaints (headache, abdominal pain, menstrual cramping, back or extremity pain) may be reasonable causes for limited participation on occasion, but persistent problems should prompt medical evaluation for an accurate diagnosis and recommended management strategies. Students with refractory complaints should also undergo medical evaluation for possible avoidance of physical activity. Bullying (by peers or teachers), concerns regarding personal appearance (hair, body habitus, hygiene/odor), physical ability, or anxiety/depression should be considered.[25] Identification and treatment of such issues often prove invaluable not only in returning the student to physical activity but also in helping them attain overall health benefits.

Modified and Adapted PE Programs

Participation in PE classes with one's peers should be the goal for every child. The Individuals with Disabilities Education Act (IDEA) was reauthorized in 2004 to bring it in line with the No Child Left Behind Act. IDEA states in section 300.108(b) that "each child with a disability must be afforded the opportunity to participate in the same PE program available to nondisabled children unless: (1) the child is enrolled full time in a separate facility; or (2) the child needs specially designed curriculum, as prescribed in the child's Individualized Education Program (IEP)."

PE should be considered an important part of the IEP, augmenting services provided elsewhere and preparing the child for a lifetime of activity in the community. Individual state education agencies and each school district often interpret eligibility for adapted PE within the mandate of the federal law differently, so resources vary and formal assessments of physical function may or may not be required. In some cases, adaptive PE specialists participate in the evaluation and development of an IEP. These specialists have experience and training in physical and motor development and communicate with other school personnel in a multidisciplinary manner.[26] In other cases, the general PE instructor is solely responsible for the development of this curriculum. Input from the child's medical caregivers (therapists, audiologist, physician) assists in creation of the IEP in many circumstances. The IEP should provide specific measurable goals and objectives for the students that are reassessed regularly to determine successful achievement or any need for modification. For example, many children, whether with physical or behavioral issues, are able to participate in regular PE with the assistance of an aide. Some children may be able to achieve the goals of the rest of the class, and others may require goals addressing social interaction or behavioral redirection. Children with more significant limitations (eg, muscular dystrophy or nonambulatory cerebral palsy) may require more extensive adaptations, such as 1-on-1 PE in the pool to allow increased movement in a water-suspended environment with the assistance of suitable flotation devices. Goals for students in these circumstances might include achievement of an activity with (or without) a given level of assistance, such as transfer to an adaptive device or into the water, floating for a specific duration, completion of a length of the pool, or even just putting their face in the water, depending on their ability and developmental needs. The Adapted Physical Education National Standards are available at: **www.apens.org**.

Role of the Physician in Adaptive Physical Education Programs

Physicians often identify children with a disability or developmental delay and refer them for further evaluation and treatment by specialists. Eligibility for special education services, including adapted PE, usually relies on diagnoses provided by a physician. Additionally, this physician should be available to serve as a consultant to the IEP team to advocate for the needs of the individual student, in writing or in person.[27] Specific documentation of visual, behavioral, physical, auditory, and psychological issues are instrumental for educators in determining the needs and adaptations required in the school, especially in the absence of adaptive specialists. A review of the IEP goals for specific and measurable criteria to enhance benefits for the affected child is another degree to which some practitioners may participate. Children and youth with special health care needs require daily exercise as much or more than their able-bodied peers.[2] The physician can advise schools how to modify PE program according to each student's underlying disability.

Other Opportunities to Increase Physical Activity at School

The Society of Health and Physical Educators (formerly National Association for Sport and Physical Education) recommends a comprehensive school physical activity program that incorporates physical activity before, during, and after school. Although not a substitute for PE, other physical activity programs are important. These should include bouts of physical activity in the classroom, such as integrating movement into academic content using TAKE 10 structuring (**www.take10.net**). Incorporating such physical activities directly into the classroom and the maximization of PE and recreation time may be vital for children and youth living in some environments where safe outdoor places to play and active transportation may be limited.

The Society of Health and Physical Educators also recommends at least 20 minutes/day of recess for elementary students. Recess allows children the necessary periods of interruption during the school day to improve attention in subsequent classroom sessions. In addition to the physical health benefits, it encourages peer interaction, where important communication skills (negotiation, sharing, problem solving, and self-control) are gained.[28] These benefits also apply to middle and high schools students, who should be provided free time during lunch or other drop-in sessions that promote lifestyle physical activity. Intramural activities can include sports, self-directed activities (jogging), classes (yoga), and activity clubs (hiking) that appeal to all students. Interscholastic school sports offer opportunity to more skillful students. These school-related activities appear to have a positive association with better health outcomes in addition to cognitive skills and academic achievements while facilitating social development.

Active transportation (walking, biking) to school should be facilitated by following guidelines in Safe Routes to School and the Walking School Bus program. For many children and families, schools represent the primary community resource for physical activity through access to playgrounds, gymnasiums, and meeting spaces. Increased prevalence of play structures contributes to increased physical activity by children both in and out of school.[29]

School-Based Athletic Programs

School-related sports teams, clubs, and physical activity programs at all levels of schooling provide additional ways to enhance fitness and social interaction. These opportunities appear to increase future physical activity after graduation, regardless of the number of activities in which a child participated during schooling.[30] Unfortunately, the time of transition into secondary school represents a period of decline in physical activity and participation in sports.[31] Reasons cited include socioeconomic status (lack of community resources and family financial constraints), advancing skill levels and decreased team sizes limiting ability or opportunities to participate, and competing time commitments for academics and other extracurricular activities. The emphasis should not be solely on the school to provide these opportunities but rather allowing the school to support and foster program development through parent and community-partner commitment. This benefits not only the student but also the families in neighborhoods around the school. Physicians should encourage parents to become involved with schools to develop programs in support of child and youth fitness through community engagement.

Physical Assessments Related to Physical Activity

Optimally, medical assessments should be required annually or every 2 years for all students. This is not strictly practiced in all US schools, but many districts require a medical assessment before student involvement in PE or other athletic activities. Medical assessments allow earlier detection of underlying chronic medical conditions, which may affect safe exercise participation. Detailed information on many disorders can be found elsewhere, but a brief review of a few are included in this chapter.[32,33]

Asthma

Many students with asthma have low physical activity levels and poor cardiovascular fitness because they fear exercise will exacerbate their disease. However, most can be physically active as long as their symptoms are well controlled. Students should keep an accurate history of their symptoms, triggers, and treatments. Most children with asthma experience "exercise-induced bronchospasm," which can be diagnosed by a drop in forced expiratory volume in 1 second (FEV1) by 10% to 15% after a 6- to 8-minute exercise challenge and a positive response to beta-2 agonist medication. Inhaled beta-2 agonists should be readily available for use 15 to 30 minutes before exercise to manage symptoms. Students in middle school and higher grades are usually responsible enough to carry their own quick-acting metered-dose inhalers. It is helpful if the PE teacher, classroom teacher, or school nurse reminds younger students to take their preexercise medications. Pediatricians can inform families and school staff of a particular student's needs by including specific warm-up exercise instructions and optimal hydration along with the student's medication instructions through the development an individual asthma action plan (**www.cdc.gov/asthma/actionplan.html**).[21,32-34]

Insulin-Dependent Diabetes Mellitus

Students with diabetes mellitus type 1 should be encouraged to be physically active to reduce some long-term complications of this disease. They can participate in most activities, provided they demonstrate good metabolic control through the adherence to recommended nutrition and insulin replacement.

They should also monitor blood glucose during and after exercise to avoid episodes of low blood sugar. Teachers should be taught how to recognize the signs of hypoglycemia, and ready sources of fast-acting sugars, such as milk or orange juice, should be available. Protective padding and extra layers of clothing are important for diabetic students wearing an insulin pump during body contact-related sports or outdoor events in the cold.[21,32,33]

Seizure Disorders

Parents of children with seizure disorders commonly impose restrictions on sports participation for safety reasons, but seizures are rarely triggered by physical activity. Exercise has been shown to be beneficial to those affected with epilepsy by improving self-esteem. It can also activate several seizure-inhibitory components, which may reduce seizure susceptibility.[34] A neurologist should assess affected students regularly, but provided their disease is well controlled, they maintain fluid and electrolyte balance, and adhere to safe play guidelines, they can fully participate in PE and other athletics. Those with suboptimal seizure control risk injury in contact sports, swimming, strength training, and activities involving heights. School staff should be extra vigilant under these circumstances and be aware of basic first aid seizure management.[21,32,33]

Hemophilia

Fitness and strength are lower in students with hemophilia, possibly because of excessive restrictions placed on physical activity. Exercise may have a beneficial effect on coagulation, and high-impact activity has been shown to improve bone health. A pediatric hematologist should assess affected students to determine appropriate factor prophylaxis to reduce bleeding risks. Those with prior bleeding into joints may have lower muscle strength and endurance. A physician should assess joint and muscle function before PE and sport involvement to ensure safe participation. The risk of bleeding depends on the individual's level of clotting factor and their prophylactic treatment. The National Hemophilia Association offers guidance on appropriate sports (**www.hemophilia.org/sites/default/files/document/files/PlayingItSafe.pdf**) for children with hemophilia. The school should have a written plan (**www.hemophiliafed.org/resource-library/back-to-school-toolkit**) including descriptions of protective clothing and equipment, the need for quick access to cold compresses after an injury, and a plan to transport the student promptly to a facility where clotting factor can be replenished.[21,32,33,35]

Preparticipation Physical Examination

The preparticipation physical examination (PPE) serves a number of purposes for the student-athlete prior to participation in sports. The overall purpose is not to exclude participation in physical activity but to optimize health and safety. The PPE includes sports-specific history and assessment of the appropriate fitness level of the child. Importantly, completed forms assist in the coordination of care and awareness of underlying medical conditions.[22] Administratively, forms provide documentation for clearance to participate in sport and exercise by a physician and may meet legal and liability requirements for the sponsoring organization. Although studies have not shown that the PPE decreases mortality in youth sports, important roles include the identification of "medical and orthopedic conditions that might affect an athlete's ability to participate safely in sports".[22,36] Because the PPE is ideally performed in a primary care physician's office, it also provides an opportunity to establish the medical home, where immunizations, management of chronic conditions, and anticipatory guidance are can be provided.[22]

The PPE includes a 54-point history questionnaire to identify a relevant family history as well as personal history of cardiac issues, menstrual problems, musculoskeletal injury, and other health conditions that may affect participation (**https://www.aap.org/en-us/about-the-aap/Committees-Councils-Sections/Council-on-sports-medicine-and-fitness/Documents/PPE-4-forms.pdf#search=PPE**). Additionally, it promotes a head-to-toe physical examination, with the potential for a detailed joint examination if there are specific concerns. Although required by many organizations for sports participation, the tenants of the PPE apply to any child pursuing physical activity. Most issues identified on the PPE still allow modified sports participation, with complete exclusion occurring only 2% to 3% of the time.[21,22,36] Cardiac conditions are most frequently implicated in exclusion from sports, but case-by-case prohibitions may occur when a disorder places the student at risk of further injury or death. Children with special health care needs present unique considerations, but a modified history form is available within the PPE to serve as an appropriate evaluation tool.[22]

Nutrition and Exercise

Adequate nutrition is important for optimal physical activity participation. Usual PE classes and recess have a short duration; hence, additional intake beyond regular meals and snacks is unnecessary, except for water. For after-school athletes, lunch provides the primary opportunity for energy intake. Recommendations for preexercise carbohydrates include: 4 g/kg, 3 to 4 hours before, and an additional 0.5 to 1 g/kg of easily digested carbohydrates 1 hour before exercise.[37-39] If lunch is more than 4 hours before exercise, more carbohydrate may be required, provided the student does not overeat to the detriment of athletic performance. Eating during practice is not required for most school-related sports.[37] Generally, intake of water (3–8 ounces every 20 minutes for 9- to 12-year-olds, up to 34–50 ounces/hour for teenagers) is enough to minimize sweat-induced body-water deficits during exercise, as long as the preactivity hydration status is good.[40] Pre- to postactivity body-weight changes can provide more specific insight into the student athlete's rehydration needs. Although water is often sufficient, long-duration (at least 1-hour) or repeated same-day sessions of strenuous exercise, or rigorous sport and intense physical activity, might warrant rehydration with electrolyte-supplemented beverages (sport drinks) that emphasize sodium replacement. This is especially justified in warm to hot weather conditions, when sweat loss is extensive.[40] School personnel and parents should educate students that energy drinks, which pose potential significant health risks, primarily because of stimulant content, should never be consumed.[37] Postexercise intake of 1 to 1.5 g/kg of carbohydrates within 30 to 45 minutes of the event is important to replenish glycogen stores, and protein is also required for muscle development in these athletes. The ingestion of a meal or snack containing both protein and carbohydrate usually suffices, but fluid replacements providing a ratio of 3 carbohydrates to 1 protein, such as chocolate milk, may serve as convenient alternatives.[37,41]

Nutritional Deficiencies in Athletes

Youth often experience nutrition deficiencies, especially females, if they decide to stop eating meat without adding alternative sources of iron. The US recommended daily allowance for female adolescents is 15 mg of iron, which many female athletes do not achieve. The addition of menstrual losses can increase risks of iron deficiency with and without anemia. The physician should initiate appropriate investigations, nutritional counseling, and iron treatment when such deficiencies are detected.[42]

Calcium and vitamin D deficiencies may occur in students across America from lack of sufficient solar exposure and significant dietary restrictions. The current recommendation for vitamin D intake for 9- to 18-year-olds is 1300 mg calcium/day and 600 IU/day. Some athletes have underlying unintentional or intentional disordered eating in an attempt to improve appearance or athletic performance. They are at higher risk of developing low bone mineral density and stress fractures. Although more common in females, often associated with the "female athlete triad" of anorexia, amenorrhea, and osteoporosis, male athletes are also frequently affected.[42,43] Bone mineral density and lateral thoracolumbar spine radiographs should be obtained, and if abnormal, increasing dietary calcium should be considered (1500 mg calcium/day).[42] Athletes should be monitored closely for eating disorders and intentional weight loss issues, which should be discussed to identify those requiring further treatment. Conversely, other athletes may be more focused on weight gain, which should also occur in a healthy manner rather than by just overconsumption of calories.

> The National Program for Playground Safety has introduced S.A.F.E. factors as part of their national action plan for the prevention of playground injuries: supervision, age-appropriate, fall surfacing, and equipment.

Student Safety and Injury Prevention

Playgrounds provide a resource for children to be active while at school, as well as for the community at large. Unfortunately, playgrounds also present an opportunity for injury, depending on the apparatus used. Swings are responsible for the majority of traumatic brain injuries occurring on playgrounds, and monkey bars contribute to most fractures.[44] The National Program for Playground Safety has introduced S.A.F.E. factors as part of their national action plan for the prevention of playground injuries: supervision, age-appropriate, fall surfacing, and equipment. Children should always be supervised when using school playgrounds to promote age-appropriate use of the equipment. The American Society for Testing and Materials (ASTM) sets standards on surfacing and equipment, and the Consumer Products Safety Commission (CPSC) issues guidelines on the construction and design of safe playgrounds.

Extrinsic factors, such as weather conditions and playing field surface, influence injury in school sports. The field of play for sports should be maintained to optimal conditions, and the referee or governing organization should advise when weather conditions preclude participation or require adaptations to minimize risk of injury[37] (see section on Dehydration, Heat, and Cold). Endurance sports are associated with overuse problems, whereas contact and collision sports have a higher risk of acute injury, especially if protective equipment is not adequate or safety rules are not enforced. The use of protective equipment is in a period of rapid change as athletes, parents, and officials desire safe sport participation to minimize the risk of injury without drastically changing the fundamental nature of the individual sport.

Sports-related concussions are common, especially for those youth participating in collision and contact events. On-field assessment by knowledgeable athletic trainers or coaches facilitates early removal of affected students from the playing field. Symptoms are varied and the recovery course is longer than for adult athletes; hence, assessment by a physician with concussion experience is warranted and mandated in many states.[45] These students require physical and cognitive rest until symptoms resolve with rest and exertion; hence, physicians may require teachers to modify student workloads. Education of school staff, parents, and students about this condition is integral to helping improve awareness, recognition, and management.[46]

Intrinsic factors specific to the athlete that play a role in injury include general health, fitness, psychological makeup, and anatomic and biomechanical factors.[46] Smaller athletes may sustain more injury in contact sports, and girls are at higher risk of anterior cruciate ligament (ACL) injuries. Unfit and overweight individuals may develop soft tissue strains and heat illness. Incomplete rehabilitation of previous injuries increases the risk of subsequent injury. Neuromuscular training occurs during preactivity warm-up that includes stretching, strengthening, balance exercises, sports-specific maneuvers, and techniques to prevent common injuries. This has been shown to be protective across all age ranges, for multiple sports, and for both genders.[47]

Rules and regulations are designed to minimize injury or deter risk-taking behaviors that may injure others. Examples include pitch counts for baseball pitchers, use of protective equipment (eg, helmets, pads, mouth guards), and penalties.[46,48] Physicians play an important role in introducing and supporting injury prevention policy because of their general medical knowledge and professional expertise. Opportunities for advocacy may occur at the local, state, and even national level through schools, the AAP (and its state chapters), community organizations, and legislative testimony.

Suggested Sport and Activity Injury-Related Policy

- Encourage students to report pain to a responsible adult. Assure young athletes their team position is not in jeopardy because of injury.
- Prohibit students in pain from continued participation in any activity that might exacerbate the injury. If pain relievers are required to continue playing, the activity should not be permitted and the student should be encouraged to see his or her primary care provider if unable to discontinue pain relievers within 5 to 7 days.
- Develop alternative activities that help maintain fitness or develop skills without involving an injured limb or body system for students who temporarily cannot participate.
- Require parent notification about injuries immediately. Do not rely on a student's self-report, especially with head, chest, and abdominal injuries.
- Record all injuries, including data on time of day, nature of the sport, site of injury, nature of collision or other circumstance, level of supervision, age and sex of the injured student, and the geographic location within the school or off-campus activity.
- Routinely monitor the:
  - Student's level of conditioning and nutritional practices, particularly hydration;
  - Status of previous injuries, particularly those that might not have completely healed;
  - Student's psychological and motivational status;
  - Number of available, experienced adult supervisors with cardiopulmonary resuscitation (CPR) and first aid training;
  - Availability, status, and use of personal protective equipment; and
  - Status of district equipment and field facilities.
- Establish an effective communication system with emergency paramedic assistance.

Protective Equipment

The use of approved equipment to prevent injury is essential. Bicycle helmets endorsed by the Snell Memorial Foundation have been shown to prevent 69% of head injuries and 65% of injuries to the face.[49] Similarly approved helmets for skiers and snowboarders can reduce concussion and head injuries, in general, by 35%, especially children younger than 13 years.[45,50] Football helmets meeting National Operating Committee on Standards for Athletic Equipment requirements and approved hockey helmets reduce impact forces to the head and protect against skull fracture, but a reduction in concussion is not consistently seen.[45,51] All headgear should be fitted and worn properly, and damaged equipment should be replaced promptly according to manufacturers' recommendations. Eye guards approved by the ASTM and other protective equipment may reduce eye injuries. Eye protection is mandatory for athletes with a single functional eye (corrected vision less than 20/40). Boxing and full-contact martial arts are not recommended, especially for students with a single functional eye, because ocular protection is impractical and/or not permitted.[21,22] Mouth guards approved by the American Dental Association can reduce dental injury but have not been shown to be effective in the prevention of concussion to date.[51] For athletes with a single functioning kidney, flak-jackets are an option, although they are unproven in their degree of protection against injury. The exclusion of athletes with solitary organs from sports with a risk of injury to the remaining functional organ is controversial, but many are allowed to play after extensive discussion regarding risks. Likewise, male athletes with a single testicle may choose to wear a protective cup.[21] Ankle braces have been shown to prevent injuries in football and basketball.[52]

Injury Reports

The National High School Sports Injury Surveillance System, the University of North Carolina National Center for Catastrophic Sports Injury Research, the US Consumer Product Safety Commission, the Centers for Disease Control and Prevention (CDC), and other federal agencies collect data regarding sports-related injuries. These injury databases are critical to the identification of catastrophic and noncatastrophic injury patterns and can affect future decisions about recommended or required equipment modifications, sports surfaces, coach and athlete preparation, and education.[53]

Dehydration, Heat, and Cold

Recent studies suggest similarly fit and heat-acclimatized children and adults exposed to equal exercise intensity in a hot environment have similar rectal temperatures and cardiovascular responses.[40] It is undue exertion, insufficient recovery time between bouts of exercise, underlying illness, and heavy clothing and protective equipment that play a major role in heat retention. Indeed, exertional heat illness is usually preventable. Most healthy children and youth can safely participate in a hot environment with appropriate preparation, modifications, and monitoring. These include adequate fitness and acclimatization (10-14 days), avoidance or limiting physical activity if ill recently or obese, suitable hydration (before, during, and after activity), longer recovery time between sessions, and ensuring personnel and facilities for effective heat illness treatment are available on site. The PPE is an effective way to identify recent illnesses (fever, gastroenteritis), underlying chronic diseases (diabetes, hyperthyroidism, cystic fibrosis, sickle cell disease and trait) or medications that might affect thermoregulation (dopamine-reuptake inhibitors for attention-deficit/hyperactivity [ADHD]).[22,40]

Pediatricians should educate school staff, parents, and students on heat illness reduction strategies and the recognition of signs of heat stress and develop and implement an emergency action plan. Heat cramps are painful muscle contractions associated with intense exercise, muscle fatigue, dehydration, and electrolyte disturbances. The body temperature is normal and treatment is limited to rest, massaging and stretching affected muscles, and rehydration with cold water or sport drink. Heat exhaustion is a moderate heat illness resulting from strenuous exercise, acute dehydration and low energy levels, and an inability to maintain blood pressure and sustain adequate cardiac output. Youth are weak and dizzy, suffer syncope and nausea, and have red facial flushing and an elevated core body temperature that is under 40°C. These students should stop participating and seek medical attention. Exertional heat stroke is characterized by delirium, convulsions or coma, circulatory failure with a core body temperature over 40°C, and often, organ failure. Emergency medical services (EMS) must be notified immediately, and affected students should have heavy clothing and equipment removed and undergo rapid cooling using ice packs (avoiding direct sun exposure) while awaiting evacuation to a treatment facility.[40,54]

The 2 most common cold-related illnesses include hypothermia and frostbite. Frostbite is a localized cold injury in which crystallization of fluids in the skin occurs on exposure to below-freezing temperatures. School staff should initiate treatment by removing the student from the cold, detaching any wet clothing, warming the extremities against an unaffected body part while avoiding vigorous massage of the affected skin, and putting on dry protective clothing. These athletes should not be allowed to return to the cold to avoid refreezing and should be referred to the pediatrician or to an emergency department for subsequent medical care. Hypothermia can occur from severe cold exposure or immersion in cold water, and symptoms can vary from shivering and faster heart rate (mild) to altered level of consciousness or coma and an absence of shivering (severe). School officials should activate EMS while removing the athlete carefully from the field, unfastening wet clothes, and covering him or her with insulating material. These athletes need to be transferred to a suitable medical facility for further treatment.[54]

> The most common pediatric causes of sudden cardiac arrest are hypertrophic cardiomyopathy, congenital coronary artery anomalies, aortic stenosis, myocarditis, and dysrhythmias.

Automated External Defibrillators

Sudden cardiac arrest is the leading cause of death in adults but it is uncommon in children and teenagers. The most common pediatric causes of sudden cardiac arrest are hypertrophic cardiomyopathy, congenital coronary artery anomalies, aortic stenosis, myocarditis, and dysrhythmias. A cardiologist should assess all athletes with any of these conditions before sports participation is allowed, because most of these conditions carry significant risk of sudden death with intense exercise. Many adult cardiac arrests are precipitated by lethal arrhythmias that can be reversed by rapid use of an automated external defibrillator (AED). The role of AEDs in response to a cardiac arrest in children is not as clear, because cardiac arrest in children is often precipitated by respiratory arrest and not related to lethal arrhythmias. Nonetheless, numerous lives have been saved by the use of AEDs in airports, stadiums, and schools. The American Heart Association supports AED placement in schools and recommends CPR training and familiarization with AEDs in secondary school curricula. However, the cost of these devices, at several thousand dollars each, is beyond the reach of many school districts.[55,56]

Potential Problems Associated With
Physical Activity and Sports

Stress

Physical activity improves mood, and organized sports as well as unstructured physical activity can stimulate character development and confidence if competent adult supervision by coaches and parents is in place. Pediatricians should educate parents about the negative effects of them being over- or underinvolved in their child's sport. Overinvolvement can lead to stress from criticism, interference in practices, and pressuring their child to win. Underinvolvement can reduce the child's motivation to participate and parents lacking knowledge about the coach's ability to provide a positive learning environment. Avoidance of early sport specialization and forced sport participation are good strategies to reduce the likelihood of sport dissatisfaction and burnout by the child. The pediatrician should also look for signs of depression, anorexia, bulimia, and substance abuse, which often require referral to appropriate mental health experts.[57,58]

Substance Abuse

Students who participate in regular physical activity and athletic programs tend to engage less in substance abuse than their nonactive peers.[59,60] The Youth Risk Behavior Survey (YRBS) of students in grades 9 through 12 demonstrated that approximately 40% had used marijuana, 11% had sniffed glue or other inhalants, 9% had used hallucinogenic drugs, 8% had abused ecstasy, and about 3% had abused heroin one or more times.[5] However, athletes gravitate toward certain (ergogenic) substances to increase endurance, speed, muscle strength, and performance. Students may be less likely to take these agents if appropriately educated. Physicians, along with PE teachers and coaches, have an important role in preventing substance abuse, and a useful free resource is *The Coach's Playbook Against Drugs*.

Stimulants

Stimulants increase alertness and delay fatigue. The YRBS revealed that 6.8% of high school students had used cocaine and 4% had used methamphetamines at least once.[5] Athletes may be less likely to abuse these drugs, but other stimulants are available. Caffeine is the most widely obtainable stimulant but also acts as a diuretic, leading to reduced strength and endurance and greater risk of heat illness. Energy drinks are especially dangerous, containing large quantities of caffeine and other stimulants that may lead to catastrophic events. Cigarette smoking was prevalent in the YRBS, with 18% of students considered current smokers.[5] Although athletes smoke less than their nonathletic peers, nicotine is also found in smokeless tobacco, which is used among baseball players. Some athletes abuse ephedrine (herbal teas, cold medications, and weight loss supplements) or amphetamines (including methylphenidate for AHDH), which can cause tachycardia and lead to disastrous outcomes and are prohibited from international competition.[61,62]

Creatine

Often found in dietary supplements that are loosely regulated by the Dietary Supplement Health and Education Act of 1994, creatine has been touted as a performance-enhancing supplement. Although small improvements in brief exercise activity have been demonstrated in some athletes, those in endurance sports (cycling, swimming, distance running) experience performance degradation. Students may be at higher risks of dehydration and heat illness.[62-65] It is also recommended that youth at risk of renal dysfunction (diabetes, hypertension, impaired glomerular filtration rate) and those with established renal disease avoid creatine supplementation.

Anabolic Steroids

Anabolic steroids are banned substances (androgens) that can increase muscle size and strength when combined with adequate caloric intake and strength training. Although athletes have been known to abuse anabolic steroids, their nonathlete peers sometimes also take these agents to enhance physical appearance. Adverse effects include high blood pressure, aggression, possible cardiomyopathy, and liver tumors.[62,65]

Other Agents

Adrenocorticotropic hormone, human growth hormone, and human chorionic gonadotropin are usually used to increase height, muscle mass, and body weight. They are expensive and not readily available. However, counterfeits of these substances are widely advertised. Beta-2 agonists like clenbuterol (used to treat asthma) can have stimulant and anabolic effects. Albuterol and salbutamol (abused by some athletes) require medical evidence of reactive airways disease to allow use in international competition.[62,65-68]

How to Work With Schools

A useful mechanism to promote healthy eating and physical activity is a coordinated school health framework, which provides integrated school-affiliated strategies designed to promote the optimal physical, emotional, social, and educational development of students. A coordinated school health framework is directed by a multidisciplinary "wellness advisory committee" and integrates multiple components of the school environment that influence student health. Such a committee should involve school personnel, students, families, and community stakeholders, including health care providers.[69]

Wellness Advisory Committees and School Physical Education and Physical Activity Policies

The *Child Nutrition and WIC Reauthorization Act of 2004* required that school districts participating in the National School Lunch Program establish a local wellness policy by the 2006-2007 school year. By 2008, most had a wellness policy, but the quality varied, and many lacked implementation planning. The *Healthy, Hunger-Free Kids Act of 2010* updated the requirements of school wellness policies to include at least goals to promote healthy eating and physical activity, engagement of school and community stakeholders in the development and implementation of the wellness policy, regular evaluation of the policy, and communication of this information to the public.

> Local school wellness policies have provided an unprecedented opportunity to mold the school environment in terms of nutrition and physical activity. Pediatricians looking to be involved in their own child's school should consider joining the school wellness committee.

A multidiscipline wellness advisory committee should be formed and use resources like the National Association of State Boards of Education's *Fit, Healthy and Ready to Learn* to develop policy using language consistent with state, district, and school visions for student learning and health. Process (if program was implemented as intended) and outcome (changes in school environment or behaviors) evaluation should be included using resources like the CDC's *Framework for Program Evaluation in Public Health*. The committee should strive to create a school environment that ensures safe facilities and equipment, safe routes to school, access to extracurricular physical activity programs that are safe and age appropriate, acceptance of diverse abilities, and no bullying. A useful resource is the *Consumer Product Safety Commission Handbook for Public Playground Safety*. The committee should implement a comprehensive health education and a physical activity program (K-12) that meets the needs of all students, with a quality daily PE curriculum that follows national standards. The Physical Education Curriculum Analysis Tool (PECAT) can help enhance school curriculum, and the Society of Health and Physical Educators has various resources to evaluate student performance. Fitness testing, using a reliable resource like the Fitnessgram, can encourage students to adhere to their personal activity goals, especially if scores are kept confidential.[70] The wellness advisory committee should establish a formal agreement between schools and community organizations to increase access to PA facilities and programs. A free resource to address liability issues can be found in the *National Policy and Legal Analysis Network to Prevent Childhood Obesity*. The PE curriculum should encourage full student participation in noncompetitive active games and lifestyle activities like dancing and jumping rope. Policy should require other means of physical activity, like daily recess; physical activity breaks in the classroom; intramural sports and lifestyle physical activity; and active transportation to school using resources like the National Centre for Safe Routes to School.

The wellness advisory committee should ensure all students are taught health education meeting national standards; CDC's Health Education Curriculum Analysis Tool (HECAT) can help schools develop suitable curricula. Students should also have access to needed physical and mental health and social services, which may require community partnerships. Policy should include open lines of communication to motivate families and community partners to promote involvement and address cultural diversity. The CDC *School Health Index* can help using suitable communication tools.[71] The committee should develop and implement a school employee wellness program with annual professional development opportunities and require the hiring of certified physical education, health education teachers, and nutrition services staff.[69]

Local school wellness policies have provided an unprecedented opportunity to mold the school environment in terms of nutrition and physical activity. Pediatricians looking to be involved in their own child's school should consider joining the school wellness committee.

Recommendations for Pediatricians

School health is not dictated by national school health laws but rather through the state or local district. This should not discourage pediatricians from becoming a school physician, because growth and development, disease processes, and health maintenance in children and youth are the backbone of pediatric training.[72] The school nurse is often the health care representative within the school and is the natural ally for physician involvement. Physicians can play a major role in the promotion of health through physical activity and PE. Responsibilities might include school injury prevention, including concussion management; recognition of underlying medical conditions through the PPE, which may disqualify students from participation; and providing guidance on hydration and extremes of climate and emergency preparedness. Additional roles can include involvement in an adaptive PE program. Ultimately, the school physician has an opportunity to be a leading member of a coordinated school health model through which links between health and learning are stressed and relationships between the families and community can be made. The AAP Council on School Health Web site (**http://www2.aap.org/sections/schoolhealth/**) provides additional guidance on how pediatricians can work with schools.

Unfortunately, most states do not mandate school physicians, despite recommendations by the American Medical Association and the AAP.[72] Nonetheless, doctors can have a professional relationship with schools as full-or part-time employees, in an independent consultant role, or as a volunteer on a school wellness advisory committee. Some may choose to volunteer as team physicians, but a good understanding of state laws addressing district obligations to hire a medical director is important. It is also critical that physicians contact their medical liability insurance company to be sure coverage is guaranteed.[72]

Pediatricians can be involved with schools in many other ways. Nationally, the AAP and its Council on School Health contribute policy statements and advocacy positions that have helped to promote strong national active healthy living school policies. In daily practice, pediatricians can encourage families and patients to adopt healthy lifestyles.

Pediatricians and other health care professionals are encouraged to support districts in their efforts to promote physical activity and fitness by:

- assisting districts in adapting physical education programs to meet the physical activity needs of acutely injured or chronically disabled students;
- encouraging school boards to implement effective kindergarten through grade 12 curricula that provide information and skills for lifetime fitness;
- advocating for the creation of a school wellness advisory committee;
- supporting policies that require students to use appropriate safety equipment for sports and physical activities in all settings;
- helping to create medical emergency and weather extremes policies relating to exercise and sport participation;
- developing policies addressing mixed gender competition, the use of physical activity as a punishment, and antibullying;
- overseeing preparticipation examination and safe return to exercise and sports following illness or injury;
- acting as an athletic advisor and or team physician;

- educating members of the school community about current activity patterns, obesity and other chronic illnesses linked to physical inactivity, and strategies for increasing daily activity levels;
- creating appropriate health education curriculum;
- empowering children, youth, and family members to engage in physical activities together;
- promoting the funding and hiring of personnel resources that would offer opportunities for all students to be physically active and to receive appropriate direction and supervision from well-trained, knowledgeable adults;
- joining school health advisory boards and advocating for more pe during the school day in addition to increased physical activity opportunities before, during, and after school;
- endorsing the creation and implementation of staff wellness policies;
- recommending accessible community sports/recreation programs through which school gymnasiums or local facilities are open after regular school hours to provide all children and youth physical activity opportunities at low to no cost;
- sustaining the implementation of policies addressing safe recreational facilities, playgrounds, parks, bike paths, sidewalks, and crosswalks; and
- adopting a physically active lifestyle—physicians who exercise regularly are more likely to promote it to their patients.

Recommendations for Program Directors and Trainees

Schools are complex systems that are able to offer students and pediatric residents a unique perspective on how we seek to optimize child health through policies, programs, practices, education, and measures. Although the school nurse is the appropriate link between health professionals and students, the school PE teacher is the best contact when looking into modifying physical activity and PE programs. Review of school policies, compared with national "best practices," can be enlightening for trainees and can help promote competence in practice-based learning and improvement and systems-based practice. Likewise, sideline or training room management of athletes under the supervision of a staff physician provides experiences that may translate to later career opportunities or involvement in schools. The economics of facilities and equipment, the pressures to minimize recess, regular daily activity, and PE are all topics that trainees can experience. Examining the pros and cons of the many controversial issues surrounding schools is an exercise that sharpens a student's sensitivity to the nuances of policy making for schools. PE in schools can be an excellent opportunity to train sports medicine fellows to manage injuries on the field. In addition, trainees in pediatrics can serve as consultants to PE teachers when it comes to evaluating medical conditions requiring exclusion from play such as infections, concussions, sprains, and strains as well as medical conditions exacerbated by sports, such as asthma.

Take-Home Points

- The increasing obesity epidemic has focused medical, recreational, and public health communities on the link between sedentary behavior and inadequate physical activity and adverse health outcomes.
- National childcare and preschool physical activity policies that require the teaching of fundamental movement skills is essential to the life-long implementation of an active, healthy lifestyle.
- National physical activity and PE standards play an important role in directing school programs. These have been shown to be effective in meeting the health and academic needs of US students.
- Creative in-school planning and partnerships with community facilities can help staff, parents, and students reach needed physical activity goals.
- The school physical education specialist is poised to create appropriate PE and physical activity curricula to meet the needs of all students. Their work should be strongly supported by the health care community.
- Physical activity and PE policies and standards directly affect not only students' health and well-being but also their behavior and academic performance.
- Community professionals can have a direct effect on local school wellness through participation on school wellness advisory committees.

> **Resources**
>
> For additional school health related resources, visit www.aap.org/schoolhealthmanual.

References

1. Ogden CL, Carroll MD, Kit BK, Flegal KM. Prevalence of obesity and trends in body mass index among US children and adolescents, 1999-2010. *JAMA*. 2012;307(5):483–490

2. Lipnowski S, LeBlanc CM; Canadian Paediatric Society, Healthy Active Living and Sports Medicine Committee. Healthy active living: physical activity guidelines for children and adolescents. *Paediatr Child Health*. 2012;17(4):209–229

3. US Department of Health and Human Services. *2008 Physical Activity Guidelines for Americans*. Washington, DC: US Department of Health and Human Services; 2008. Available at: http://www.health.gov/paguidelines/guidelines/. Accessed April 13, 2015

4. US Department of Health and Human Services. *Healthy People 2020*. Washington, DC: US Department of Health and Human Services; 2010. Available at: http://www.healthypeople.gov/2020. Accessed April 13, 2015

5. Centers for Disease Control and Prevention. Youth risk behavior surveillance – United States, 2011. *MMWR Morb Mortal Wkly Rep*. 2012;61:(SS-4):1–168

6. Kann L, Brener ND, Wechsler H. Overview and summary: School Health Policies and Programs Study 2006. *J Sch Health*. 2007;77(8):385–397

7. Rasberry CN, Lee SM, Robin L, Laris BA, Russell LA, Coyle KK, Nihiser AJ. The association between school-based physical activity, including physical education, and academic performance: a systematic review of the literature. *Prev Med*. 2011;52(Suppl 1):S10–S20

8. Janssen I, Leblanc AG. Systematic review of the health benefits of physical activity and fitness in school-aged children and youth. *Int J Behav Nutr Phys Act*. 2010;7:40

9. Janz KF, Burns TL, Levy SM, et al. Everyday activity predicts bone geometry in children: the Iowa bone development study. *Med Sci Sports Exerc*. 2004;36(7):1124–1131

10. Larun L, Nordheim LV, Ekeland E, Hagen KB, Heian F. Exercise in prevention and treatment of anxiety and depression among children and young people. *Cochrane Database Syst Rev*. 2006;19(3):CD004691

11. Stock S, Miranda C, Evans S, et al. Healthy Buddies: a novel, peer-led health promotion program for the prevention of obesity and eating disorders in children in elementary school. *Pediatrics*. 2007;120(4):e1059–e1068

12. Landry GL. Benefits of sports participation. In: Anderson SJ, Harris SS, eds. *Care of the Young Athlete*. 2nd ed. Elk Grove Village, IL: American Academy of Pediatrics; 2010:3–7

13. Centers for Disease Control and Prevention. Physical activity levels of high school students – United States, 2010. *MMWR Morb Mortal Wkly Rep*. 2011;60(23):773–777

14. National Association for Sport and Physical Education. *What Constitutes a Quality Physical Education Program?* Position statement. Reston, VA: National Association for Sport and Physical Education; 2003

15. National Association for Sport and Physical Education, American Heart Association. *2012 Shape of the Nation Report: Status of Physical Education in the USA*. Reston, VA: American Alliance for Health, Physical Education, Recreation and Dance; 2012. Available at: http://www.shapeamerica.org/advocacy/son/2012/upload/2012-Shape-of-Nation-full-report-web.pdf. Accessed April 13, 2015

16. American Academy of Pediatrics, Council on Sports Medicine and Fitness, Council on School Health. Active healthy living: prevention of childhood obesity through increased physical activity. *Pediatrics.* 2006;117(5):1834–1842

17. Lagarde F, LeBlanc CMA. Policy options to support physical activity in schools. *Can J Public Health.* 2010;101(Suppl 2):S9–S13

18. Harris SS. Readiness to participate in sports. In: Anderson SJ, Harris SS, eds. *Care of the Young Athlete.* 2nd ed. Elk Grove Village, IL: American Academy of Pediatrics; 2010:9–15

19. Long BJ. Promoting physical activity. In: Anderson SJ, Harris SS, eds. *Care of the Young Athlete.* 2nd ed. Elk Grove Village, IL: American Academy of Pediatrics; 2010:25-34

20. McCambridge TM, Stricker PR; American Academy of Pediatrics, Council on Sports Medicine and Fitness. Strength training by children and adolescents. *Pediatrics.* 2008;121(4):835–840. Reaffirmed June 2011

21. Rice SG; American Academy of Pediatrics, Council on Sports Medicine and Fitness. Medical conditions affecting sports participation. *Pediatrics.* 2008;121(4):841–848. Reaffirmed June 2014

22. Bernhardt DT, Roberts WO, eds. *PPE: Preparticipation Physical Examination.* 4th ed. Elk Grove Village, IL: American Academy of Pediatrics; 2010

23. Anderson SJ. Return-to-play decisions. In: Anderson SJ, Harris SS, eds. *Care of the Young Athlete.* 2nd ed. Elk Grove Village, IL: American Academy of Pediatrics; 2010:124–129

24. Anderson SJ. Principles of rehabilitation. In: Anderson SJ, Harris SS, eds. Care of the Young Athlete. 2nd ed. Elk Grove Village, IL: American Academy of Pediatrics; 2010:303-314

25. Pate RR, Saunders RP, O'Neill JR, Dowda M. Overcoming barriers to physical activity: helping youth be more active. *ACSM's Health & Fitness Journal.* 2011;15(1):7–12

26. Developing the individual education program. In: Auxter D, Pyfer J, Huettig C, eds. *Principles and Methods of Adapted Physical Education and Recreation.* McGraw-Hill Higher Education; 2010

27. American Academy of Pediatrics, Committee on Children With Disabilities. The pediatrician's role in development and implementation of an individual education plan (IEP) and/or an individual family service plan (IFSP). *Pediatrics.* 1999;104(1 Pt 1):124–127

28. Murray R, Ramstetter C; American Academy of Pediatrics, Council on School Health. The crucial role of recess in school. *Pediatrics.* 2013;131(1):183–188

29. Taylor RW, Farmer VL, Cameron SL, Meredith-Jones K, Williams SM, Mann JI. School playgrounds and physical activity policies as predictors of school and home time activity. *Int J Behav Nutr Phys Act.* 2011;8:38

30. Fuller D, Sabiston C, Karp I, Barnett T, O'Loughlin J. School sports opportunities influence physical activity in secondary school and beyond. *J Sch Health.* 2011;81(8):449–454

31. Johnston LD, Delva J, O'Malley PM. Sport participation and physical education in American secondary schools: current levels and racial/ethnic and socioeconomic disparities. *Am J Prev Med.* 2007;33(4 Suppl):S195–S208

32. Orenstein DM, Landry GL. Exercise, asthma and anaphylaxis. In: Anderson SJ, Harris SS, eds. *Care of the Young Athlete.* 2nd ed. Elk Grove Village, IL: American Academy of Pediatrics; 2010:221–226

33. LeBlanc CMA. Chronic conditions. In: Anderson SJ, Harris SS, eds. *Care of the Young Athlete.* 2nd ed. Elk Grove Village, IL: American Academy of Pediatrics; 2010:233-244

34. Arida RM, Scorza FA, Terra VC, Scorza CA, de Almeida AC, Cavalheiro EA. Physical exercise in epilepsy: what kind of stressor is it? *Epilepsy Behav.* 2009;16(3):381–387

35. Philpott J, Houghton K, Luke A. Physical activity recommendations for children with specific chronic health conditions: juvenile idiopathic arthritis, hemophilia, asthma and cystic fibrosis. *Paediatr Child Health.* 2010;15(4):213–218

36. Peterson AR, Bernhardt DT. The preparticipation sports evaluation. *Pediatr Rev.* 2011;32(5):e53–e65

37. American Academy of Pediatrics, Committee on Nutrition and the Council on Sports Medicine and Fitness. Sports drinks and energy drinks for children and adolescents: are they appropriate? *Pediatrics*. 2011:127(6):1182–1189

38. American Academy of Pediatrics, Committee on Nutrition. Sports nutrition. In: Kleinman RE, Greer FR, eds. *Pediatric Nutrition*. 7th ed. Elk Grove Village, IL: American Academy of Pediatrics; 2014:265–287

39. Holway FE, Spriet LL. Sport-specific nutrition: practical strategies for team sports. *J Sports Sci*. 2011;29(Suppl 1):S115–S125

40. Bergeron MF, Devore C, Rice SG; American Academy of Pediatrics, Council on Sports Medicine and Fitness, Council on School Health. Climatic heat stress and exercising children and adolescents. *Pediatrics*. 2011;128(3):e741–e747. Reaffirmed February 2015

41. Pritchett K, Pritchett R. Chocolate milk: a post-exercise recovery beverage for endurance sports. *Med Sport Sci*. 2012;59:127–134

42. Johnson MD. Female athletes. In: Anderson SJ, Harris SS, eds. *Care of the Young Athlete*. 2nd ed. Elk Grove Village, IL: American Academy of Pediatrics; 2010:137–144

43. Sundgot-Borgen J, Torstveit MK. Prevalence of eating disorders in elite athletes is higher than in the general population. *Clin J Sport Med*. 2004;14(1):25–32

44. Loder RT. The demographics of playground equipment injuries in children. *J Pediatr Surg*. 2008;43(4):691–699

45. Halstead ME, Walter KD; American Academy of Pediatrics, Council on Sports Medicine and Fitness. Sport-related concussion in children and adolescents. *Pediatrics*. 2010;126(3):597–615. Reaffirmed August 2014

46. Brenner J, Anderson SJ, Harris SS. General principles of injury prevention. In: Anderson SJ, Harris SS, eds. *Care of the Young Athlete*. 2nd ed. Elk Grove Village, IL: American Academy of Pediatrics; 2010:111–120

47. Herman K, Barton C. Malliaras P, Morrissey D. The effectiveness of neuromuscular warm-up strategies that require no additional equipment, for preventing lower limb injuries during sports participation: a systematic review. *BMC Med*. 2012;10:75

48. Rice SG, Congeni JA; American Academy of Pediatrics, Council on Sports Medicine and Fitness. Baseball and softball. *Pediatrics*. 2012;129(3):e842–e856

49. American Academy of Pediatrics Committee on Injury and Poison Prevention. Bicycle helmets. *Pediatrics*. 2001;108(4):1030–1032. Reaffirmed November 2011

50. Russell K, Christie J, Hagel BE. The effect of helmets on the risk of head and neck injuries among skiers and snowboarders: a meta-analysis. *CMAJ*. 2010;182(4):333–340

51. Purcell LK, Canadian Paediatric Society, Healthy Active Living and Sports Medicine Committee. *Paediatr Child Health*. 2012;17(1):31–34

52. McGuine TA, Hetzel S, Wilson J, Brooks A. The effect of lace-up ankle braces on injury rates in high school football players. *Am J Sports Med*. 2012;40(1):49–57

53. Rice SG. Risks of injury during sports participation. In: Anderson SJ, Harris SS, eds. *Care of the Young Athlete*. 2nd ed. Elk Grove Village, IL: American Academy of Pediatrics; 2010:101–108

54. Feinstein R. Thermoregulation. In: Anderson SJ, Harris SS, eds. *Care of the Young Athlete*. 2nd ed. Elk Grove Village, IL: American Academy of Pediatrics; 2010:65–70

55. Washington RL. Cardiac conditions. In: Anderson SJ, Harris SS, eds. *Care of the Young Athlete*. 2nd ed. Elk Grove Village, IL: American Academy of Pediatrics; 2010:179–184

56. Cave DM, Aufderheide TP, Beeson J, et al. Importance and implementation of training in cardiopulmonary resuscitation and automated external defibrillation in schools: a science advisory from the American Heart Association. *Circulation*. 2011;123(6):691–706

57. Gould D, Medbery R. Psychological issues. In: Anderson SJ, Harris SS, eds. *Care of the Young Athlete*. 2nd ed. Elk Grove Village, IL: American Academy of Pediatrics; 2010:91–97

58. Brenner JS; American Academy of Pediatrics, Council on Sports Medicine and Fitness. Overuse injuries, overtraining, and burnout in child and adolescent athletes. *Pediatrics.* 2007;119(6):1242–1245. Reaffirmed June 2014

59. Collingwood TR, Sunderlin J, Reynolds R, Kohl HW III. Physical training as a substance abuse prevention intervention for youth. *J Drug Educ.* 2000;30(4):435–451

60. MacKinnon DP, Goldberg L, Clarke GN, et al. Mediating mechanisms in a program to reduce intentions to use anabolic steroids and improve exercise self-efficacy and dietary behavior. *Prev Sci.* 2001;2(1):15–28

61. Graham TE. Caffeine, coffee, and ephedrine: impact on exercise performance and metabolism. *Can J Appl Physiol.* 2001;26:S103–S119

62. Griesemer BA. Performance-enhancing substances. In: Anderson SJ, Harris SS, eds. *Care of the Young Athlete.* 2nd ed. Elk Grove Village, IL: American Academy of Pediatrics; 2010:82–89

63. Metzl JD, Small E, Levine SR, Gershel JC. Creatine use among young athletes. *Pediatrics.* 2001;108(2):421–425

64. Lawrence ME, Kirby DF. Nutrition and sports supplements: fact or fiction. *J Clin Gastroenterol.* 2002;35(4):299–306

65. Maughan RJ, Greenhaff PL, Hespel P. Dietary supplements for athletes: emerging trends and recurring themes. *J Sports Sci.* 2011;29(S1):S57–S66

66. Labre MB. Adolescent boys and the muscular male body ideal. *J Adolesc Health.* 2002;30(4):233–242

67. Irving LM, Wall M, Newmark-Sztainer D, Story M. Steroid use among adolescents: findings from Project EAT. *J Adolesc Health.* 2002;30(4):243–252

68. Rogol AD. Sex steroid and growth hormone supplementation to enhance performance in adolescent athletes. *Curr Opin Pediatr.* 2000;12(4):382–387

69. Centers for Disease Control and Prevention. School health guidelines to promote healthy eating and physical activity—United States, 2011. *MMWR Morb Mortal Wkly Rep.* 2011;60(5):1–76

70. Meredith MD, Welk GJ, eds. *FitnessGram and ActivityGram Test Administration Manual.* 4th ed. Dallas TX: The Cooper Institute; 2014

71. Centers for Disease Control and Prevention. School Health Index. A Self-Assessment and Planning Guide. Middle School/High School Version. Atlanta, GA: Centers for Disease Control and Prevention, US Department of Health and Human Services; 2012. Available at: http://www.cdc.gov/Healthyyouth/SHI/pdf/Middle-HighTotal-2014-Tagged_508.pdf. Accessed April 13, 2015

72. Devore CD, Wheeler LS, American Academy of Pediatrics Council on School Health. Role of the school physician. *Pediatrics.* 2013;131(1):178–182

CHAPTER

6

Mental Health and Social Services

SECTION 1
Special Education

Nathaniel S. Beers, MD, MPA, FAAP
Manuel E. Jimenez, MD, MS, FAAP

Although many developmental and behavioral conditions are identified in the medical setting, therapies and treatments often take place in school or the community through early intervention or special education. The different institutional cultures, funding mechanisms, and regulations between the health care system and these community resources can result in severe fragmentation of care. Yet, children's access to appropriate accommodations and services plays a critical role in their health and well-being.

The American Academy of Pediatrics (AAP) encourages pediatricians to play an active role in the early intervention and special education processes as part of the family-centered medical home.[1] Armed with basic knowledge, pediatricians can support families through these processes and be powerful advocates for children throughout the life course. In particular, pediatricians can play an important role in identifying developmental concerns, linking families to services and helping families advocate for optimal services once they are in place. This chapter aims to provide pediatricians with basic background and tools to achieve these goals.

Legislative Background

Four key legislative achievements are of critical importance for children with developmental disabilities and/or special health care needs (Table 6.1.1). The Americans with Disabilities Act (ADA) and Section 504 of the Rehabilitation Act are civil rights laws that prevent discrimination on the basis of a disability. The ADA protects individuals with disabilities from discrimination in the workplace, government services, public accommodations, and telecommunications. Section 504 protects individuals with disabilities from exclusion by any entity receiving federal funds, including schools. The Individuals with Disabilities Education Improvement Act (IDEA), most recently reauthorized in 2004, guarantees a free and appropriate public education in the least restrictive environment for children with disabilities age 0 through 21 years. Children age 3 through 21 years receive special education services through Part B of IDEA. Infants and toddlers age 0 to 3 years and their families receive early intervention services through Part C of IDEA. The federal government provides a portion of these funds for states to implement IDEA programs. Variability in implementation exists because of the extent of state and local funding of Part B and C of IDEA. Finally, of note, the Elementary and Secondary Education Act was enacted by Congress to promote equity and accountability in education for all children. When reauthorized in 2002 as the No Child Left Behind Act, the legislation included provisions that apply accountability standards for the education of children with disabilities. This chapter will focus mostly on the implications of IDEA and Section 504.

Table 6.1.1. Key Legislative Achievements for Children with Disabilities

Legislation	Brief Summary
Section 504 of the Rehabilitation Act	Civil rights legislation that prevents discrimination on the basis of a disability
The Americans with Disabilities Act	Civil rights legislation that prevents discrimination on the basis of a disability
Individuals with Disabilities Education Act	Guarantees a free and appropriate education and provides funding to states to implement programs
No Child Left Behind	Sets accountability standards for children with disabilities

> The AAP also recommends pairing developmental surveillance with developmental screening at the 9-, 18-, and 24- to 30-month visits using a validated screening tool as well as autism specific screening at the 18- and 24-month visits.[9,10]

Birth to Three

Part C of IDEA provides financial assistance to states to deliver early intervention (EI) services to infants and toddlers with developmental delay. Currently, all states participate in Part C of IDEA. Individual states set eligibility standards. States may also provide services to infants and toddlers at risk of developmental delay, but not all states offer this option.

EI services are designed to be family centered and should occur in the natural environment, which means they typically occur in the family's home or another location designated by the family. Therapists (eg, speech, occupational, and/or physical) help families build capacity to promote optimal development during their daily routines. In some states, services are free to the family, although states are able to apply a sliding scale based on income. Programs like EI have been shown to improve developmental outcomes, reduce secondary behavioral problems, and help families effectively advocate for their children.[2-5] However, many potentially eligible children do not receive needed EI services.[6] In fact, fewer than half of children with developmental delays are identified before school age,[7] and even when children are identified with developmental concerns, many are not linked to services.[8]

IDEA requires that states have a mechanism to identify, locate, and evaluate all children with disabilities. This requirement is known as "Child Find," and its implementation varies by state. Pediatricians can play a key role in the identification of infants and toddlers with developmental delay and linking them to EI services. The AAP recommends developmental surveillance at all well-child visits from age 0 to 5 years.[9] Surveillance is defined as "a flexible, longitudinal, continuous, and cumulative process whereby knowledgeable health care professionals identify children who may have developmental problems."[10] According to this definition, developmental surveillance includes 5 key components: (1) eliciting and attending to parents' concerns, (2) maintaining a developmental history, (3) making accurate and informed observations about the child, (4) identifying the presence of risk and protective factors, and

(5) complete documentation. The AAP also recommends pairing developmental surveillance with developmental screening at the 9-, 18-, and 24- to 30-month visits using a validated screening tool as well as autism-specific screening at the 18- and 24-month visits.[9,10]

If a pediatrician elicits a developmental concern through surveillance or screening, he or she should refer the child to the local EI provider for evaluation for services. Although the exact process varies by locality, pediatricians can alert families to expect an intake process followed by a multidisciplinary evaluation. The EI service provider assigns each family to a service coordinator who helps to facilitate the EI process. If the child is found eligible for services, families and EI staff develop an individualized family services plan (IFSP). The IFSP documents the goals set by families and EI staff regarding the identified developmental concerns as well as services to address these goals. Families and EI staff review the IFSP on a regular basis, and it remains in effect until the family chooses to discontinue services, the goals are met, or when the child transitions to preschool special education services that can range by state from age 3 to 5 years. For children transitioning to preschool services, the transition process should begin at least 6 months in advance with input from the parents, school staff, and ideally EI staff to ensure a seamless transition. In some states, EI continues beyond 3 years of age and may continue up until a child is of mandatory school age or 5 years old. Pediatricians can act as an important safety net to ensure the transition process is taking place if necessary. They can also make helpful suggestions such as encouraging parents to visit preschools in advance or meet staff or linking parents to other experienced parents or support groups.

Three to Five

As previously noted, developmental surveillance continues to be an integral part of well-child visits through age 5 years.[9] As suggested in *Bright Futures,* pediatricians can elicit developmental concerns from families by starting with a question such as "Do you have any specific concerns regarding your child's development, learning, or behavior?" The pediatrician can then transition into more focused questions regarding social emotional, cognitive, communicative, and physical development.[9] Concerns can be managed through additional medical workup and/or referral to subspecialists as necessary (eg, developmental pediatrician). Referral and evaluation for special education services should take place concurrently. Pediatricians can link families to the local Child Find office, which may be the neighborhood school or a centralized office in the region, to arrange for an evaluation for preschool special education services. The referral process varies by locality. A directory of state-specific information can be located by exploring the resources at the end of this chapter.

For children found eligible for preschool special education, service plans transition from an IFSP to an individualized education program (IEP). Families will likely notice the shift from the family-centered approach to EI for 0- to 3-year-olds to a more child-centered approach in preschool. The other major change is that starting at 3 years old, to be eligible for special education, there must be an effect of the disability on education. This means there may be some children eligible under EI who are no longer eligible for special education. This is particularly true for children with isolated motor delays. Pediatricians can support parents as the setting of services and their role as advocate for their child evolves. An in-depth discussion of IEPs is presented below.

Five to Sixteen

Pediatricians continue to play an important role promoting optimal child development and school success in middle childhood and adolescence. Through developmental surveillance at each well visit, pediatricians continue to be well positioned to identify children with developmental problems and those at risk of school difficulty or school failure. There are validated screeners for behavioral and mental health concerns that can help a pediatrician identify children and adolescents who may need additional support or evaluations. Pediatricians can also be a knowledgeable resource for families regarding their legal rights. Finally, pediatricians can play an active role ensuring services meet the child and families' needs and advocating for the rights of families. Working knowledge of the IEP process and Section 504 plans are prerequisites to achieve these goals. Equally important is the ability to link families to educational advocates and legal resources when necessary.

Individualized Education Program

IDEA requires that children who receive special education have an IEP. Although the IEP is a complex legal document that can seem overwhelming at first glance, the IEP process is structured and governed by law. As a result, pediatricians can help families detect departures from the process and ensure their concerns and goals are being addressed.

Under IDEA, parents have a legal right to request an evaluation for special education services by their school district. As previously noted, pediatricians play a key role in the identification of children with special education needs through developmental screening. Parents can initiate an evaluation for special education services simply by raising their concerns with their teacher or guidance counselor or, if necessary, contacting their school district. Teachers can also refer children for evaluation for special education, but parents must consent to the evaluation. Schools cannot require parents to have a doctor make a referral for services or evaluation. However, some jurisdictions do ask for a physician's order to be able to bill Medicaid for these services.

Every child with a suspected disability has a right to a comprehensive evaluation through IDEA. For the purposes of IDEA, a child with a disability is a child evaluated and found to be in 1 of 13 diagnostic categories (Table 6.2.2) that require special education and related services. Related services are defined in IDEA as:

> " transportation and such developmental, corrective, and other supportive services as are required to assist a child with a disability to benefit from special education, and includes speech-language pathology and audiology services, interpreting services, psychological services, physical and occupational therapy, recreation, including therapeutic recreation, early identification and assessment of disabilities in children, counseling services, including rehabilitation counseling, orientation and mobility services, and medical services for diagnostic or evaluation purposes. Related services also include school health services and school nurse services, social work services in schools, and parent counseling and training."

IDEA lists a 60-day timeframe for an evaluation to take place after parent consent. However, states may vary from this timeline with approval from the US Department of Education. The evaluation begins with a review of existing information about the child. The school district can decide that the existing

Table 6.2.2. Disability Categories in IDEA

- Autism
- Deaf-blindness
- Deafness
- Emotional disturbance
- Hearing impairment
- Intellectual disability
- Multiple disabilities
- Orthopedic impairment
- Other health impaired
- Specific learning disability
- Speech or language impairment
- Traumatic brain injury
- Visual impairment including blindness

information is sufficient to make a decision on placement. Some school districts are using response to interventions as an outcome to determine whether students need to progress to assessments or if they simply need some minor intervention. If the school district decides that further assessment is not necessary, families still have a right to request that an assessment take place. Assessments involve several disciplines and may include psychologists, therapists, and educators, depending on the specific concern. IDEA further specifies that assessments must include a variety of methods and instruments used must be evidence based. After the evaluation has taken place, parents participate in the group that determines eligibility. If a child is found eligible, an IEP should be written within 30 days.

Pediatricians can play an important role in the writing and implementation of an IEP. Although attending an IEP meeting may not be feasible given the time demands of a pediatrician, pediatricians can still contribute to the IEP process. IDEA states that the IEP team should consist of the parents, a regular education teacher, a special education teacher, a school district representative, an individual who can interpret the evaluation results, others with special expertise about the child, and when appropriate, the child. Importantly, pediatricians can counsel parents that they may invite someone with special expertise regarding the child to the IEP meeting. This may include an educational advocate, therapist, other specialist, or even the pediatrician. If the pediatrician cannot attend the meeting in person, he or she can still work with the parents by providing reports or written recommendations for consideration by the IEP team.

The IEP is a highly structured document that outlines the school experience for the child. Although there may be some variation in the structure and content of IEPs between states, key information, such as information about the child's evaluations, annual goals, services, accommodations, ongoing assessments, and related services, should be included. Information regarding the setting and exposure to typically developing children must also be included. IDEA clearly indicates that children with disabilities should not be removed from the regular classroom unless the severity of the disability prevents the child's educational needs from being met in a regular classroom with the maximum supports and services. This defines the "least restrictive environment." Even if children are not in the regular classroom for academics, they should still be given an opportunity to interact with typically developing children throughout the day to the maximum extent possible (eg, recess, gym, art, music). Once written, the IEP should be reviewed at least once a year, but parents have the right to request a review at any time. As discussed below, the IEP cannot be implemented without the consent of the parent. In addition to the annual review of the IEP, an eligibility determination must take place every 3 years, including a review of progress and any new assessments.

Safeguards

IDEA outlines several procedural safeguards for parents. Although a full discussion of all safeguards is beyond the scope of this chapter, a brief summary of key rights is included. Parents and pediatricians are encouraged to use the resources at the end of this chapter and/or to work with educational advocates to gain more detail. Perhaps, most salient, pediatricians can reinforce that parents must provide informed written consent before implementation of the IEP and that they have a right to refuse or revoke their consent at any time.

Under IDEA, parents must have the opportunity to participate in the IEP meeting and to review all educational records with respect to identification, evaluation, and educational placement and the provision of a free and appropriate public education. They also have the right to participate in the group that makes placement decisions. Parents have the right to obtain an independent educational evaluation, potentially at the public's expense. In the event of a disagreement between the parent and the school district, IDEA carefully outlines a process that includes mediation, a due process complaint, resolution process, and due process hearing. Mediation provides an opportunity for the parent and school district to avoid a due process complaint through the use of an impartial mediator. The mediation process must be voluntary and should not be used to deny parents their right to a due process complaint. Parents can file a due process complaint alleging violations of their child's rights. After filing a due process complaint, there is an opportunity for a resolution meeting in which representatives from the school district and the parent and his or her representative attempt to resolve the issue. If the issue is not resolved within 30 days, the due process hearing occurs. Parents must receive a procedural safeguard notice at least on an annual basis.

Section 504 Plan

Consistent with the fact that every child with a disability is unique, some children with a disability do not need special education services. These children's rights to a free and appropriate education are still protected under Section 504 of the Rehabilitation Act. Section 504 protects children with disabilities from exclusion in schools accepting federal funds. As a result, accommodations for children with disabilities must be made so that they can participate in school activities just as their typically developing peers or to the extent that meets their own unique needs. Accommodations for these students are outlined in a Section 504 plan. Accommodations can range from preferred seating and sensory breaks for children with ADHD to wheelchair-accessible ramps for children with physical disabilities. Pediatricians have an important role in helping families understand their right to request Section 504 accommodations. In addition, pediatricians can help schools translate the student's medical needs into actual accommodations for school, as many school districts lack a medical professional to help explain the implications of medical conditions on the school. The Section 504 plan should be reviewed regularly; in most jurisdictions, this means at least annually. For children needing special education, any necessary accommodations should be included in their IEP. Pediatricians can monitor their patients' progress to ensure that their needs are being adequately met. An easy distinction between the student who would require an IEP versus the student who would need a Section 504 plan is that a student in need of modification of instruction (specialized instruction) or direct related services needs an IEP, whereas a student needing accommodations to access instruction or only consultative related services should receive a Section 504 plan. Under Section 504, parents are afforded the right to disagree with the school, although they do not have the same procedural protections under IDEA.

> Pediatricians can play an important role by ensuring that transition planning is in place and that the adolescent is being included in the process.

Sixteen to Twenty-Two

Transition from childhood to adulthood is a particularly vulnerable time for children with disabilities and their parents/caregivers. Pediatricians can help families through this challenging period not only by assisting in their health care transition to adult providers, but also their transition from special education into the community as an adult. During this transition, young adults leave a highly structured, centralized service system and enter into a system of services that can seem nebulous and fragmented. Successful transition requires careful planning, with a goal of achieving the level of independence appropriate for the young adult. According to IDEA, transition planning should begin no later than age 16 and should be included in the student's IEP. Under transition services, IDEA specifies that the IEP should include (1) information regarding the student's postsecondary education goals (this may include career and technical training and school-to-work programs), and (2) the necessary services to help the student achieve those goals. Pediatricians can play an important role by ensuring that transition planning is in place and that the adolescent is being included in the process. Further, pediatricians can link parents to support groups and other experienced parents who are familiar with the transition process.

Although postsecondary schools do not fall under the jurisdiction of IDEA, provisions from Section 504 and the ADA still apply. However, once the student passes grade 12, the onus falls on him or her to ensure accommodations are in place. Ideally, students and their families should investigate accommodations for students with disabilities before selecting a college or other postsecondary school or employment opportunity. At the very least, students transitioning to college should contact the designated support office for individuals with disabilities early in the semester, if not earlier, to arrange for accommodations or services.

Special Circumstances

Private Schools

The level of protection offered by IDEA and the special education process differs for children in private schools.[11] IDEA distinguishes between children who are placed in a private school by their parents versus children placed in a private school by the school district. For children placed in private school by the school district, there is no difference from children who are enrolled in the school district's public schools. However, children enrolled by their parent in a private school do not benefit from the same level of protection as children who are enrolled by their parents in public schools. Child Find requirements, as described earlier, still apply to children in private schools. In these circumstances, pediatricians can play an important role by identifying children with special education needs through developmental surveillance. Pediatricians can also inform parents about the child's right to an evaluation by the school district where the private school is located, if a disability is suspected. If a child is identified as having a disability, a service plan must be developed and implemented. Service plans are developed with representatives from the school district, the private school, and the parents. The service plan is not required to be as comprehensive as an IEP and is only required to provide equitable services. Services can also be limited by the funding available to cover such services.

If the private school receives federal funds, it is obligated to provide accommodations under Section 504. However, it has no obligations through IDEA and can remove a child administrators believe the school is unable to serve. It is important to note that although parents can file a due process complaint with regards to Child Find activities (evaluation and eligibility), parents cannot file a due process complaint with regards to the provision of services.

Recommendations for Pediatricians

Pediatricians do not need to be special education lawyers. However, pediatricians can help facilitate the EI and/or special education process for families. Although schools and EI programs cannot require that the referral be made by the pediatrician, additional weight may be given to the referral made by a pediatrician. A note on a prescription expressing concern about a child's development can reinforce the request of a parent for assessment or program modification. Pediatricians do play an important role in advising parents and schools when children have health issues affecting their development or learning, such as behavioral health disorders or congenital disorders. Schools may lack health experts to advise on how to care for a student or what the effect may be on learning. Pediatricians also may recommend additional services above and beyond what is offered by the school. This is particularly important for children with motor delays that may not be eligible for services or receive direct services from the school. Most important, parents are looking for pediatricians to be a sounding board and for assistance in connecting with other support services, such as parent groups, additional services not covered by schools, or educational advocates. Pediatricians can also play an important role in helping schools understand medical diagnoses that may affect development, including the potential life course of a disease or syndrome and the medical differential for some school difficulty or behavior.

Recommendations for Program Directors and Trainees

Regardless of the long-term professional plans of a trainee, all pediatricians will interface with the special education system in some way. With this in mind, ensuring adequate exposure to special education is important, including exposure to schools and professionals working in special education and EI. Part of this exposure may come during a developmental behavioral pediatrics rotation or during continuity clinic experience. There is a value in being able to be part of an IEP meeting to understand how parents may feel during the process and the overwhelming amount of information that is shared during IEP meetings. Many educational advocacy organizations have parent trainings on a regular basis on the IEP process and parent's rights during that process. These can provide a useful background and help connect trainees with educational advocates to assist their families during training. Special education should also be an integral part of the training experiences of developmental and behavioral pediatric fellows as well as psychology students' internships and field experiences. The coordinated multidisciplinary effort that goes into the design and implementation of an IEP or Section 504 plan reinforces the trainees' systems-based practice competency.

Take-Home Points

- Early intervention provides services for children ages 0 to 3 years and up to 5 years in some states.
  - States set the eligibility criteria.
  - Services are provided in the natural environment, often at home or in child care.
  - Transition to special education services in the school should start at least 6 months before the third birthday.
- Special education provides services for children and adolescents ages 3 to 22 years.
- To be eligible, the child must have a disability that has an effect on his or her education.
- Initial referrals can be made by anyone, although the parent must consent to the evaluation.
- From initial referral, schools have 60 days to complete an eligibility determination, unless the state has an exemption to extend that timeline. In states that are using response to intervention as an outcome, the timeline may be extended to allow time to determine whether the intervention may be effective.
- An IEP must be developed within 30 days of determining a child is eligible for special education and must be reviewed at least once a year.
- Planning for the transition to adult services should begin by the time the adolescent is 16 years old and should involve the adolescent.

Resources

For additional school health related resources, visit www.aap.org/schoolhealthmanual.

References

1. American Academy of Pediatrics, Committee on Children With Disabilities. The pediatrician's role in development and implementation of an Individual Education Plan (IEP) and/or an Individual Family Service Plan (IFSP). *Pediatrics.* 1999;104(1 Pt 1):124–127

2. Shonkoff JP, Hauser-Cram P. Early intervention for disabled infants and their families: a quantitative analysis. *Pediatrics.* 1987;80(5):650–658

3. National Research Council, Committee on Integrating the Science of Early Childhood Development. Shonkoff JP, Phillips D, eds. *From Neurons to Neighborhoods: The Science of Early Child Development.* Washington, DC: National Academies Press; 2000

4. Nordhov SM, Ronning JA, Ulvund SE, Dahl LB, Kaaresen PI. Early intervention improves behavioral outcomes for preterm infants: randomized controlled trial. *Pediatrics.* 2012;129(1):e9–e16

5. Bailey DB Jr, Hebbeler K, Spiker D, Scarborough A, Mallik S, Nelson L. Thirty-six-month outcomes for families of children who have disabilities and participated in early intervention. *Pediatrics.* 2005;116(6):1346–1352

6. Rosenberg SA, Zhang D, Robinson CC. Prevalence of developmental delays and participation in early intervention services for young children. *Pediatrics.* 2008;121(6):e1503–1509

7. Developmental monitoring and screening. Centers for Disease Control and Prevention Web site. Available at: http://www.cdc.gov/ncbddd/childdevelopment/screening.html. Accessed April 13, 2015

8. King TM, Tandon SD, Macias MM, et al. Implementing developmental screening and referrals: lessons learned from a national project. *Pediatrics.* 2010;125(2):350–360

9. Hagan JF, Shaw JS, Duncan PM, eds. *Bright Futures: Guidelines for Health Supervision of Infants, Children, and Adolescents.* 3rd ed. Elk Grove Village, IL: American Academy of Pediatrics; 2008

10. Identifying infants and young children with developmental disorders in the medical home: an algorithm for developmental surveillance and screening. *Pediatrics.* 2006;118(1):405–420

11. National Dissemination Center for Children with Disabilities. *Building the Legacy for Our Youngest Children with Disabilities: A Training Curriculum on IDEA 2004's Part C.* Available at: http://www.parentcenterhub.org/repository/legacy-partc/. Accessed April 13, 2015

SECTION 2

Mental Health

Olga Acosta Price, PhD
Kenneth Tellerman, MD, FAAP

Background

Mental, emotional, and behavioral health concerns in children and adolescents are widespread. These problems can interfere with healthy development and learning and pose a significant challenge to school personnel, mental health professionals, and pediatric primary care clinicians (pediatricians) who care for youth. It is estimated that 14% to 20% of children and teenagers experience the signs and symptoms of a serious emotional disturbance, with a median estimate of approximately 12%.[1] Yet, only a small proportion of children experiencing mental health conditions receive adequate treatment.[2,3] The gap in services is even greater for ethnic minority and low-income families,[4] a factor that contributes to the mental health disparities present among these already disadvantaged groups.[2] Half of adults in the United States with a diagnosed mental health disorder report having had symptoms by age 14, and 75% report having had symptoms by age 24, indicating that early intervention and prevention programs coordinated among various caregivers and providers offer an opportunity to reduce the burden of these conditions.[1,5]

Not only do children and adolescents with mental health problems experience emotional, behavioral, or social consequences related to their disorders, but they often also experience lower educational achievement, have higher truancy levels, and are more likely to be suspended or expelled than children with other disabilities, such as learning, developmental, or physical disabilities.

> Although not as widely understood as other risky behaviors, there is growing concern that self-injurious behavior is becoming increasingly prevalent among adolescents and young adults without associated developmental disabilities.

Research confirms that when youth are removed from the classroom, there is a significant probability that they will repeat a grade, drop out, or become involved in the juvenile justice system.[6]

US prevalence rates by disorder reveal that a significant number of youth experience mental health problems that warrant clinical intervention:

- 8% of youth meet criteria for attention-deficit/hyperactivity disorder (ADHD), with boys (11%) being about twice as likely as girls (6%) to have a diagnosis of ADHD.[7]
- 32% of adolescents have some type of anxiety disorders, with girls having higher rates than boys across all subtypes of anxiety.[8]
- 3.8% of female adolescents and 1.5% of male adolescents have an eating disorder.[8]
- 10% of 12- to 17-year-olds are illicit drug users, 13% report current alcohol use, and 7% are current marijuana users.[9]
- Of youth with at least 1 diagnosed disorder, more than 40% meet criteria for an additional disorder.[8]
- 14% of adolescents meet criteria for depression, with twice as many girls as boys experiencing depression.[8]
- Girls are at higher risk of developing depression as they get older. National figures show that major depression triples for girls between the ages of 12 and 15 (from 5.1% to 15.2%).[9]
- 16% of students in grades 9 through 12 have seriously considered suicide and 7% have made an attempt in the previous 12 months.[10] Untreated depression is the leading cause of suicide among teenagers.
- National statistics indicate that across all races and both sexes, suicide is the third leading cause of death among 10- to 19-year-olds.[11] The majority of adolescents with suicidal ideation or who have a plan or made an attempt had no contact with a mental health specialist in the past year.[12]
- Studies estimate a lifetime prevalence of nonsuicidal self-injury (NSSI) to range from 13% to 23% among adolescents.[13]

With easy-to-use measures, evidence-based screening tools, clear practice guidelines, and referral networks in place, pediatricians can be effective partners in the implementation of strategies to address unmet mental health problems among at-risk youth.

Although not as widely understood as other risky behaviors, there is growing concern that self-injurious behavior is becoming increasingly prevalent among adolescents and young adults without associated developmental disabilities. Self-harm, or NSSI, can be described as deliberate and voluntary physical self-injury, which often involves cutting of oneself with a knife or razor, that is not life-threatening and is without any conscious intent to die.[13]

Community-based providers strive to build a system of care that addresses the multiplicity of needs among the youth population, but the current prevalence rates of emotional and behavioral problems suggests that strengthening the collaboration and integration of services, resources, and expertise is necessary if we hope to see improvements in health and education outcomes. Research indicates that primary care providers need to take greater advantage of opportunities for initiating conversations and screening for adolescent emotional distress.[14] Relying on parental disclosure of emerging mental health problems may also yield limited results, despite the fact that most parents report that their children have regular contact with a doctor or other health professional. Data show that only 41% of parents who have psychosocial concerns about their children discuss them at a pediatric visit, and only 61% of mental health referrals made by pediatricians are completed.[15] Youth who are from poor households are particularly vulnerable to "suffer in silence" because they are less likely to make contact with a primary care provider than youth from families with income above the poverty threshold, with insurance coverage accounting for much of the difference in rates of treatment use.[9] For example, 20% of adolescents in families below the poverty level have no health insurance,[16] and insured children are 4 to 6 times more likely to have visited a physician than a child who is uninsured.[7] Yet, armed with easy-to-use measures, evidence-based screening tools, clear practice guidelines, and referral networks in place, pediatricians can be effective partners in the implementation of strategies to address unmet mental health problems among at-risk youth. Strengthening collaboration between primary care and education systems has emerged as one of the most promising avenues for preventing risk and promoting health among children and adolescents.

School Mental Health: Definitions and Models

Almost 50 million school-aged children attend public schools in the United States.[17] Children and teenagers spend a large portion of their lives attending school, and in many communities, particularly where there is a shortage of community-based clinical providers, schools have become the largest provider of mental health services to children and adolescents.[18]

A number of school-connected approaches for addressing mental health concerns among students have emerged over the last 30 years, but a clear definition of or expert consensus about a conceptual model for school mental health does not yet exist.[19] The more traditional avenue for providing mental health services and supports occurs through school-hired pupil service professionals, generally school psychologists, school social workers, and school counselors. Depending on student demand, competing priorities, and staff responsibilities, school-hired mental health professionals may work with the population of students in general education or they may be dedicated exclusively to providing mandated services (ie, assessment or counseling services) to students who have been identified as having special needs and who are receiving special education services.

To enhance their capacity to serve students in need, a growing number of schools have executed formal agreements with public or private mental health providers to offer comprehensive mental health services and programs in schools that complement the interventions offered by school-hired mental health professionals.[20] The array of interventions available includes screening, behavioral observations, consultation, assessment, counseling, and crisis response services, and these arrangements often extend access to mental health care without the need for a medical diagnosis. In addition, a variety of prevention and promotion activities are implemented to enhance skills and competencies among children and strengthen the health of the school population. Some schools and school districts have forged collaborative relationships with community health and mental health providers to operate school-based health centers offering a variety of pediatric health services on-site to students enrolled in those schools. School-based health centers blend medical care with preventive and psychosocial services and organize broader school-based and community-based health promotion efforts on site in partner schools. Typically staffed with nurse practitioners and health aides, they increasingly include mental health professionals (see Center for Health and Health Care in Schools [**www.healthinschools.org**] or the School-Based Health Alliance [**http://www.sbh4all.org**] and refer to the American Academy of Pediatrics (AAP) policy statement "School-Based Health Centers and Pediatric Practice" **http://pediatrics.aappublications.org/content/129/2/387.full**).

Some types of school-hired mental health professionals are as follows:

- School psychologists are trained in both psychology and education at the graduate level and complete training in mental health and educational interventions, child development, learning, behavior, motivation, curriculum and instruction, assessment, consultation, collaboration, school law, and systems. School psychologists must be certified and/or licensed by the state in which they work and may be nationally certified by the National School Psychology Certification Board (**http://www.nasponline.org/about_sp/whatis.aspx**).

- School counselors are certified/licensed educators with a minimum of a master's degree in school counseling and are required to meet their state certification/licensure standards. School counselors address students' academic, personal/social, and career development needs by designing, implementing, evaluating, and enhancing a comprehensive school counseling program that promotes and enhances student success (**http://www.schoolcounselor.org**).

- School social work is a specialized area of practice within the broad field of the social work profession. School social workers are trained in mental health concerns; behavioral concerns; positive behavioral support; academic and classroom support; consultation with teachers, parents, and administrators; and with individual and group counseling techniques. The majority of school social workers hold a master's degree in social work, which is the prescribed entry level in most states. Some states, however, do allow entry level at the bachelor's level. Certification requirements are developed by each state and vary accordingly (**www.sswaa.org/?page=1**).

Approximately half of all US adolescents with serious mental health problems have never had contact with a mental health provider. Experts agree that systematic voluntary mental health screening can be effective, especially if the screening facilitates a referral for follow-up service options within the school or with mental health providers outside of the school.[24]

Continuum of Care and Support

The number of school-wide programs with evidence of positive effect on child and adolescent health and learning has grown tremendously. School personnel and community providers who partner with them are in a unique position to provide a wide range of effective mental health interventions and programs in and around schools.

Universal Interventions

Universal interventions in schools are designed to benefit *all* students, regardless of a student's individual risk level, and can be delivered in a variety of settings, including in classrooms, at recess or in lunchrooms, or school-wide. Types of universal interventions include:

- **Classroom-based curricula:** A variety of programs have been designed to reduce the prevalence of risky behaviors by focusing on raising awareness, improving knowledge, or changing behavior associated with negative outcomes, such as substance abuse, aggression/violence, or unsafe sexual behavior. School-based violence prevention programs, a common universal intervention across K-12 schools, have been shown to affect individual student behavior and performance but also improve the general school environment.[21] (Visit the following sites for information on evidence-based universal prevention programs: **http://www.nrepp.samhsa.gov**, **http://www.hhs.gov/ash/oah/oah-initiatives/tpp_program**, **http://www.colorado.edu/cspv/blueprints**, and **http://casel.org/guide/**.)

- **Screening:** A valuable universal activity conducted in school settings involves screening youth for emotional or behavioral problems so that appropriate interventions can be initiated as early as possible. Age-appropriate validated screening instruments can be used within the context of a health care visit to accurately identify youth at risk of developing full-blown disorders.[2] A number of reliable screening tools are available for health professionals to use with youth and/or with their families.[22,23] Best practices dictate that mental health screening is conducted when systems are in place to ensure appropriate follow-up care.

Approximately half of all US adolescents with serious mental health problems have never had contact with a mental health provider. Experts agree that systematic voluntary mental health screening can be effective, especially if the screening facilitates a referral for follow-up service options within the school or with mental health providers outside of the school.[24]

- **School climate interventions:** More and more schools are successfully implementing programs to foster a positive *school climate*. School climate refers to the social and environmental atmosphere present in a school and reflects the values, interpersonal relationships, and teaching and learning practices of that environment. A positive climate is achieved when parents, students, and school personnel view the school as a safe, welcoming, caring, and respectful place and where policies, practices, and organizational structures are all in alignment with these stated values. Research has illuminated the link between improved school climate and positive student outcomes, such as better school attendance, reduced drug use, and enhanced emotional health,[25] and improvements in teacher retention, stress, and job satisfaction levels.[26]

- **Positive Behavioral Interventions and Supports (PBIS):** PBIS is a framework to guide the implementation of a coordinated set of evidence-based interventions within a multitiered system to support the academic and behavioral success of all students in a school. (Visit **http://www.pbis.org** for more information.) Although PBIS was originally developed to address the concerns of children with behavioral disorders, it is currently being implemented as a school-wide approach to promote better classroom management, safe school climates, and individual student success. Schools that utilize a PBIS approach have reported significant decreases in student behavioral and concentration problems and improvements in social-emotional functioning and prosocial behavior.[27]

- **Social and emotional learning (SEL):** SEL is a process that promotes the development of life skills such as recognizing and managing emotions, developing caring and concern for others, establishing positive relationships, making responsible decisions, and handling challenging situations constructively and ethically. Effective SEL programs help students develop social and emotional competencies such as self-awareness, social awareness, responsible decision making, and self-management and relationship skills but are also associated with significant improvements in school performance.[28] (Visit **www.casel.org** for more information.)

Targeted or Selective Interventions

Selective interventions focus on early identification and intervention for students who exhibit any number of personal or environmental risk factors (such as academic underachievement, disruptive behaviors, high mobility, family discord, exposure to community violence, etc.) that make them more vulnerable to developing a disorder. The aim of selective interventions is to delay or help prevent the onset of a behavioral or emotional disorder by focusing on skill building in an individual or addressing an environmental risk factor. Types of targeted interventions include:

- **School-wide interventions:** A number of evidence-based programs are used in schools to reduce the incidence or prevent the occurrence of a variety of problems, including bullying, violence, and suicide. In addition to being a school-based universal intervention program, the Olweus Bullying Prevention Program includes components in their curriculum targeted for students who are identified as bullies or victims of bullying. (Visit **http://www.violencepreventionworks.org/public/index.page**.)

- **Multi-faceted programs:** Some school administrators and staff implement comprehensive programs for individual students assessed to be at higher risk than their peers. For example, the Incredible Years Series promotes social competence and is a curriculum for parents, teachers, and elementary school-aged children who are displaying behavior problems and deemed at risk of developing conduct disorders. (Visit **http://www.incredibleyears.com**.)

- **Pediatricians and targeted interventions:** The pediatrician plays an important role in the early identification and interventions for physical health conditions that may contribute to the worsening of emotional or behavioral functioning. In addition, the pediatrician plays an important role in the early identification of mental health disorders, substance abuse disorders, and emotional issues related to family chaos and dysfunction. Medical conditions such as *sleep deprivation, poor nutrition,* and *obesity* have been shown to be associated with increases in mental health problems:
  - Screening for snoring and sleep problems and underlying obstructive sleep apnea and appropriate interventions can be an effective early intervention.[29] Adequate sleep is essential for memory consolidation and learning enhancement. Sleep deprivation can adversely affect grades, decision-making skills, executive functioning, and behavioral inhibition and can lead to increases in depressed mood as well as academic and mental health problems.[30] Habitual snoring can also contribute to problematic outcomes, because it is significantly associated with hyperactive and inattentive behaviors and peer problems.[31]

- Inquiring about nutrition and balanced eating habits offer another window of opportunity to reduce the severity of mental health symptoms. A high quality breakfast has been shown to improve mental health in adolescents.[32] Iron supplementation may have a role in managing some patients with ADHD and optimizing stimulant therapy, while PUFA (poly-unsaturated fatty acids) dietary supplements have resulted in improvements in some patients with ADHD.[33]

- In addition to the physical health benefits, identification and early intervention for obesity may have some protective mental health effects. Studies show that children with higher body mass index (BMI) at 4 to 5 years of age have more peer problems and more teacher reported emotional problems at 8 to 9 years of age.[34] Teasing about body weight is associated with low self-esteem, depressive symptoms, and suicidal ideation.[35] Additional studies have also linked being overweight to emotional and behavior problems.[36]

Tertiary or Indicated Interventions

Indicated interventions target specific students who are experiencing mental health symptoms and are implemented to treat a condition or reduce the severity of symptoms. Mental health care provided in schools can involve numerous components:

- **Assessment:** Some school mental health professionals and primary care clinicians can effectively evaluate and diagnose mental illness among students who have been identified with behavioral or mental health symptoms. Screening and diagnostic tools are available that include observational, self-report, and/or collateral report data.

- **Treatment:** Counseling provided in schools may involve individual, family, and group therapy sessions with a focus on symptom reduction or the enhancement of functioning. Curricula or manualized interventions informed by evidence-based research are available and should be conducted by trained personnel in schools. Many of these interventions are derived from behavioral, cognitive-behavioral, solution-focused, or interpersonal therapies as they lend themselves more readily to implementation in school settings. One example of a school-based mental health curriculum is CBITS (Cognitive Behavioral Intervention for Trauma in Schools), a group and individual intervention designed to reduce the symptoms of post-traumatic stress disorder (PTSD) and depression among middle and high school students. (Visit **http://cbitsprogram.org** for more information.)

▪ **Medication management in schools:** For some youth with mental health conditions that have a biological underpinning, pharmacologic interventions are often necessary and effective. Pediatricians who prescribe medication can maintain contact with the school staff to monitor for physical adverse effects, track indicated laboratory data, and ultimately establish efficacy of treatment.

▪ **Case management:** Coordination of care can be provided for students with more complex problems. Case management may entail referral to school-based providers, to community mental health organizations, or to other social services for students who require additional wrap-around or social supports.

Diagnostic and Statistical Manual of Mental Disorders (DSM) is the standard classification of mental disorders used by mental health professionals in the United States and contains a listing of diagnostic criteria for every psychiatric disorder recognized by the US health care system. The fifth edition (DSM-5) is used by numerous professionals in a wide variety of settings, including psychiatrists and other physicians, psychologists, social workers, nurses, occupational and rehabilitation therapists, and counselors (**http://www.dsm5.org/Pages/Default.aspx**). Another relevant resource for pediatricians is the *Diagnostic and Statistical Manual of Mental Disorders: Primary Care Version* (DSM-IV-PC).

Crisis Intervention

Crisis intervention is intended to stabilize individual students with severe problems such as acute depression or suicidal ideation, active eating disorders, or violent behavior. Such students may require referral to mental health professionals outside of the school or brief hospitalization on a psychiatric inpatient unit. Mobile crisis teams are often deployed by school districts or local mental

National studies have shown that many adolescents, especially males, who experience suicidal ideation do not receive specialized mental health services. When care is offered, it is more likely to be delivered by a mental health specialist in health care or school settings than by general medical providers.[12]

health agencies to assist with these crisis situations. School-wide crisis intervention programs have been successfully implemented when schools have experienced both natural and manmade emergencies such as hurricanes, tornadoes, gang violence, and school shootings. School-wide crisis intervention teams, often composed of school staff and community providers, typically incorporate a 4-stage approach including mitigation and prevention, preparedness, response, and recovery. (Refer to AAP policy statement "Disaster Planning for Schools" **http://pediatrics.aappublications.org/content/122/4/895.full**).

Advantages and Limitations of School Mental Health Programs

National studies have shown that many adolescents, especially males, who experience suicidal ideation do not receive specialized mental health services. When care is offered, it is more likely to be delivered by a mental health specialist in health care or school settings than by general medical providers.[12]

School mental health programs address a wide array of mental health concerns including a variety of behavioral problems, problems related to trauma and violence exposure, poor academic performance and learning disabilities, depression and suicidal ideation, anxiety disorders, stressors related to sexual orientation, substance abuse, child abuse, delinquency, gang–related problems, aggression, and bullying, just to name a few. A number of benefits are associated with providing mental health services and supports to students in need. (Refer to AAP policy statement "School-Based Mental Health Services" **http://pediatrics.aappublications.org/content/113/6/1839.full**). Advantages include:

- Mental health services are provided to students on site, reducing barriers to services and facilitating access to care.
- Parents may be more easily engaged if they live close to the school. Services provided at the school also minimize loss of parental work time.
- Providing mental health care in the school obviates the stigma that many families feel about seeking and receiving community mental health services.
- On-site care allows for ease of monitoring and providing follow-up care. The school environment provides a rich opportunity to observe students longitudinally and in multiple settings to improve the accuracy of diagnoses.

- Working collaboratively with teachers, administrators, and other school health staff maximizes the likelihood of positive benefits, because the needs of the "whole child" (ie, emotional, behavioral, physical, social, and academic) can be attended to in 1 setting with input from a multidisciplinary team.

- Financial constraints to the delivery of mental health care are also minimized, because school mental health services are often free or delivered at considerable discount to families.

- The integration of medical and mental health screening and services offered through school-based health centers are related to positive school performance (Refer to AAP policy statement "School-Based Health Centers and Pediatric Practice" **http://pediatrics.aappublications.org/content/129/2/387.full**).

- Finally, high-quality implementation of multilevel mental health prevention and intervention services in schools has been associated with improvements in emotional, behavioral, and academic outcomes.[37]

Major limitations and challenges of school mental health programs involve issues of understaffing and long-term sustainability, especially in light of the enormous fiscal constraints currently facing school districts and state agencies. Even though the volume of students with mental health needs may be offset by identifying additional health and mental health personnel who are available to provide services in schools, colocation of providers is fraught with potential pitfalls if attention to planning and organizational management is shortchanged.[38] School administrators must work hard to ensure that outside mental health services are not simply colocated but actively integrated into the school day and that best clinical practices are maintained. Medication management, coordination of care (such as making sure that a policy exists about where to obtain care when schools are closed), and communication among providers and educators are paramount.

The Family Educational Rights and Privacy Act (FERPA) is the federal law that protects the privacy of students' educational records if that student is enrolled in any school (public or private) that receives funds from the Department of Education (see 20 USC § 1232g; 34 CFR Part 99).

Community providers may also be unaware of the unique ethical and legal concerns that occur when health or mental health services are delivered in school settings.[39] (Refer to AAP policy statement "Confidentiality in Adolescent Health Care" **http://aapnews.aappublications.org/cgi/reprint/5/4/9**.) Ensuring privacy and confidentiality of mental health services remains an additional concern in schools, including the need to be clear about the informed consent and exchange of information processes, the management of clinical files, and the delivery of services in confidential spaces. Although primary care providers are aware of regulations associated with the Health Insurance Portability and Accountability Act of 1996 (HIPAA), pediatric primary care providers who collaborate with school professionals must also familiarize themselves with the Family Educational Rights and Privacy Act (FERPA), especially in light of the fact that some health information (such as immunization records maintained by a school nurse or services provided to special education students) may be considered part of the "educational record" and may, therefore, be subject to FERPA and not HIPAA.[40] The distinction between FERPA and HIPAA becomes particularly important in states where a minor may be legally allowed to consent for services and, therefore, determines when and with whom information from the clinical record can be shared, whereas schools, authorized by FERPA, may release any information to parents without the consent of the eligible student.

FERPA is the federal law that protects the privacy of students' educational records if that student is enrolled in any school (public or private) that receives funds from the Department of Education (see 20 USC § 1232g; 34 CFR Part 99).

Financing School Mental Health Programs

School mental health programs may be financed through a combination of federal and state funding, private grants, Medicaid, private health insurers, and direct payment by families (often at reduced cost). These programs are more likely to be sustained long-term when close collaboration between school, community mental health providers, and local mental health departments is attained. A number of programs around the United States have developed successful business models for sustainable services by maximizing reimbursement from Medicaid and other insurers.[41]

Lessons from in-depth case studies note the importance of:

- Maximizing all possible sources for support, including insurers and in-kind contributions from the school system and both private and public grants to subsidize nonbillable services.
- Using "clout" through connections with local power brokers to bring insurance providers to the table to negotiate.
- Adapting clear productivity expectations for clinicians maintaining a balance of billable- versus nonbillable services. Acknowledging the need for a strong fiscal foundation is imperative to sustaining services to all students in need regardless of ability to pay.
- Investing in billing infrastructure to successfully verify eligibility, bill, track payments, and collect co-pays and deductibles.
- Establishing the 3 E's essential to third party reimbursement: knowledge of *eligible* services, *eligible* clients and *eligible* providers to optimize insurance coverage of the student population.

Cultural Diversity Issues

The demographic shift evidenced in classrooms has been quite dramatic,[42] and many educators feel ill prepared to address the unique needs of diverse students or to effectively engage their caregivers in their child's learning. Cultural attributes (such as race, ethnicity, religious beliefs, language, sexual orientation, disability, and socioeconomic status), influence many aspects of mental health, including the definitions of illness and health, the expression of symptoms, the nature of help-seeking behaviors, the acceptability of treatment, and levels of disclosure.[43] It is critical that pediatricians remain attuned to cultural diversity and particularly its effect on behavior. Cultural attitudes toward sleep, discipline, the importance of education, the roles of fathers and mothers in the family, and family hierarchy as well as perceptions of health and mental health may vary. Behaviors and interventions must, therefore, be considered within the context of the child's cultural background.[44] (Refer to AAP policy statement "Ensuring Culturally Effective Pediatric Care" **http://pediatrics. aappublications.org/content/114/6/1677**.)

> It is important for pediatricians to gain the parental perspective on behavior problems when communicating with families of different cultural backgrounds.[44]

Pediatricians should also remain attuned to the unique challenges facing immigrant and refugee families. Children from immigrant and refugee families live in communities across the country and make up over 20% of the total school-aged population.[45] Immigrant and refugee children represent a group that is at higher risk of psychosocial and learning problems. Preimmigration experiences, trauma experienced during migration, issues of resettlement, and substandard living conditions in the host country may all factor into the development of mental health problems.[43]

It is important for pediatricians to gain the parental perspective on behavior problems when communicating with families of different cultural backgrounds.[44] "What are your concerns?" "Why do you think your child has this problem?" "Have you spoken to other people about these concerns and what do they say?" "Sometimes there are other ways to treat a problem that physicians do not know about—have you tried anything else to help solve this?"

Although a number of reliable screening and assessment measures are used today, few have been validated for use with non-English–speaking individuals.[46] Assessment procedures need to take the language abilities of immigrant children and their families into account to obtain an accurate accounting of the children's abilities and achievements.[47] Public schools, because of their legal mandate to provide a free and appropriate public education to all students, must make resources available to educate students of foreign-born or non-English–speaking families. Schools often also provide support to family members who have low proficiency in English as a means to improve communication bilaterally, either through interpreters, translation, or even cultural liaisons who can provide assistance to immigrant students and their families.

Section 504 of the Rehabilitation Act of 1973 requires school districts to provide a "free appropriate public education" to all students and protects the rights of students with disabilities by entitling them to specific related aids and services to ensure an appropriate educational setting. Pediatricians can be involved in the formulation of Section 504 plans that provide children in need with helpful classroom accommodations.

Common Mental Health Problems

There are many mental health issues likely to be noted by school personnel and pediatricians, including:

- depression and suicide;
- bipolar disorders;
- anxiety;
- ADHD;
- eating disorders;
- aggression and bullying;
- substance abuse;
- sexual orientation concerns; and
- childhood stress and trauma (physical and psychological abuse).

Please refer to the AAP Council on School Health Web site (**http://www2.aap.org/sections/schoolhealth/**) for a more in-depth examination of these issues and some practical clinical tools that can be used to screen and engage children, adolescents, and families in a discussion about these concerns.

Depression and Suicide

Depression in children and teenagers often presents differently than it does in adults. Feelings of sadness and loneliness are common, but moodiness or irritability may be more predominant expressions of these underlying feelings. Additional symptoms may include loss of appetite or overeating, and sleep disturbances such as excessive sleeping, insomnia, or day-night reversal. Depressed children and adolescents often exhibit social withdrawal or changes in school performance and may engage in self-destructive and risk-taking behaviors such as cutting, substance use, driving while impaired, sexual promiscuity, and running away. Clinicians should be direct in asking patients who appear depressed whether they are having suicidal thoughts or have specific plans to hurt themselves.

Administering depression screens such as the KADS (Kutcher Adolescent Depression Scale), the CDS (Columbia Depression Scale), the CES-DS (Center for Epidemiological Studies- Depression Scale for Children), or the PHQ9 (Patient Health Questionnaire[50]) (visit **http://www.mdaap.org/biped.html** for more information) can be helpful tools in identifying problematic symptoms early and taking swift action to provide a more in-depth evaluation and an accurate diagnosis. Information from school partners, with regard to the presence of behavioral problems, withdrawal from social activities or friends, or changes in academic performance will provide validation of the screening results and will help individualize the intervention approach.

Bipolar Disorder

Bipolar disorder, a mood disorder, is characterized by intense mood swings ranging from depression to mania. This manic phase can be associated with impulsive and reckless behavior, feelings of grandiosity, agitation, or frenzied activities. Resources, such as the STABLE toolkit, are available to assist with screening, assessment, and monitoring of patients suspected of having bipolar disorder. (Visit http://**www.integration.samhsa.gov/images/res/STABLE_toolkit.pdf**.)

Anxiety

Anxiety is manifested by students who worry a great deal, are nervous, and may be considered high strung or perfectionist. Separation issues from parents and school refusal are often indicative of underlying anxiety disorders, particularly among younger children. Children and teenagers may also display fears that get in the way of their daily activities, social anxiety marked by avoidance of social gatherings, and outright panic attack marked by diaphoresis, tachycardia, and hyperventilation. Obsessive-compulsive behaviors such as repeated rituals and recurring thoughts and recurrent somatic symptoms including headaches, abdominal pain, and sleep disturbances such as insomnia may also be manifestations of anxiety. Screening tools such the SCARED or the Spence Anxiety Scale can be helpful adjuncts in making a diagnosis.

ADHD

Children with ADHD often present with behaviors such as diminished attention span, daydreaming, difficulty following directions, and distractibility. These children may be excessively active, impulsive, fidgety, or talkative, with symptoms that are present for at least 6 months and with impairment noted in more than 1 domain of the child's life. Children with ADHD may be socially awkward displaying a poor sense of physical and social boundaries, touching other children inappropriately, or getting too close to their peers. Organizational difficulties in space (losing things, disordered notebooks and bedrooms, forgetting to hand in assignments) and in time (difficulty with planning for long-term projects or studying for exams) are common as well. Administration of screening tools such as the Vanderbilt[22] to teachers and parents can be helpful adjuncts in making a diagnosis. Information that is shared with pediatricians, such as rating scales completed by teachers or parents, can be very helpful in making a differential diagnosis between ADHD and anxiety. First-line psychopharmacologic interventions and referral for counseling also fall into the domain of the pediatrician.

Eating Disorders

Patients with anorexia nervosa are significantly underweight, do not fully perceive the severity of their condition, and suffer from intense fear of weight gain. Patients with bulimia nervosa present with recurrent binge eating and subsequent attempts to compensate by vomiting, fasting, using laxatives, severely dieting, or excessively exercising. Eating disorders can be life threatening and more difficult to recover from the later they are detected.[51]

Eating disorders should be suspected in children and adolescents who are rapidly losing weight, who refuse to eat in public, who wear baggy clothing to hide their weight loss, or who constantly use the bathroom during or after meals. Physical signs include dizziness, fatigue, headaches, heartburn, dehy- dration, irregular heartbeat, menstrual irregularities (in girls), calluses on fingers from induced vomiting (bulimia), damaged gums, and discoloration of the teeth and nails. Girls and boys who are heavily involved in activities such as dance, gymnastics, or wrestling may be at higher risk than other students because of the pressure or requirement in these sports to maintain a certain weight. The SCOFF Questionnaire is 1 tool that could be administered to students suspected of having an eating disorder. Referral to an experienced eating disorder multidisciplinary team is key when an eating disorder is recognized. (Visit **www.aedweb.org** for more information.)

SCOFF Questionnaire (2 or more "Yes" answers indicate risk of anorexia nervosa or bulimia nervosa):

Do you make yourself Sick (vomit) because you feel uncomfortably full?
☐ Yes ☐ No

Do you worry that you have lost Control over how much you eat?
☐ Yes ☐ No

Have you recently lost more than One stone (6.3 kg or 14 lb) in a 3-month period?
☐ Yes ☐ No

Do you believe yourself to be Fat when others say you are too thin?
☐ Yes ☐ No

Would you say that Food do minates your life?
☐ Yes ☐ No

Reproduced from Morgan JF, Reid F, Lacey JH. The SCOFF questionnaire: assessment of a new screening tool for eating disorders. *BMJ*. 1999;319:1467, with permission from BMJ Publishing Group, Ltd.

Aggression/Violence/Bullying

Aggressive behavior can be a symptom of a variety of problems and can be differentiated by subtypes.[52] Reactive aggression can be an angry, defensive response to a threat or provocation. Children with ADHD or oppositional defiant disorder (ODD) may demonstrate this type of aggression. Proactive aggression is premeditated and calculated with an end goal in mind. This type of aggression may occur in children with ODD or conduct disorder (CD). Children with an ODD may be aggressive toward peers or authority figures. Severe violence and aggression and antisocial behaviors may be signs of a CD or gang affiliation, but consideration of imminent threats within the environment is important in making an accurate diagnosis.

Bullying is a form of aggression in which one or more children repeatedly and intentionally intimidate, harass, or physically harm a victim. Bullying includes actions such as making threats, spreading rumors, attacking someone physically or verbally, and excluding someone from a group on purpose. (Visit **http://www.stopbullying.gov** for more information.)

Victims of bullying report more sleep disturbances, enuresis, headaches, and feeling sadder than children who are not bullied.[53] Recent studies also report that youth who have been both bullied and who have bullied others are at increased risk of suicidal ideation and suicide attempts.[54]

Substance Abuse

Substance abuse may be a manifestation of depression but is best viewed as a primary disease rather than a symptom. (Refer to AAP policy statement "Substance Use Screening, Brief Interventions, and Referral to Treatment for Pediatricians" **http://pediatrics.aappublications.org/content/128/5/ e1330.full.**) Substance use can be viewed along of continuum of experimentation, beginning with nonproblematic use, problem use, abuse, and ultimately dependence.[44] Teachers and parents may note suspicious behaviors such as dizziness, lightheadedness, somnolence, mood swings, or erratic behaviors, and parents may complain about missing money at home. Changes in style of clothing, donning of sunglasses, suddenly affiliating with a new peer group, or changes in school performance may be warning signs of drug or alcohol use. Additional risk-taking behaviors such as sexual promiscuity may also be associated with substance use.

Pediatricians also need to be aware of the recent increase in use of synthetic cannabinoid products ("K2" or "spice") and synthetic cathinones ("bath salts"), which can be easily obtained in the community or on the Internet.[55] These so-called "designer drugs" can produce symptoms of euphoria, tachycardia, headaches, hallucinations, panic attacks, and seizures. Synthetic cathinones have been associated with insomnia, aggression, paranoia, and violent and psychotic behaviors. Many of these drugs are not identified on routine drug testing, so clinicians need to remain vigilant. The pediatrician can also play an important role in openly encouraging abstaining from drug/alcohol use, cutting back (eg, on weeknights), and avoiding dangerous situations such as substance use and driving.

Screening tools such as the CRAFFT are helpful in identifying a substance abuse problem and differentiating between substance use and abuse:[56]

Part B

1. Have you ever ridden in a <u>CAR</u> driven by someone (including yourself) who was "high" or had been using alcohol or drugs?
   ☐ No   ☐ Yes

2. Do you ever use alcohol or drugs to <u>RELAX</u>, feel better about yourself, or fit in?
   ☐ No   ☐ Yes

3. Do you ever use alcohol or drugs while you are by yourself, or <u>ALONE</u>?
   ☐ No   ☐ Yes

4. Do you ever <u>FORGET</u> things you did while using alcohol or drugs?
   ☐ No   ☐ Yes

5. Do your <u>FAMILY</u> or <u>FRIENDS</u> ever tell you that you should cut down on your drinking or drug use?
   ☐ No   ☐ Yes

6. Have you ever gotten into <u>TROUBLE</u> while you were using alcohol or drugs?
   ☐ No   ☐ Yes

*Two or more YES answers on the CRAFFT suggest a serious problem and need for further assessment.

Pediatricians can also gauge their patient's readiness for change by asking some of the following questions[57,58]:

"Is this a problem for you?"
☐ No   ☐ Yes

"How does drinking or using drugs interfere with other things that you hope to accomplish?"
☐ No   ☐ Yes

"How ready are you to make a change?"
☐ No   ☐ Yes

"What is your time frame?"
☐ No   ☐ Yes

Sexual Orientation

Adolescence is a natural time for the development of sexual identity and for students to become more self-aware of their emerging sexual orientation. Some youth may experience confusion about their sexual orientation and have questions about identity and sexual behavior that a pediatrician can discuss in the context of a health visit. Other youth may comfortably identify as lesbian, gay, bisexual, or transgender (LGBT) but have realistic concerns about their safety or their emotional well being given the stigma that may exist in their community. The stigma and stress associated with feeling isolated or victimized may lead to a number of destructive behaviors such as substance abuse, suicide attempts, or sexual risk-taking behaviors.[59]

Screening questions that are neutral open the door to further dialogue.

"Have you ever wondered if you are gay or bisexual?"

"Have you ever had a romantic relationship with a boy or a girl?"

"When you think of people to whom you are sexually attracted, are they boys, girls, both, neither, or are you not sure yet?"[59]

"Have you discussed any concerns you may have about your sexuality with your parents or another adult or with your friends or siblings?"

Discussion should also focus on whether the adolescent is prepared to disclose his or her nonheterosexuality to his or her parents. Schools may have support groups, or community organizations may be available to adolescents in their desire to navigate the circumstances around "coming out." Referral for counseling is appropriate for teenagers who are seeking assistance or if students are depressed or suicidal or engaging in substance abuse or risky sexual activities.

LGBT youth report higher levels of bullying and poor school climates, often contributing to higher prevalence rates of mental disorder than youth in national samples,[60] but research has shown that gay-straight alliances in schools offer critical support and reduce the risk of suicide attempts in lesbian, gay, and bisexual youth.[61]

Childhood Stress and Trauma

Familial poverty, parental substance use or untreated mental illness, and exposure to chronic community violence or abuse can all have profound effect on a child's emotional, social, and cognitive development. Poverty is associated with a number of negative physical health, cognitive, educational, and emotional/behavioral outcomes.[4] For example, 1 subgroup, homeless children, have higher rates of developmental and academic delays and mental health issues such as depression, anxiety, stress, and aggression than their peers.[62]

Chronic stressful conditions can contribute to higher incidence of various types of child abuse and neglect. Families with significant internal conflict, adult mental health problems, and parental substance abuse are at high risk of psychological maltreatment. Indicators of child maltreatment may manifest in schools, requiring school and health personnel to be acutely aware of risk factors and signs of abuse. Studies have also shown that the exposure to traumatic childhood experiences is linked to multiple health risk factors and psychiatric disorders in adulthood (ACES study).[63] Abuse and emotional trauma can lead to profound structural, functional, and molecular alterations of the brain and to poor future psychosocial functioning.

Overt signs of physical abuse include bruising, unexplained injuries, and delays in seeking medical attention. Pain, redness, or discharge from genitals or rectum, urinary frequency, or loss of bowel control can also be signs of sexual abuse. Recent studies suggest that harsh physical punishment in the absence of child maltreatment has serious mental health implications.[64] Psychological or emotional maltreatment is the most prevalent form of child abuse and neglect.[65] Psychologically abusive behavior may entail a chronic pattern of belittling, threatening, isolating the child, modeling or encouraging antisocial behavior, detachment, and/or limiting a child's access to health care. Children and teenagers enduring abuse may present with depression, substance abuse, and aggressive and bullying behaviors.

Pediatricians are in an optimal position for early intervention by identifying mothers who are experiencing postpartum depression and for identifying parents with a history of substance abuse or mental health problems, all conditions that place children at higher risk of abuse. Pediatricians can also proactively teach appropriate discipline techniques to parents in place of corporal punishment and partner with schools to conduct parenting workshops. (Visit **http://www.mdaap.org/biped.html** for more information.)

When to Refer

Pediatricians should refer children and teenagers for mental health consultation under the following circumstances:

- The problem is refractory to primary care interventions.
- The problem is out of the comfort zone of the pediatrician.
- The family requests a referral to a mental health specialist.
- Significant psychopathology is suspected.
- Significant marital and family discord/domestic violence/parental substance abuse.

Assessment of Strengths and Assets

In the course of assessing child and adolescent mental health problems, it is critical to identify the child's strengths, positive coping strategies, and key positive influences in his or her support network. Increased attention is being given to the importance of assessing not only the level of dysfunction that may exist in a young person's life, but also to the strengths and developmental assets that protect and buffer that person from the effects of individual, social, or environmental risks. Research indicates the value of assessing strengths and its connection to psychosocial functioning.[66] The empirical evidence on the efficacy of strength-based approaches in practice continues to grow, but many agree that a complimentary focus on individual and group strengths enhances opportunities for student growth. (For more information on the Developmental Assets, visit **http://www.search-institute.org/ developmental-assets**, or for the Strengths and Difficulties Questionnaire [SDQ], visit **http://www.sdqinfo.com/a0.html**.)

How to Work With Schools

A positive relationship between pediatricians and the school community is critical in addressing childhood mental health problems. Pediatric practitioners are an important link in the continuum of care for students with emerging, acute, or chronic mental health problems. There are a number of roles that pediatricians can effectively play and key objectives they can advance to support the emotional and behavioral well being of young people.

Collaboration

Sharing information between pediatricians and school personnel is of key importance. Pediatricians can often provide important family contextual information as a professional who has had a long-standing relationship with the student and family. School mental health specialists can in turn provide the pediatrician with rich longitudinal information about the student's academic performance and school behaviors. Communication typically is mediated by telephone, via e-mail, or through standardized checklists. Pediatricians may also elect to participate directly on the student support team by being physically present or by teleconference when their patients are being evaluated by school personnel. Pediatricians can perform a diagnostic evaluation or health assessment that may facilitate the design and implementation of student accommodations and resources through a Section 504 plan individualized education program (IEP).

The student support team (SST) process (in some cases these teams might also be referred to as teacher assistance teams or child study teams) involves a multidisciplinary team of school-based professionals who engage in a problem-solving approach to address learning, attendance, behavior, or social-emotional concerns for all children within the general education setting. Specific areas of concern are identified; information is gathered through a variety of methods (ie, observation, interview, review of school records, and informal assessment) and interventions are developed and monitored for their efficacy in addressing the identified need. The SST may be the portal of entry to determine the need for more specialized educational services, but it should not be equated with the team that designs a student's IEP for students deemed to have special needs.

Section 504 of the Rehabilitation Act of 1973 requires school districts to provide a "free appropriate public education" to all students and protects the rights of students with disabilities by entitling them to specific related aids and services to ensure an appropriate educational setting. Pediatricians can be involved in the formulation of Section 504 plans that provide children in need with helpful classroom accommodations (**http://www2.ed.gov/about/ offices/list/ocr/docs/edlite-FAPE504.html**).

Community Health Resource

Pediatricians can be critical resources to school staff that are trying to identify primary care providers for their students. The AAP supports this approach of practitioners serving as a *medical home* for children and teenagers in the community. (Refer to AAP policy statement "The Future of Pediatrics: Mental Health Competencies for Pediatric Primary Care" **http://pediatrics.aappublications. org/content/124/1/410**.) In addition, pediatricians can provide valuable assistance in facilitating patient referrals to mental health providers or other specialists in the community. Some pediatricians provide mental health services within the medical home through colocation with a mental health provider or through integrated and collaborative primary care and mental health services within their office setting.[48,49] (Refer to American Academy of Child and Adolescent Psychiatry policy statement "Improving Mental Health Services in Primary Care: Reducing Administrative and Financial Barriers to Access and Collaboration" **http://pediatrics.aappublications.org/content/123/4/1248**.)

Education and Consultation

Parental education is an important means of reducing the stigma associated with mental health issues that serves as a barrier to obtaining help for their children. Pediatricians can conduct in-services and workshops to school personnel and to parents on developmental and mental health topics. Parents may also feel less resistant to advice offered by pediatricians, because they are not directly involved in assessing student performance and do not determine educational outcomes. Pediatricians can volunteer or work at community school-based health centers or supervise pediatric nurse practitioners that work in schools. Pediatricians may also elect to serve as medical consultants to schools or serve on the school health advisory council, an important group that can influence local school policies and practices.

Advocacy

Schools, although familiar, may be intimidating places for parents, especially for parents whose children are having difficulties. Because of their preexisting relationship with families, pediatricians can serve as a bridge between the parent/caregiver and the school and advocate for students who may require evaluation and mental health interventions in school. Pediatricians can help patients to obtain a Section 504 accommodation plan and counsel parents about behavioral management strategies that can be effective. (Visit **http://www. mdaap.org/biped.html** for more information.) In addition, pediatricians can serve as advocates for policy on a local, state, or national level to help ensure that the mental health needs of children and teenagers are met through adequate funding and the provision of resources particularly for the underserved. Pediatricians can work toward the reduction of financial barriers to mental health care by lobbying for reimbursement by insurance providers for mental health care delivered in a primary care or school setting.

> Pediatricians can use open-ended screening questions as a means to initiating dialog about mental health concerns.

Recommendations for Pediatricians

Pediatricians often have a trusting relationship with patients and families and offer family-centered care while demonstrating an understanding of the social, emotional, and educational problems in the context of child development. The pediatrician, therefore, has a unique opportunity to prevent and treat mental health problems through proactive guidance, early identification, and primary care mental health interventions. Pediatricians, pediatric nurse practitioners, and nurses who work in school settings as well as community-based pediatric primary care centers are important members of the school mental health team. The AAP has called for the development of mental health competencies by pediatricians to enhance medical knowledge and develop interpersonal and communication skills.[15] (Refer to AAP policy statement "The Future of Pediatrics: Mental Health Competencies for Pediatric Primary Care" **http://pediatrics. aappublications.org/content/124/1/410.full.**)

Pediatricians are in an advantageous position to screen for behavioral and mental health problems and to link youth and their families to appropriate treatment.[67] Pediatricians who work in school settings or in community practice can perform brief mental health assessments[15,57,58] using a model of the 4 C's: connect, concerns, create, and conclude. The pediatrician initially *connects* with the patient through a process of reflective listening. The pediatrician can use open-ended questions to elicit *concerns*. The clinician works with the patient or family to *create* a plan. Such a plan may entail crisis intervention, referral to a mental health consultant, or follow-up with the school-based practitioner or student's pediatrician for further assessment and management. The encounter *concludes* by summarizing or having the patient/family summarize the chosen plan of action. School-based pediatric practitioners and primary care pediatricians may wish to bring the patient back for a more comprehensive evaluation. Using a behavioral template to conduct the interview can facilitate this process. (Visit **http://www.mdaap.org/biped.html** for more information.) Diagnoses can be further corroborated using standardized focused screening tools such as those outlined throughout this chapter.

When mental health problems are identified, close communication between school mental health personnel and the community-based pediatrician is critical. Pediatricians, nurse practitioners, and mental health professionals who work directly in schools as well as those who work in the community are essential links in the identification, diagnosis, and management of mental health problems. Children and adolescents can present with a constellation of diagnostic symptoms, and the identification of dysfunctional behaviors is key in preventing or reducing the development of a full-blown mental illness. Jensen and his colleagues suggest that the use of "action signs," or symptom profiles may be an effective method for identifying the frequency, duration, and severity of impairing disorders early and facilitating evaluation and treatment.[68] Once a concern is identified, pediatricians can consult with health or mental health providers in the school about additional manifestations of the problem. Pediatricians can inquire about school-based services or programs that may be available for the student or his or her family, jointly design interventions that can ameliorate the symptoms, and assist in implementing methods for tracking symptom changes or treatment progress.

Pediatricians can use open-ended screening questions as a means to initiating dialog about mental health concerns (Refer to AAP policy supplement "Enhancing Pediatric Mental Health Care" **http://pediatrics.aappublications. org/content/pediatrics/125/Supplement_3/S75.full.pdf**):

"Tell me, in general, how you think things have been going for you lately?"

"What are the things that are most stressful for *you* these days? How do you manage stress?"

"How would you describe your mood over the past few weeks? Does this seem any different from usual for you?"

"Does it seem that you've been feeling more irritable or angry lately?"

"What changes have you noticed lately in your sleeping?"

Recommendations for Program Directors

The Accreditation Council for Graduate Medical Education (ACGME) states that "pediatrics encompasses the study and practice of health promotion, disease prevention, diagnosis, care, and treatment of infants, children, adolescents and young adults during health and all stages of illness." Guidelines are provided for pediatric residents to receive training in behavioral and developmental pediatrics and to learn to "communicate effectively with patients, families…across a broad range of socioeconomic and cultural backgrounds." The guidelines also stipulate working with interprofessional teams and learning to "advocate for quality patient care and optimal patient care systems." The AAP has endorsed the development of mental health competencies by pediatricians in the care of children with ADHD, anxiety, depression, and substance abuse. (Refer to AAP policy statement "The Future of Pediatrics: Mental Health

Competencies for Pediatric Primary Care" **http://pediatrics.aappublications. org/content/124/1/410.full**.)

Children and adolescents spend significant amounts of time in a school setting. Observing children in schools is an essential component of training, allowing the trainee to understand children in the context of their community. Participation in a school is a valuable educational experience that provides trainees with exposure to a variety of developmental and mental health problems needed to develop core mental health competencies. Trainees at schools can also witness the implementation of mental health interventions, including the opportunity to directly observe classroom-based behavioral management.

Attending schools during a behavioral and developmental pediatrics rotation is one way to expose the trainee to community experience outside of the hospital, and observing a student support team in particular can provide the trainee with a model of the interprofessional team approach to problem solving. An optimal experience would allow trainees to observe students in school settings across the age continuum from preschool to high school. Visiting schools in a variety of socioeconomic communities can be enlightening in exposing the trainee to educational disparities and cultural diversity. Visiting schools that feature special education provides the trainee with exposure to children with a variety of needs. Rotating through schools also provides the trainee with a snapshot of the abilities and limitations of schools in providing for the mental health needs of students.

Participating in a school experience can also help trainees define their relationship to the community and provide them with an opportunity to consider how they may serve as advocates for their patients. Trainees can witness the needs of the school and community and begin to define their role as child advocates on a local, state or national level through the support of programming and budgeting for child mental health services and fulfilling the pediatric training objective of serving as an "advocate for quality patient care and optimal patient care systems." (Visit **http://www.acgme.org** for more information.)

Recommendations for Trainees

Exposure to school settings is an important experience for the pediatric trainee during the behavioral and developmental pediatrics rotation in meeting expected core competencies of training (Refer to AAP policy statement "The Future

of Pediatrics: Mental Health Competencies for Pediatric Primary Care"
http://pediatrics.aappublications.org/content/124/1/410.full.) The experience provides the trainee with a snapshot of how young patients spend a large percentage of their time. Trainees are also offered a picture of the community outside of the hospital setting. Trainees can be exposed to children across all developmental ages and learn to distinguish between normal and abnormal development.

Schools also provide trainees with an opportunity to observe children from diverse socioeconomic and cultural backgrounds. Trainees will learn about the abilities and limitations of schools to educate as well as to address the many types of mental health concerns that present in a school setting. Trainees will likely be exposed to diverse mental health problems such as autism spectrum disorder, ADHD, depression, anxiety, aggression, and substance abuse. In addition, the trainee has the opportunity to observe how these problems may present in a classroom setting, the value of early identification, and the need for multidisciplinary collaboration. Observation of school mental health professionals provides the trainee with insight into mental health interventions and classroom management techniques. Opportunities to visit schools also allows trainees to begin the process of identifying their role in the general community as well as their role as a child advocate for individual students and for local, state, and national policy issues.

Take-Home Points

- Prevalence rates of childhood mental illness warrant a continued emphasis on the individual, family, and social determinants of mental health and on the implementation of effective "place-based" strategies that include schools and medical homes. Pediatricians are urged to continue to develop competencies in the identification and first-line interventions for children and adolescents with behavior and mental health problems.
- Expanding pediatrician involvement from a focus on early intervention or treatment of mental illness to a broader focus on prevention and promotion of mental health will benefit a larger population of children and adolescents and will foster better use of limited local resources. Acknowledging both the challenges as well as the strengths evident in a child and his or her family will encourage motivation and engagement and ultimately promote psychological well-being.

- Reliable and valid screening and assessment tools are available to help identify a variety of childhood mental, emotional, and behavioral problems. Information and data acquired by the pediatric provider during office visits can be supplemented by valuable information obtained from school personnel, such as how the student interacts with peers and authority figures, how the student transitions between settings, how the student performs under pressure, and how the student learns and acquires new information. Together, the information provides a more complete picture of a student's deficits as well as his or her areas of strength.

- Pediatric primary care providers should become familiar with the staff, resources, and programs available in neighboring schools and in the surrounding community. Identifying contact people in a few key mental health organizations will reduce the burden and stress on the primary care provider later when a patient is in immediate need of mental health services.

- Active collaboration and the intentional pursuit of open communication between primary care providers and school personnel is essential if positive student outcomes are to be expected. Pediatricians need to remain mindful that education professionals may not readily identify opportunities to advance student health if it is not in the service of improving academic achievement or educational outcomes. Although health and education professionals bring differing perspectives to bear on the complex issues facing students, interventions that reflect the expertise of multiple disciplines offer the greatest promise for effectively managing emerging mental health problems.

- The vast number of children with mental health problems, the well-documented risk of chronicity into adulthood, and the relative paucity of adequate services available in many communities places the pediatrician in a critical role of advocating for the funding and sustainability of comprehensive and integrated child mental health prevention, early intervention, and treatment services on a local, state, and national level.

Resources

For additional school health related resources, visit www.aap.org/schoolhealthmanual.

References

1. Costello JE, Egger H, Angold A. 10-year research update review: the epidemiology of child and adolescent psychiatric disorders: I. Methods and public health burden. *J Am Acad Child Adolesc Psychiatry.* 2005;44(10):972–986

2. Institute of Medicine. *Preventing Mental, Emotional, and Behavioral Disorders Among Young People: Progress and Possibilities.* Washington, DC: The National Academies Press; 2009 Available at: http://www.iom.edu/Reports/2009/Preventing-Mental-Emotional-and-Behavioral-Disorders-Among-Young-People-Progress-and-Possibilities.aspx. Accessed April 13, 2015

3. Kataoka SH, Zhang L, Wells K. Unmet need for mental health care among U.S. children: Variation by ethnicity and insurance status. *Am J Psychiatry.* 2002;159(9):1548–1555

4. Yoshikawa H, Aber JL, Beardslee WR. The effects of poverty on the mental, emotional, and behavioral health of children and youth: implications for prevention. *Am Psychol.* 2012;67(4):272–284

5. Kessler RC, Berglund P, Demler O, et al. Lifetime prevalence and age-of-onset distributions of DSM-IV disorders in the National Comorbidity Survey Replication. *Arch Gen Psychiatry.* 2005;62(6):593–602

6. Fabelo T, Thompson MD, Plotkin M, Carmichael D, Marchbanks MP, Booth EA; Justice Center, Public Policy Research Institute. Breaking schools' rules: a statewide study of how school discipline relates to students' success and juvenile justice involvement. July 18, 2011. Available at: http://csgjusticecenter.org/youth/publications/breaking-schools-rules-a-statewide-study-of-how-school-discipline-relates-to-students-success-and-juvenile-involvement-2/ . Accessed April 13, 2015

7. Bloom B, Cohen RA, Freeman G; National Center for Health Statistics. Summary health status for US children: National Health Interview Survey, 2010. *Vital Health Stat.* 2011;10(250):1-89

8. Merikangas KR, He JP, Burstein M, et al. Lifetime prevalence of mental disorders in U.S. adolescents: results from the National Comorbidity Survey Replication—Adolescent Supplement (NCS-A). *J Am Acad Child Adolesc Psychiatry.* 2010;49(10):980–989

9. Substance Abuse and Mental Health Services Administration. Results from the 2012 National Survey on Drug Use and Health: Summary of National Findings, NSDUH Series H-46, HHS Publication No. (SMA) 13-4795. Rockville, MD: Substance Abuse and Mental Health Services Administration; 2013

10. Eaton DK, Kann L, Kinchen S, et al. Youth risk behavior surveillance—United States, 2011. *MMWR Surveill Summ.* 2012;61(4):1–162

11. Heron M. Deaths: leading causes for 2008. *Natl Vital Stat Rep.* 2012;60(6):1–94

12. Husky MM, Olfson M, He J, et al. Twelve-month suicidal symptoms and use of services among adolescents: results from the National Comorbidity Survey. *Psychiatr Serv.* 2012;63(10):989–996

13. Jacobson CM, Gould M. The epidemiology and phenomenology of non-suicidal self-injurious behavior among adolescents: a critical review of the literature. *Arch Suicide Res.* 2007;11(2):129–147

14. Ozer EM, Zahnd EG, Adams SH, et al. Are adolescents being screened for emotional distress in primary care? *J Adolesc Health.* 2009;44(6):520–527

15. Wissow L, Gadomski A, Roter D, et al. Improving child and parent mental health in primary care: a cluster-randomized trial of communication skills training. *Pediatrics.* 2008;121(2):266–275

16. MacKay AP, Duran C; National Center for Health Statistics. Adolescent Health in the United States, 2007. Atlanta, GA: National Center for Health Statistics; 2008. Available at: http://www.cdc.gov/nchs/data/misc/adolescent2007.pdf. Accessed April 13, 2015

17. US Department of Education, National Center for Education Statistics. Digest of Education Statistics 2011. Available at: http://nces.ed.gov/pubs2012/2012001.pdf. Accessed April 13, 2015

18. Foster S, Rollefson M, Doksum T, Noonan D, Robinson G, Teich J. School Mental Health Services in the United States, 2002-2003. DHHS publication (SMA) 05-4068. Rockville, MD: Substance Abuse and Mental Health Services Administration; 2005. Available at: http://store. samhsa.gov/shin/content/SMA05-4068/SMA05-4068.pdf. Accessed April 13, 2015

19. Kutash K, Duchnowski AJ, Lynn N; The Research and Training Center for Children's Mental Health. School-Based Mental Health: An Empirical Guide for Decision Makers. Available at: http://rtckids.fmhi.usf.edu/rtcpubs/study04/SBMHfull.pdf. Accessed April 13, 2015

20. Acosta OM, Tashman NA, Prodente C, Proescher E. Establishing successful school mental health programs: guidelines and recommendations. In: *Providing Mental Health Services to Youth Where They Are: School and Community-Based Approaches.* Ghuman HS, Weist MD, Sarles RM, eds. New York, NY: Brunner-Routeldge; 2002:57–74

21. Hahn R, Fuqua-Whitley D, Wethington H, et al. Effectiveness of universal school-based programs to prevent violent and aggressive behavior: a systematic review. *Am J Prev Med.* 2007;33(Suppl 2):S114–S129

22. Jellinek M, Patel BP, Froehle MC, eds. *Bright Futures in Practice: Mental Health—Volume I, Practice Guide.* Arlington, VA: National Center for Education in Maternal and Child Health; 2002

23. Jellinek M, Patel BP, Froehle MC, eds. *Bright Futures in Practice: Mental Health—Volume II, Toolkit.* Arlington, VA: National Center for Education in Maternal and Child Health; 2002

24. Husky MM, Sheridan M, McGuire L, Olfson M. Mental health screening and follow-up care in public high schools. *J Am Acad Child Adolesc Psychiatry.* 2011;50(9):881–891

25. Kidger J, Araya R, Donovan J, Gunnell D. The effect of the school environment on the emotional health of adolescents: a systematic review. *Pediatrics.* 2012;129(5):925–949

26. Cohen J, Pickeral T, McCloskey M. Assessing school climate. *Education Digest: Essential Readings Condensed for Quick Review.* 2009;74(8):45–48

27. Bradshaw C, Waadsorp TE, Leaf PJ. Effects of school-wide positive behavioral interventions and supports on child behavior problems. *Pediatrics.* 2012;130(5):e1136–e1145

28. Durlak JA, Weissberg RP, Dymnicki AB, Taylor RD, Shellinger KB. The impact of enhancing students' social and emotional learning: a meta-analysis of school-based universal interventions. *Child Dev.* 2011;82(1):405–432

29. Quach J, Hiscock H, Ukoumunne OC, Wake M. A brief sleep intervention improves outcomes in the school entry year: a randomized control trial. *Pediatrics.* 2011;128(4):692–701

30. Amos L, D'Andrea L. The sleepy teenager: waking up to the unique sleep needs of adolescents. *Contemp Pediatr.* 2012;29(10):34–45

31. Beebe DW, Rausch J, Bayars KC, Lanphear B, Yolton K. Persistent snoring in preschool children: Predictors and behavioral and developmental correlates. *Pediatrics.* 2012;130(3):382–389

32. O'Sullivan TA, Robinson M, Kendall GE, et al. A good-quality breakfast is associated with better mental health in adolescence. *Public Health Nutr.* 2009;12(2):249–258

33. Millichap J, Yee MM. The diet factor in attention-deficit/hyperactivity disorder. *Pediatrics.* 2012;129(2):330–337

34. Sawyer M, Harchak T, Wake M, Lynch J. Four-year prospective study of BMI and mental health problems in young children. *Pediatrics.* 2011;128(4):677–684

35. Eisenberg ME, Neumark-Sztainer D, Story M. Associations of weight-based teasing and emotional well-being among adolescents. *Arch Pediatr Adolesc Med.* 2003;157(8):733–738

36. BeLue R, Francis LA, Colaco B. Mental health problems and overweight in a nationally representative sample of adolescents: effects of race and ethnicity. *Pediatrics.* 2009;123(2):697–702

37. Rones M, Hoagwood K. School-based mental health services: a research review. *Clin Child Fam Psychol Rev.* 2000;3(4):223–241

38. Weist MD, Proescher E, Prodente C, Ambrose MG, Waxman RP. Mental health, health, and education staff working together in schools. *Child Adolesc Psychiatr Clin North Am.* 2001;10(1):33–43

39. Prodente CA, Sander MA, Grabill C, Rubin M, Schwab N. Addressing unique ethical and legal challenges in expanded school mental health. In: Weist MD, Evans SW, Lever NA, eds. *Handbook of School Mental Health: Advancing Practice and Research.* New York, NY: Kluwer Academic/Plenum Publishers; 2003:363–374

40. US Department of Health and Human Services. Joint guidance on the application of the Family Educational Rights and Privacy Act (FERPA) and the Health Insurance Portability and Accountability Act of 1996 (HIPAA) to student health records. Rockville, MD: US Department of Health and Human Services; 2008. Available at: http://www.hhs.gov/ocr/privacy/hipaa/understanding/coveredentities/hipaaferpajointguide.pdf. Accessed April 13, 2015

41. Behrens D, Lear JG, Price OA; The Center for Health and Health Care in Schools, The George Washington University. Developing a business plan for sustaining school mental health services: three success stories. Washington, DC: The Center for Health and Health Care in Schools; 2012. Available at: http://www.healthinschools.org/School-Based-Mental-Health/Sustaining-School-Mental-Health-Services.aspx. Accessed April 13, 2015

42. Camarota SA. Center for Immigration Studies. Immigrants in the United States, 2007: A profile of America's foreign-born population. Washington, DC: Center for Immigration Studies; November 2007. Available at: http://www.cis.org/articles/2007/back1007.pdf. Accessed April 13, 2015

43. Acosta Price O, Ellis BH, Escudero PV, Huffman-Gottschling K, Sander MA, Birman D. Implementing trauma interventions in schools: addressing the immigrant and refugee experience. In: Notaro SR, ed. *Health Disparities Among Under-served Populations: Implications for Research, Policy, and Praxis.* Wagon Lane, Bingley, UK: Emerald Group Publishing Limited; 2012:95–119

44. Augustyn M, Zuckerman B, Caronna EB. *The Zuckerman Parker Handbook of Developmental and Behavioral Pediatrics for Primary Care.* 3rd ed. New York, NY: Wolters Kluwer/Lippincott Williams & Wilkins; 2011

45. Forum on Child and Family Statistics. Current population survey, annual social and economic supplements. Children of at least one foreign-born parent. Forum on Child and Family Statistics Web site. Available at: http://www.childstats.gov/americaschildren/family4.asp. Accessed July 17, 2015

46. Birman D, Chan WY; Center for Health and Health Care in Schools. Screening and assessing immigrant and refugee youth in school-based mental health programs. Washington, DC: Center for Health and Health Care in Schools; May 2008. Available at: http://www.healthinschools.org/Immigrant-and-Refugee-Children/Tools-and-Documents.aspx. Accessed April 13, 2015

47. Thomas-Presswood TN, Presswood D. *Meeting the Needs of Students and Families from Poverty: A Handbook for School and Mental Health Professionals.* Baltimore, MD: Paul H Brookes Publishing Company; 2008

48. Kolko DJ, Campo JV, Kilbourne AM, Kelleher K. Doctor-office collaborative care for pediatric behavioral problems: a preliminary clinical trial. *Arch Pediatr Adolesc Med.* 2012;166(3):224–231

49. Perrin E, Sheldrick RC. The challenge of mental health care in pediatrics. *Arch Pediatr Adolesc Med.* 2012;166(3):287–288

50. Zuckerbrot RA, Cheung AH, Jensen PS, et al. Guidelines for Adolescent Depression in Primary Care (GLAD-PC): I. Identification, assessment, and initial management. *Pediatrics.* 2007;120(5):e1299–e1312

51. Rome, ES, Ammerman, S, Rosen, DS, et al. Children and adolescents with eating disorders: the state of the art. *Pediatrics.* 2003;111(1):e98–e108

52. Lohr WD, Honaker JT. Pathology and evaluation of childhood aggression. *Contemp Pediatr.* 2012;29(4):20–27

53. Vreeman RC, Carroll AE. A systematic review of school-based interventions to prevent bullying. *Arch Pediatr Adolesc Med.* 2007;161(1):78–88

54. Hepburn L, Azrael D, Molnar B, Miller M. Bullying and suicidal behaviors among urban high school youth. *J Adolesc Health.* 2012;51(1):93–95

55. Saha S, Wilson DJ, Hoover AR. K2, spice and bath salts: Commercially available drugs of abuse. *Contemp Pediatr.* 2012;29(10):22–28

56. Knight JR, Sherritt L, Shrier LA, Harris SK, Chang G. Validity of the CRAFFT substance abuse screening test among adolescent clinic patients. *Arch Pediatr Adolesc Med.* 2002;156(6):607–614

57. Tellerman K. Catalyst for change: motivational interviewing can help parents to help their kids. Part 1 of 2. *Contemp Pediatr.* 2010;27(12):26–38

58. Tellerman K. Catalyst for change: motivational interviewing can help parents to help their kids. Part 2 of 2. *Contemp Pediatr.* 2011;28(1):47–54

59. Frankowski BL; American Academy of Pediatrics, Committee on Adolescence. Sexual orientation and adolescents. *Pediatrics.* 2004;113(6):1827–1832

60. Mustanski BS, Garofalo R, Emerson EM. Mental health disorders, psychological distress, and suicidality in a diverse sample of lesbian, gay, bisexual and transgender youths. *Am J Public Health.* 2010;100(12):2426–2432

61. Hatzenbuehler M. The social environment and suicide attempts in lesbian, gay, and bisexual youth. *Pediatrrics.* 2011;127(5):896–903

62. Thomas-Presswood TN, Presswood D. *Meeting the Needs of Students and Families from Poverty: A Handbook for School and Mental Health Professionals.* Baltimore, MD: Paul H Brookes Publishing Company; 2008

63. Felitti VJ, Anda RF, Nordenberg D, et al. Relationship of childhood abuse and household dysfunction to many of the leading causes of death in adults. The Adverse Childhood Experiences (ACE) Study. *Am J Prev Med.* 1998;14(4):245–258

64. Afifi TO, Mota NP, Dasiewicz P, MacMillan HL, Sareen J. Physical punishment and mental disorders: results from a nationally representative US sample. *Pediatrics.* 2012;130(2):184–192

65. Hibbard R, Barlow J, Macmillian H, et al. Psychological maltreatment. *Pediatrics.* 2012;130(2):372–378

66. Goodman A, Goodman R. Population mean scores predict child mental disorder rates: Validating SDQ prevalence estimators in Britain. *J Child Psychol Pyschiatry.* 2011;52(1): 100–108

67. Boydston L. Pediatric depression detection methods. *Pediatr Ann.* 2011;40(10):512–518

68. Jensen PS, Goldman E, Offord D, et al. Overlooked and underserved: "action signs" for identifying children with unmet mental health needs. *Pediatrics.* 2011;128(5):970–979

CHAPTER

7

Nutrition and Schools

Robert D. Murray, MD, FAAP

Background

Nutrition in schools represents not only the foods and beverages associated with the formal meal programs but also products sold in competition to those meal programs as well as the wide variety of foods brought into the school by students, parents, teachers, and other staff. This chapter focuses on the food programs that constitute the US Department of Agriculture (USDA) nutrition safety net for school children, their basis in the US Dietary Guidelines, and their nutritional impact as well as the challenges facing the school dietary service staff. Preschool and child care nutritional policies and practices have become an important target for improving early life nutrition and activity.

USDA School Meal Programs

School meals ensure a foundation for good nutrition among all children, but especially poor or food insecure children. School meals augment other federal programs that constitute the nutrition safety net. The National School Lunch Program (NSLP) in 1946 and the School Breakfast Program in 1975 established nutrition as a permanent component of public schooling. A series of other national programs serve specific populations and fill in dietary gaps. The USDA oversees a series of programs for school children through its Food and Nutrition Service (FNS), including:

- The NSLP;
- The School Breakfast Program (SBP);
- Afterschool Snack Program;
- The Special Milk Program;
- The Fresh Fruit and Vegetable Program;

- The Child and Adult Care Food Program;
- The Summer Meal Program and Seamless Summer Option; and
- Team Nutrition.

THE USDA SCHOOL MEAL PROGRAMS: A SAFETY NET FOR CHILDREN

- A typical child spends as much as 6 hours per day in school and consumes more than 35% of his or her daily energy at school, compared with 56% at home.

- A healthy, well-fed child is a better student academically, particularly those who face economic or social disadvantages.

The Reach of School Meals
- In 1946, 7.1 million students participated in school lunch. Now, 60 years later, 32 million students participate daily in more than 100,000 schools, public and private.

- Over 224 billion lunches have been served since inception of the National School Lunch Program.

Source: www.usda.gov

US Dietary Guidelines

Nutritional targets for all the school meal programs are based on the Dietary Guidelines for Americans (DGAs). The 2010 DGAs were written following the recommendations of an independent panel of experts after their review of the literature on nutrition and health, addressing 130 specific topical questions. New guidelines will be issued in 2015.

DGAs stress energy balance and nutrient density within our diet. Core recommendations for individuals older than 2 years include:

- **Balance** calories to maintain weight
  - Prevent or reduce overweight and obesity
  - Control total calories
  - Increase physical activity and reduce sedentary behaviors
- **Increase** certain foods and nutrients
  - fruits and vegetables
  - dark-green, red, yellow vegetables plus beans and peas
  - whole grains
  - fat-free or low-fat milk and dairy products
  - protein-rich foods (eg, eggs, nuts, seeds, soy, seafood, lean meats)

- – use oils to replace solid fats
- – choose foods rich in fiber, calcium, vitamin D and potassium
- – special populations:
  - • pregnant females: increase iron, iron enhancers (vitamin C), and folic acid
  - • pregnant and breastfeeding: take iron supplements, 8 to 12 oz seafood per week (avoiding certain fish; see **www.usda.gov**)
  - • elderly: increase foods with B_{12} or take a multivitamin
- ▪ **Reduce** certain foods and nutrients
  - – Sodium limits
    - • 2300 mg normal population older than 2 years
    - • 1500 mg if older than 51 years, African-American, hypertensive, or have diabetes or kidney disease
  - – Saturated fats (10% of calories or less)
  - – Cholesterol (300 mg or less)
  - – Trans fats – avoid
  - – Solid fats and added sugars – limited
  - – Refined grains – limited
- ▪ **Build** a healthy eating pattern
  - – Consume a diet that balances nutrient needs over time within an appropriate calorie range
  - – Assess how every food and beverage fits into an overall healthy eating pattern
  - – Follow food safety recommendations for food preparation

---

CONSUMER TIPS FOR USING THE DGAs

- • Enjoy your food, but eat less
- • Avoid oversized portions
- • Make half your diet fruits and vegetables
- • Switch to fat-free or low-fat (1%) milk
- • Choose lower-sodium varieties of foods like soup, bread, and frozen meals
- • Drink water or milk instead of sugary drinks

National Nutrition Standards for School Meals

Preschool and school nutrition programs are addressed through the Child Nutrition Reauthorization Act. The latest reauthorization was the Healthy, Hunger-Free Kids Act of 2010. The USDA FNS then developed new rules to adhere to the reauthorization. School meals are based on the 5 basic food groups with specified frequency and serving sizes, as well as minimum and maximum caloric intake targets by age and grade.

HEALTHY, HUNGER-FREE KIDS ACT OF 2010, NEW PROVISIONS:

- Additional $0.06 per reimbursed meal to improve nutritional quality

- Helps communities establish local farm-to-school networks

- Augments USDA efforts to improve the nutritional quality of commodity foods for school meal programs

- Expands access to drinking water in schools, particularly during meal times

- Gives USDA the authority to set nutritional standards for all foods regularly sold during the school day, including vended and a la carte items and those sold in school stores

- Sets basic standards for school wellness policies, including goals for nutrition, education, and physical activity

- Promotes nutrition and wellness in child-care settings through the Child and Adult Care Food Program

- Improves access to food by increasing eligibility and simplifying the process by which a child can meet requirements, while allowing for more universal access in high poverty communities through eligibility based on census data

- Enhances food safety and nutritional standards by mandating school audits every 3 years

- Gives USDA the authority to support more meals for high-risk children through after-school programs

- Provides more training for school nutrition staff to support these provisions

- The final USDA rule was published in the Federal Register Vol 79 No. 2 on January 3, 2014.

Food Patterns: Recommended meal patterns provide more fruit at breakfast, more vegetables at lunch, and more whole grains at both meals. Salad bars and other innovations are encouraged to increase vegetable consumption and decrease plate waste. Trans fats are stringently curtailed, and sodium is reduced by 25% in school breakfast and 50% in school lunches over 10 years, a substantial hurdle for food scientists and industry. The minimum and maximum calorie recommendations represent the average for a 5-day school week and not a per-meal or per-day basis. For certain age groups, such as adolescent males, the needed daily calories may be high enough to challenge school food service. To address this, limited discretionary sources of calories (solid fats and added sugars) may be added to the meal pattern provided that they are within the specifications for calories, saturated fat, trans fat, and sodium. Alternatives for meat servings and for fluid milk are offered. This approach reflects the emphasis of the Dietary Guidelines for Americans (DGAs) on *patterns of food intake* for healthy eating. Using the suggested approach, students will meet the Daily Recommended Intakes (DRIs) for 24 nutrients.

Infrastructure of School Food Service

Congress mandates and funds the school meal programs. The USDA FNS directs how the menu should be designed and provided to students. In schools, the food service staff produces meals that are palatable and economical and can be delivered within a strict time frame set aside in the school day. The school nutrition director guides the staff in training, food safety standards, menu planning, quantity food preparation, budgeting, and organizational management. The national School Nutrition Association offers credentialing, certification, resources, and advocacy to aid school nutrition staff by helping with meal quality and safety, along with educational opportunities for those in the field. Nationally, the School Food Service has a remarkable record of diet quality despite having to produce 45 million meals per day.

Economics of School Meals

The USDA provides subsidies to schools to allow them to provide meals at no cost or low cost to children from families meeting financial criteria. The income and eligibility requirements are based on the federal poverty guidelines updated annually by the Department of Health and Human Services. The income cutoff for those eligible for free school meals is 130% of the defined poverty cut-point and for reduced-price meals is 185% of the poverty cut-point. From its inception, school food programs have needed to augment the meal reimbursement to schools with food stocks from the nation's agricultural surplus. The Commodity School Program is a critical supplement to help schools meet nutritional guidelines and maintain a reasonable cost. Commodities provide approximately 15% to 20% of the food items served. More than 180 products are available to schools that cover all 5 food groups.

Federal revenues to schools are counterbalanced by costs of production. Having already invested in the infrastructure, the most effective strategy for school food services to increase revenue is to have higher student participation in school meals. In the 2010 Child Nutrition Reauthorization, a supplementary $0.06 per meal was included to aid schools in supplying the additional fruits, vegetables, whole grains, and water that were mandated in the new FNS rule, although it is unlikely to fully address the additional funds needed. Although many districts have used lucrative a la carte and vended foods to provide added revenues, the most recent reauthorization gave USDA authority to establish standards for so-called "competitive foods," those sold outside the school meal program.

Nutritional Effectiveness of the School Meal Programs

Three iterations of the School Nutrition Dietary Assessment Studies (SNDA I, II, and III) have shown rapid progress toward school meals fulfilling the Dietary Guidelines for Americans (DGAs) recommendations. Compared with packed lunches, meals sought off-campus, or foods from vending or a la carte, school meals were far more nutritious. The school lunch program was not linked with rising obesity rates, and the School Breakfast Program was associated with a decreased risk. According to SNDA III findings, intakes of protein, vitamins A and B_{12}, riboflavin, calcium, phosphorus, potassium, and zinc were higher among NSLP participants than nonparticipants.

One measure of successful outreach is the ratio of school breakfasts to school lunches served. Of the 29 largest urban US school districts, only 2 exceeded 70%, whereas many enrolled as few as 30% to 40%. The USDA established "Community Eligibility" to address the issue. Individual or collective schools having a free and reduced meal population over 40% can qualify to provide free school meals to all children without individual student income verification (http://www.fns.usda.gov/school-meals/community-eligibility-provision). As a result, rates of meal participation have risen rapidly.

Perhaps the most difficult responsibility for food service managers is balancing the dual challenges of operating costs versus federal nutrition requirements. To assist school food service, software is made available to help with menu planning: the nutrient analysis method (nutrient standard menu planning and assisted nutrient standard menu planning for nutrients and energy) and the food-based menu method (traditional or enhanced menu planning for specific meal patterns). Previous standards did *not* specify levels of cholesterol, sodium, carbohydrate,

> School breakfast aims to provide 25% and school lunch 33% of a student's
> average nutrient needs balanced over the course of a week.

or dietary fiber, although over the past decade, school food service programs
across the United States have addressed these nutrients to a varying extent.
This methodology proved highly effective in improving the nutritional quality
of school meals on the basis of SNDA I, II, and III.

The Lunch and Breakfast Programs: As a result of steady improvements,
the NSLP has been shown to be one of the nation's most powerful nutrition
interventions. Nearly every public school (99%) in the country participates—
more than 100,000 schools. Of the 31 million lunches served daily, 49% are
provided free and another 10% are provided at reduced cost to children from
low-income families. Similarly, more than 10 million children per day—almost
one-quarter of all students—participated in the School Breakfast Program in
2007. More than 70% of breakfasts are provided free and another 10% are provided at a reduced price. Yet, this represents only one third of those participating
in the NSLP, a missed opportunity for raising nutrition quality.

Universal Breakfast: In the United States in 2007, nearly 70% of schools
offered some form of breakfast to students. Two-thirds of schools participated
in the USDA reimbursable School Breakfast Program, while 11.9% offered other
breakfast options to students. Many schools are starting to offer universal breakfast to take advantage of the benefits of this meal for all children. For districts with
a high population of eligible students, universal breakfast eliminates much of the
challenge of verification while offering schools a tremendous financial benefit.

School breakfast aims to provide 25% and school lunch 33% of a student's
average nutrient needs balanced over the course of a week.

Breakfast in the Classroom: Several national organizations, including the
School Nutrition Association, Food Research and Action Center and others,
are promoting breakfast in the classroom as a simple means to achieve highest
breakfast participation rates. School administrators often voice worries about
breakfast in the classroom, including:

- cuts into class time;
- transportation issues;
- personnel needs;
- children consuming double meals;
- supervision during breakfast; and
- infestations of the school.

All of these objections have been addressed successfully through a prepre-pared, grab-and-go format. Daily breakfast in the classroom offers substantial benefits, not only for diet quality, but also for many measures of psychosocial functioning, including:

- improved attentiveness for complex work in the late morning;
- improved cognitive function and testing, especially memory;
- lowered tardiness and absenteeism;
- fewer visits to the school nurse; and
- improved classroom behavior.

If just the 29 largest urban districts in the United States had achieved a 70% rate of breakfasts served to eligible children, an additional 595,000 children would have been fed daily and schools would have collected an additional $151 million in available federal dollars.

Of students eligible for free or reduced price meals at school, only 1 in 10 have access to USDA meal programs in summer and on holidays, making this a remarkable opportunity to address food insecurity and nutrition quality.

Challenges for School Food Service

The Individuals with Disabilities Education Act specifies that children with disabilities are to be provided with a free and appropriate public education to prepare them for future employment and independent living. As a result, schools, school nurses, and the school food service collaborate to develop policies and practices to address a variety of nutritional challenges:

- food allergy;
- celiac disease (gluten sensitivity);
- lactose intolerance;
- special diets for genetic or medical conditions;
- religious-based diets and lifestyle preferences; and
- vegetarian or vegan diets.

> Centers for Disease Control and Prevention data show that food allergies, especially more severe cases, are on the rise.

Food Allergies: The most prevalent of the specific dietary adjustments is for food allergies. In 90% of the nation's schools, more than one child in attendance has a food allergy. Half of these schools have experienced a child having allergic reaction. Food allergies are the most common cause for anaphylaxis, representing a sudden, potentially fatal, reaction. Only 8 foods account for 90% of all food allergies in children:

- egg;
- milk;
- soy;
- wheat;
- peanuts;
- tree nuts;
- fish; and
- shellfish.

Centers for Disease Control and Prevention data show that food allergies, especially more severe cases, are on the rise. The largest study found that 8% (5.9 million children) have food allergies, and of those, 30% have allergies to multiple foods and 39% had severe forms of reaction.

Anaphylactic or Fatal Reactions: In children, these usually are caused by peanut and tree nuts (eg, walnuts, cashews, etc), milk, and seafood. Anaphylaxis is most often seen among adolescents with established asthma. But in 25% of cases involving anaphylaxis in schools, no prior diagnosis of food allergy existed. Parents of children with severe food allergies have concerns about the potential for contact with allergic trigger foods, not only in school meals, but also in packed meals of other students. Although the food service staff is trained to deal with allergy by careful food handling techniques, the cafeteria environment is difficult to control because of packed lunches, food trading among students, and contaminated surfaces. Misconceptions about food allergy prevalence, definitions, and triggers are common. Among physicians, strategies offered for approaching food allergies differ widely, making uniform dietary strategies difficult to establish.

Avoidance is the first-line strategy for all food allergies.

Allergy Management: Allergy management involves:

- strict avoidance of the allergen/food;
- recognition of symptoms (intestinal, respiratory and neurologic);
- rapid administration of epinephrine; and
- a well-designed individualized health care plan (IHCP).

The routine of keeping food ingredient lists for a few days allows the school food service director to help identify new food allergies as they arise in their student population.

The IHCP: The school nurse will require documentation from the primary care physician as follows:

- a description of the allergic reactions;
- a list of the triggers and warning signals noted previously; and
- a history of past reactions, including anaphylactic reactions.

Allergy Avoidance: Few controlled trials on avoidance measures in schools and child care centers exist, but best practice guidelines are available:

- Skin contact and routine inhalation without heat vaporization do not induce systemic reactions.
- Cleaning of hands and surfaces with soap and water or commercial wipes is effective.
- Antibacterial gels alone are not effective.
- Although the concept of an "allergen-safe table" in the cafeteria may be important for some hypersensitive children, they do not need to be physically separated from their friends or other children (provided that the others at the table are eating safe foods).
- Within the classroom environment, blanket bans of offending allergens may be warranted (particularly for younger children with a high likelihood of incidental spread or ingestion).
- Eating bans on field trips and school buses also are important means of control.
- Education is the most effective way to prevent unforeseen allergic reactions.
- Avoidance is the first-line strategy for all food allergies.

Food Safety

Inspections: Schools participating in the federal school breakfast and lunch programs must obtain 2 inspections yearly, post the inspection report, and release a copy to the public on request. Inspection parameters include food handling, hand washing, equipment, food temperature, storage, and environment. A school foodborne infection outbreak is a significant event for the dietary staff and costly for school districts, resulting in disruption of food service, loss of participation in the school meal programs, and potential liability for medical expenses, attorney fees, increased insurance rates as well as additional training or equipment to rectify food safety practices.

> Between 1990 and 1999, there were only 292 foodborne outbreaks in schools involving 16,232 children and teenagers, a remarkably low rate compared with the general public. National statistics during this same time showed that the 7 most serious food pathogens caused 325,000 hospitalizations and 5000 deaths and cost as much as $34.9 billion annual in medical costs and lost productivity.

National Standards for Competitive Foods in Schools

Despite variations in the definition of an "empty calorie," studies in recent years have shown a consistency in the influence of snack foods and beverages on the overall diet quality of youth. For instance, 30% to 40% of daily energy consumed by 2- to 18-year-olds were in the form of empty calories—433 kcal came from solid fats and 365 kcal came from added sugars. More than half of empty calories can be attributed to just the following 6 foods, most consumed away from school campus:

- sweetened soft drinks;
- fruit drinks;
- dairy desserts;
- grain desserts;
- pizza; and
- full-fat milk.

Nearly 40% of kids reported snacking at school, the frequency of which was tied directly to the number of snack machines and the school's policy affording easy availability. Parents, students, and school staff are often sources, as well, through:

- snack bars;
- school stores;
- booster sales at sporting events;
- bake sales or fund-raisers;
- in-class parties; and
- foods offered as rewards.

New Standards: A committee of the Institute of Medicine (IOM) was formed to review all available research and present recommendations for school nutrition standards for competitive foods. The IOM report concluded that to achieve dietary stability for children and at the same time maintain a financial footing for the food service, competitive foods should be strictly tied with the DGAs. These recommendations formed the basis of the new standards issued by the FNS in June 2013 titled, "Smart Snacks in School" (view USDA presentation at: **http://www.fns.usda.gov/sites/default/files/SmartSnacks2014.pdf**).

Nutrition Standards in Preschool and Child Care

Along with the powerful Special Supplemental Nutrition Program for Women, Infant, and Children (WIC) program, child care settings outside the home offer the potential for optimal, balanced nutrition that could help to shape a child's preferences and habits. More than 60% of women with children younger than 6 years are employed, the majority full time, while 75% of children younger than 6 years spend some time in organized child care. Currently, there are approximately 120,000 child care centers but an estimated additional 2.5-fold more informal child care sites, which are far less easily influenced by local, state, or national policies.

Child care settings may offer one of the best opportunities for laying a foundation of quality nutrition and routine physical activity in early life.

CHILDREN OF WORKING MOTHERS UTILIZE MANY DIFFERENT TYPES OF CARE:

- Center-based (45%)
- Child care in another family's home (14%)
- With a parent (18%)
- With a relative (17%)
- With a nanny/babysitter (6%)

The Feeding Infants and Toddlers Study (FITS) showed that total energy intake at lunch was highest in child care (332 kcal) or away from home (308 kcal), compared with home (281 kcal).

National Guidelines: Guidance to shape the nutritional quality in child care is available. A self-assessment tool was developed and tested to improve nutrition and physical activity policy in child care sites. In a position statement on nutrition in child care settings, the Academy of Nutrition and Dietetics encouraged all child care programs to align their food offerings with the 2010 DGAs. The AAP has published comprehensive standards for nutrition and physical activity in child care.[1,2] These standards provide evidence-based best practices in nutrition, physical activity, and screen time for early care and education programs. They suggest 3 eating occasions (meals and snacks) for children in child care for 8 hours and 4 eating occasions for those staying longer, essentially providing energy every 2 to 3 hours. Also, the IOM recently published guidelines for child care settings that specifically targeted the issue of obesity:

- **Physical activity:** The committee recommended a variety of activities, indoor and outside, that blend developmentally appropriate moderate and vigorous activities throughout the day.
- **Nutrition:** The IOM directed child care providers to align with national policy, such as the Child and Adult Care Food Program and the Dietary Guidelines for Americans (DGAs). A variety of foods from the 5 food groups in age-appropriate portions should form the basis of school policy.
- **Sleep:** The committee recommended that regular sleep time be provided, depending on duration of care.
- **Screen time:** The committee recommended strictly limiting access to sedentary screen time during care.
- **Staff training:** Skill development for food planning was strongly recommended.

> Local school wellness policies have provided an unprecedented opportunity
> to mold the school environment in terms of nutrition and physical activity.
> Pediatricians looking to be involved in their own child's school should
> consider joining the school wellness council.

Child care settings may offer one of the best opportunities for laying a
foundation of quality nutrition and routine physical activity in early life.

Fundamental motor skills: National Association of Sport and Physical
Education guidelines advocate structured play to promote fundamental motor
skill development. Running, jumping, throwing, and kicking are the foundation
for developing more sophisticated motor activities. More than three quarters
of disadvantaged preschoolers showed deficits in fundamental motor skills,
particularly females. Motor skills deficits hamper engagement in activity
and directly correlate with preschool obesity.

How to Work With Schools

Wellness Advisory Committees and School Nutrition Policies

Professionals outside of the school system still can contribute to improved
nutrition and physical activity. One of the most wide-reaching clauses in the
Child Nutrition and WIC Reauthorization Act of 2004 was a simple directive:
all school districts participating in the NSLP must adopt and implement a
local wellness policy by the 2006-2007 school year.

A recent comprehensive study showed that nearly all students in the United
States were under a district wellness policy. However, individual school policies
range from strong and specific to ineffective and vague. Strengthening school
wellness policies and helping to design evaluations and plans for continuous
quality improvement was a primary target of the 2010 Child Nutrition Reauthorization. Wellness councils can be extraordinary opportunities for professionals
to help shape school policies and practices. One influential national organization
with chapters in every state is Action for Healthy Kids, which has many resources
to assist physicians, dietitians, and others who participate on wellness councils.

Local school wellness policies have provided an unprecedented opportunity
to mold the school environment in terms of nutrition and physical activity.
Pediatricians looking to be involved in their own child's school should
consider joining the school wellness council.

Recommendations for Pediatricians

Pediatricians can contribute to improving nutritional quality in schools in several ways. Nationally, the AAP and its Council on School Health contribute policy statements and advocacy positions that have helped to promote strong national school policies related to nutrition and activity. Through participation on school wellness councils, pediatricians can bring to schools a holistic view of child development, health, fitness, social-emotional growth, and nutrition. Even in daily practice, pediatricians can influence student and parental choices for meals, snacks, sports snacks, parties, and fund-raising sales that contribute substantially to the overall quality of food in school. Lastly, many physicians serve as medical directors, consultants, team physicians, and advisors to schools. The school nursing staff is the health care representative within the school and the natural allies for physician involvement.

In 2015, the American Academy of Pediatrics issued a policy statement titled "Snacks, Sweetened Beverages, Added Sugars, and Schools," which highlighted advances, challenges, and controversies concerning access to low-nutrient foods and drinks as well as how to use added sugars effectively to promote diet quality (**http://pediatrics.aappublications.org/content/ 135/3/575.full.pdf+html**).[3]

Recommendations for Program Directors and Trainees

Schools are complex systems that are able to offer students and residents a unique perspective on how we seek to optimize child health through policies, programs, practices, education, and measures. Although the school nurse is the appropriate link between health professionals and school children, the school's nutrition director is the best contact when looking into the complicated arena of school food. Review of school policies, compared with national "best practices," can be enlightening for trainees. The economics of school meals, the challenges of modifying competing sources of foods and drinks throughout the school, and limits placed on physical education and recess in favor of more classroom instructional time are all topics that trainees can experience. Examining the pros and cons of the many controversial issues surrounding nutrition in schools is an exercise that sharpens a student's sensitivity to the nuances of writing policies for schools.

Take-Home Points

- Obesity has focused medical, nutrition, and public health communities on the link between the American diet and health.
- In first years of life, the WIC program, in conjunction with child care and preschool policies, offer our best opportunities to ensure diet quality and help shape the food experiences of children.
- With 55 million children and teenagers attending more than 100,000 US schools, food policies and standards directly affect not only a student's health and well-being, but also his or her behavior and academic performance.
- Food in school is a complex mix of federally subsidized meal programs, vended, and a la carte options and an array of other food sources, including contributions from parents, staff, and students.
- The school food service produces safe, economical, and high-quality meals. Its work should be strongly supported by the health care community.
- National nutrition standards directing school meal programs have been shown to be effective in meeting the nutritional needs of US children, especially those at risk of food insecurity, which is a significant factor for poor academic performance.
- Community professionals can have a direct effect on local schools through participation on school wellness councils.

Resources

For additional school health related resources, visit www.aap.org/schoolhealthmanual.

References

1. Murray R. Nutrition in school, preschool, and child care. In, *Pediatric Nutrition*. Kleinman R, Greer F, eds. 7th edition. American Academy of Pediatrics. Elk Grove Village, IL, 2014:189–218
2. American Academy of Pediatrics, American Public Health Association, and National Resource Center for Health and Safety in Child Care and Early Education. 2012. *Preventing Childhood Obesity in Early Care and Education: Selected Standards from Caring for Our Children: National Health and Safety Performance Standards; Guidelines for Early Care and Education Programs*. 3rd ed. Elk Grove Village, IL: American Academy of Pediatrics; 2012. Available at: http://cfoc.nrckids.org/WebFiles/PreventingChildhoodObesity2nd.pdf
3. Murray R, Bhatia J, Policy Statement: Snacks, sweetened beverages, added sugars, and schools. Pediatrics, 2015; 135 (3):575–583. Accessed November 18, 2015

CHAPTER

8

Healthy and Safe Environment

SECTION 1
Emergency and Disaster Preparedness in Schools

Linda M. Grant, MD, MPH, FAAP
David J. Schonfeld, MD, FAAP

Background

Children spend a large part of their time in school as well as in before- and after-school activities. In many communities throughout the United States, more children are gathered on a daily basis in school settings than in any other location, highlighting the need to be prepared that an emergency could occur during school hours. Emergency preparedness in schools represents a spectrum, from management of individual medical or mental health emergencies to integrating school emergency strategies into the larger community disaster preparedness plans. There is a fundamental link between day-to-day emergency readiness and disaster preparedness. Schools that are well prepared for an emergency involving an individual student or staff member are more likely to be prepared for complex events such as community disasters. Children may experience medical emergency situations because of injuries, complications of chronic health conditions, psychological distress, or unexpected major illnesses

Although there are no federal laws requiring all school districts to have emergency-management plans, 32 states have reported having laws or other policies that do require plans. An estimated 95% of school districts reported that they have a plan, although there is great variability in these plans.[1]

that occur during school hours. This chapter focuses on the unique needs of children in relation to the preparation for, response to, and recovery from all hazards, including major disasters and individual medical emergencies.

- Annually, 67% of schools activate emergency medical services (EMS) systems for an emergency involving a student, and 37% activate EMS for an emergency involving an adult.
- Although there are no federal laws requiring all school districts to have emergency-management plans, 32 states have reported having laws or other policies that do require plans. An estimated 95% of school districts reported that they have a plan, although there is great variability in these plans.[1]

Stages of Emergency Management

There is no one ideal school crisis plan. Each district, as well as each school, has a unique set of parameters that affect emergency planning. However, the same stages in school emergency planning occur for each type of crisis, whether an individual emergency or a larger community crisis. All school-based emergency response plans should be based on the 4 phases of emergency management: prevention-mitigation, preparedness, response, and recovery.

- **Prevention/mitigation:** Identifying potential hazards and vulnerabilities, taking the steps to prevent their occurrence when possible, and reducing the potential damage they can cause.
- **Preparedness:** Collaborating with community partners to develop plans and protocols to prepare for the possibility that the identified hazards, vulnerabilities, or emergencies will occur.
- **Response:** Working closely with first responders and community partners to effectively contain and resolve an emergency in or around a school or campus.
- **Recovery:** Teaming with community partners to assist students and staff in the recovery process and to restore a healthy and safe learning environment following an event.

These are not 4 separate, distinct phases; instead, all phases are interrelated, with success in each phase enabling success in the other 3 phases, whether for an individual or larger-scale emergency.

KEY PRINCIPLES OF DEVELOPING SCHOOL EMERGENCY PREPAREDNESS	EXAMPLES OF CRISES
• Pediatricians play an important role in emergency and disaster preparedness and response. • Schools and districts should open the channels of communication well before a crisis. • Crisis plans should be developed in partnership with other community groups, including law enforcement, fire safety officials, public health, emergency medical services, and health and mental health professionals. • Schools should tailor district crisis plans to meet individual school needs. • Training and practice are essential for the successful implementation of crisis plans.	• Natural disasters • Severe weather • Fire or explosion • Chemical or hazardous materials exposure • Radiation exposure • Bus accident • School shootings • Individual medical emergencies • Student or staff deaths (accidental, natural, suicide, homicide) • Terrorism or war • Disease outbreaks

Prevention/Mitigation

Although schools cannot eliminate all hazards, the goal of mitigation is to anticipate and minimize the effect of the hazardous event and decrease the need for response (Table 8.1.1). An important first step is for the school or community to identify situations they could be facing on the basis of geography, community trends, school incident data, and other factors. The local emergency-planning infrastructure can work with schools to address local environmental hazards or vulnerabilities and provide resources for examining the school's risk potential. The schools can then translate this information into response protocols so that appropriate essential responses of schools and students can occur.

Preparedness

During the preparedness stage, the school district, as well as the individual schools in the district, identify school crisis teams and clearly delineate the roles that staff would play during emergencies. The school crisis teams work with community stakeholders involved in overall crisis planning. The school emergency plan must be integrated into the community plan (Table 8.1.2). For information about community preparedness plan awareness, refer to **http://www.ready.gov/community-and-other-plans**.

Emergencies can be either individual, involving one child or staff, or more global, involving large portions of the school and/or greater community. Good planning facilitates an effective, coordinated response when either type of emergency occurs.

Table 8.1.1. Examples of Prevention/Mitigation Measures

- **Violent threats**
  - Establishing access control procedures
  - Gang prevention, anti-bullying, and healthy school climate initiatives
  - Intruder management procedures
- **High number of students with asthma**
  - Maintaining good air quality
  - Integrated pest management
  - Use of "green" cleaners
- **Communicable disease**
- **Syndromic surveillance and monitoring absenteeism**
- **Respiratory hygiene and etiquette procedures**
- **Community threats (weather, geography, biological, terrorism)**
  - Tornado, hurricane, earthquake building standards such as window seals, building structures, and heating, ventilation, and air conditioning systems

Table 8.1.2. Specific Steps to Create a District School Emergency Plan[a,b,c]

Step 1. Plan regular meetings with school and community stakeholders.

Step 2. Perform a needs assessment.

Step 3. Conduct a structured interview with each school principal to customize plan to the individual school.

Step 4. Conduct a site survey of every school in the district.

Step 5. Create and plan education and training modules for the school staff.

Step 6. Create 2 documents—an all-hazards emergency response manual and a school-specific emergency response handbook.

Step 7. Create a timeline for accomplishing each of the tasks in the process.

Step 8. Inform parents of the plan.

Step 9. Implement the plan.

Step 10. Conduct practice drills.

Step 11. Reevaluate the plan annually, and revise if necessary.

[a]Chung S, Danielson J, Shannon M. School-based emergency preparedness: a national analysis and recommended protocol. AHRQ Publication No. 09-0013. Rockville, MD: Agency for Healthcare Research and Quality; January 2009.
[b]Schonfeld D, Lichtenstein R, Pruett MK, Speese-Linehan D. *How to Prepare for and Respond to a Crisis.* 2nd ed. Alexandria, VA: ASCD; 2002.
[c]American Academy of Pediatrics Enhancing Pediatric Partnerships to Promote Pandemic Preparedness Web site. https://www.aap.org/en-us/advocacy-and-policy/aap-health-initiatives/Children-and-Disasters/Pages/Enhancing-Pediatric-Partnerships-to-Promote-Pandemic-Preparedness.aspx. Accessed January 6, 2016.

Although EMS traditionally is thought of as emergency medical technicians (EMTs) and ambulances, it really encompasses prehospital through emergency department management. Therefore, in the event of a medical emergency within school jurisdiction, EMS include school nurses and school staff.

General Preparation of the School

- Create policies, regulations, and protocols to address emergencies and disasters in all school settings, from classroom to playground, school-based health centers (if available), before- and after-school programs, field trips, transportation, and athletic events.
- Include algorithms for determining levels of emergencies, distinguishing minor illnesses or injuries from emergencies that require EMS activation.
  - (Refer to Illinois Emergency Medical Services for Children manual **http://www.luhs.org/depts/emsc/schl_man.htm**.)
- Clarify EMS-activation process and Incident Command for all staff.
  - (Refer to Incident Command information, Federal Emergency Management Agency **https://training.fema.gov/is/nims.aspx**.)

Although EMS traditionally is thought of as emergency medical technicians (EMTs) and ambulances, it really encompasses prehospital through emergency department management. Therefore, in the event of a medical emergency within school jurisdiction, EMS include school nurses and school staff.

- Ensure that schools have a multidisciplinary, trained school crisis team that is ready to respond to individual and school-wide emergencies and disasters. Within the team, staff roles should be specified and team members should meet regularly and receive ongoing training.
- Pediatricians (or pediatric health care providers), including the school nurse and physician, should play a key role in developing and implementing the emergency plan.
- Maintain and update sufficient supplies and equipment.
- Clarify "in loco parentis" (in-the-absence-of-parents status) policies (eg, when staff accompanies child to the hospital).
- Inform parents of reunification plans should there be need to evacuate and relocate.

During the response, and not just during recovery, it is important to identify children who are having trouble coping and address any developing mental health concerns.

Children With Special Health Care Needs

Students and staff members with chronic medical conditions or other special health care needs are more apt to have medical emergencies and require schools to have a heightened sense of readiness, not only in day-to-day management but also in preparation for a more global emergency/disaster.

All students with a special medical or mental health need should have:

- An updated individualized health care plan (IHCP) prepared by the school nurse with input from the family and the primary care clinician. Using this information, the school can then plan for accommodations for daily classroom activities, field trips, and emergency needs of the student. The IHCP can assist school teams in developing individualized education programs (IEPs) or Section 504 plans. The IHCP contains information on:
  - Medications
  - Activity levels
  - Dietary needs
  - Equipment
  - Transportation needs (or assistance)
  - Disease-specific protocols (eg, diabetes, asthma action plans, etc)
  - Other accommodations
- Individual emergency care plans (ECPs) are summaries of key treatment and management points, which are developed from information in the IHCP. These plans accompany the student should hospital treatment be required and also provide management guidelines in the event of a community-wide disaster.
  - (Refer to Emergency Information Form for Children With Special Needs, developed by the AAP and the American College of Emergency Physicians at **http://www2.aap.org/advocacy/blankform.pdf**.)

Automated External Defibrillators and Cardiopulmonary Resuscitation

Increasingly, school districts are including training in cardiopulmonary resuscitation (CPR) and automated external defibrillator (AED) deployment as part of the pre-EMS emergency management preparation. Not only must this plan interface with the overall coordinated and practiced emergency planning, but for AED use, one must also consider appropriate medical oversight, device maintenance, and an ongoing quality improvement program to monitor training and response with each use of the device.

Response

The response phase is when the planning and preparation efforts are put to use to address an individual or more global emergency. The appropriate members of the school crisis team are activated and the crisis-specific plan is followed. The ideal response involves practiced collaboration with the community response team and use of the incident command system. In this response, school nurses, teachers, and other school staff become seamless parts of EMS.

During the response, and not just during recovery, it is important to identify children who are having trouble coping and address any developing mental health concerns.

Management of Individual Medical or Mental Health Emergencies

- Assess the situation and activate the appropriate protocol(s) and determine whether EMS needs to be activated.
- Communicate school entry points to EMTs and designate a greeter.
- When possible, other students and staff members are removed from the immediate scene.
- Accurately record events to pass on to the EMTs.
- For children with special health care needs, the ECP is activated and key information is provided to the EMTs.
- Inform parents, legal guardians, or designated emergency contacts.
- Record all events for later analysis of performance and trends.

Management of Large-Scale School Emergency

▪ *Lockouts or lockdowns* are called for when a crisis occurs outside of the school and an evacuation would be dangerous. A lockdown may also be called for when there is a crisis inside and movement within the school will put students in jeopardy. All exterior and classroom doors are locked and students and staff stay in their classrooms.

▪ *Evacuation and relocation* requires all students and staff to leave the building. The evacuation plan should include backup buildings to serve as emergency shelters and include contingencies for weather conditions, transportation, accommodations for children with special health care needs and strategies for accurately identifying children with limited verbal abilities.

▪ *Shelter-in-place* is used when there is not time to evacuate or when it may be harmful to leave the building. Students and staff are held in the building and windows and doors are sealed and HVAC systems are turned off when appropriate. There can be limited movement within the building.

(Refer to "Practical Information on Crisis Planning: A Guide for Schools and Communities" (**http://www2.ed.gov/admins/lead/safety/crisisplanning.html**.)

> Communication and messaging are important components of an effective strategic response during a disaster and, therefore, are a critical component of disaster preparedness.

Communication

Clear lines of communication are crucial to a successful response to a crisis. Communication and messaging are important components of an effective strategic response during a disaster and, therefore, are a critical component of disaster preparedness.

▪ For more global emergencies, emergency communication covers all technical means and modes for public safety agencies at all levels of government (eg, law enforcement, fire services, emergency medical services) to perform their routine, daily communications. Disaster emergency communications applies to those technical means and modes required to provide and maintain operable and interoperable communication before, during, and after presidentially declared emergencies, disasters, or planned national special security events.

▪ During the response, the community needs to be prepared for a surge of external media organizations that would be providing coverage of the event.

Recovery

From the school perspective, the goal of recovery from a disaster/crisis is to restore the school's infrastructure and return to learning as soon as possible. School recovery includes physical/structural recovery of buildings and physical assets, business recovery (underscoring the importance of a continuity of operations plan), restoration of academic learning, and attention to the emotional and psychological distress of students and staff. Whenever possible after a disaster, it is best to keep the school open or at least minimize the time that children are unable to attend school. A return to the structure of school can help children adjust to personal and community crisis events, ensure that they are adequately supervised by adults in a safe setting in the aftermath of the event, and provide a context for supportive services to be offered. Academic expectations may need to be modified for individual or all students in the immediate aftermath of the event, with the goal that students will be helped to return to full academic expectations as soon as practical. All staff should be helped to understand the common reactions of children to trauma and loss and ways to provide brief psychological first aid and supportive services and know when and how to identify children who might benefit from referral to additional services within the school and/or community.

Pediatricians can play an important role in emphasizing the importance of these services, providing training or technical assistance to schools, and assisting with ensuring that school-based services are aligned with community-based services (including those offered within the medical home). Assisting others in the school and community in recognizing symptoms of posttraumatic stress is an important role of the clinician. The medical community's collective sense of the emotional effects of a disaster can help guide schools and staff in their continuing interventions. Pediatricians also may participate in those interventions, which can include trauma and grief counseling. The responsibilities of the larger community are to support schools with the necessary mental health resources and to determine which therapies are best incorporated into the school setting (eg, school-based bereavement support groups or cognitive behavioral therapy in small groups that is intended for use in schools) and which might better remain based in the community.

Mental health concerns, although a key component of the recovery phase, should be addressed in all 4 stages of disaster management.

Children experience a range of personal crises and losses, such as the death of a family member. Five percent of children will experience the death of a parent by age 16; the vast majority of children will experience the death of someone close to them by the time they finish high school.

Action Steps for Recovery

- Attempt to keep schools open whenever possible.
- Schools and districts need to keep students, families, and the media informed.
- Ensure that recovery addresses the physical/structural elements, business and finances, and academic learning, in addition to emotional recovery. Provide assessment of emotional needs of staff, students, families, and responders.
- Provide stress management during class time.
- Regularly provide staff with updates about the recovery process and plans.
- Take as much time as needed for recovery.
- Remember anniversaries of crises.
- Evaluate recovery efforts.

(Refer to AAP Promoting Adjustment and Helping Children Cope After Disaster and Crisis Web site **https://www.aap.org/en-us/advocacy-and-policy/ aap-health-initiatives/Children-and-Disasters/Pages/Promoting-Adjustment- and-Helping-Children-Cope.aspx** and National Center for School Crisis and Bereavement **www.schoolcrisiscenter.org**.)

School facilities are often designated as disaster evacuation shelter sites. These venues provide shelter for many who have lost their homes as a result of disaster and also provide an opportunity for school officials to assess family and child needs. But if schools are acting as shelters or morgues, it may seriously undermine their availability for classroom instruction.

How to Work With Schools

School preparedness for an individual student medical emergency as well as a generalized community crisis heavily depends on a team effort that involves the school administration, the individual school health and safety team and its nurse and school medical advisor, the local community (EMS, local hospital/ emergency department, community mental health providers, public health officials, emergency planners, etc), and the students' medical home/primary care clinicians. The primary care provider gains membership on this team by maintaining a strong, open, and ongoing line of communication with the school nurse and/or the school physician (when available). The school and the school nurse depend on the medical home provider's knowledge of and recommendations for a child with special health care needs. To ensure that all children's unique needs are appropriately addressed in planning for all emergencies and disasters, pediatrician representation should be integrated throughout all federal, state, and local emergency and disaster planning activities. The pediatrician can be involved with the school district's school health advisory council and provide input on health-related policies that will affect the care of individual students, including school wellness policies and emergency plans.

Recommendations for Pediatricians

Pediatricians should participate in the development of their patients' individual emergency plans as well as become familiar with the disaster plan of the patients' schools, the school resources, and staffing. Even when a practice encompasses several school districts, the pediatrician can support families in being aware of their school's preparedness plans. For the individual child and his or her family, the medical home pediatrician can provide advice on issues that might affect the student's disease management and outcome, suggesting recommendations for IEPs and Section 504 plans. After a traumatic event, the pediatrician can assess the individual student, support school staff in more effectively managing the student's response to crisis and loss, promote a safe return to school and determine whether any additional evaluation or support is indicated.

In the larger disaster planning, community-based pediatricians can be the best advocates to help a school obtain needed life-saving emergency services and advocate for policies that prevent, mitigate, and prepare for all hazard eventualities. The pediatrician can help advise parents and caregivers to be aware of and contribute to emergency planning in the school and in the home.

Recommendations for Program Directors and Trainees

Trainees largely become involved with emergency preparedness during the emergency department rotations, but the focus is on the management of the individual emergency in a controlled medical environment. Because children are likely to be at school when they have a medical emergency or when a disaster occurs, program directors can acknowledge that schools have a role in the prehospital emergency hospital system. Trainees should understand that disaster-readiness efforts must include specific components to ensure appropriate care for children of all ages and all stages of development, including those with special health care needs, in various school settings.

Take-Home Points

- The likelihood that a medical emergency or community disaster will occur during school hours is high, so schools must be prepared for all eventualities and all hazards.

- The community pediatrician has knowledge and expertise to help schools prepare for emergencies and assist in linking school preparedness to the larger community preparedness efforts.

- Children with special health care needs not only need plans for day-to-day management but also individualized plans for school-wide emergencies involving shelter-in-place, lockdown, or evacuation.

- Learning, behavior, and relationships can be affected by crises that may include the death of family members, friends, or others who are important in a child's life. School personnel, with supports and training, can promote a child's coping and adjustment.[2,3]

- To ensure that children's unique needs are appropriately addressed in planning for all emergencies and disasters, pediatrician representation should be integrated throughout all federal, state, and local emergency and disaster planning activities.[4]

Resources

For additional school health related resources, visit www.aap.org/schoolhealthmanual.

References

1. United States Government Accountability Office. Emergency management. most school districts have developed emergency management plans, but would benefit from additional federal guidance. http://www.gao.gov/new.items/d07609.pdf. June 2007. Accessed January 6, 2016

2. Schonfeld DJ, Demaria T, American Academy of Pediatrics, Disaster Preparedness Advisory Council. Providing psychosocial support to children and families in the aftermath of disasters and crises. *Pediatrics*. 2015;136(4):e1120-e1130

3. American Academy of Pediatrics, Disaster Preparedness Advisory Council. Supporting the grieving child and family. *Pediatrics*. In press

4. American Academy of Pediatrics, Disaster Preparedness Advisory Council. Medical countermeasures for children in public health emergencies, disasters, or terrorism. *Pediatrics*. 2016;137(2):e20154273

SECTION 2

The School Environment

Robert J. Geller, MD, FAAP, FACMT
Yuri Okuizumi-Wu, MD, FAAP

Background

Many studies have shown that an appropriate school environment, including good physical facility conditions, is necessary for good learning. However, many school buildings in the United States are in need of repair.[1] In the National Center of Education Statistics survey of the conditions of public school facilities in the 2012-2013 school year, 53% of public schools needed to spend money on repairs, renovations, and modernizations to put the school's onsite buildings in good overall condition,[1] at an estimated cost of $197 billion. Because children are in schools for a large part of their day and they are still growing and developing, they are especially vulnerable to the effects of environmental hazards on their well-being.[2,3] This chapter focuses on some of the major factors of the physical environment in schools necessary to provide a healthy and safe place for all children to learn and grow.

The State of US Schools

According to records of the US Department of Education[1,4] and the US General Accounting Office,[5] the average age of a public school building in the United States is 42 years, and more than one third of all US schools need extensive renovations, repairs, and renovations. The amount of money that has been spent has been unequal across and within states as well as school districts, causing wide disparities between higher and lower socioeconomic areas and between white and minority groups. Many older school buildings do not have more recent features, such as temperature/sound controls or appropriate lighting. Major factors have contributed to inadequate conditions, including school districts' decisions to defer maintenance/repair work because of funding constraints, unfunded federal and state mandates, and shifting population patterns.[1]

Crowding and Class and School Size

Overcrowding is a common problem in many schools, especially in the inner city, and has been shown to negatively affect school performance.[6] Crowded conditions within a classroom as well as within the entire school may elicit negative behavior in children, such as aggressive/disruptive behavior, social withdrawal, poor social interaction, and decreased motivation.[7] These behaviors, in turn, may directly affect academic performance. In addition, overstimulation stemming from overcrowding can result in attention overload or cognitive fatigue, both of which can lead to difficulties in students' abilities to concentrate on their schoolwork. Often, a child may "daydream" to tune out unwanted stimulation, ask to go to the bathroom to obtain some privacy, or need extended break times to escape overstimulation, all of which take away from learning time. Children with conditions such as attention-deficit/hyperactivity disorder (ADHD) or autism spectrum disorders may be especially sensitive to overcrowding.

Class size can also affect academic performance. In Tennessee, the Project STAR (Student Teacher Achievement Ratio) study on class size and academic achievement analyzed the school performance of over 12,000 students. These researchers found that children in a class size of 13 to 17 students outperformed students in classes with 22 to 26 students with and without a teacher's aide, especially in inner-city schools with minority students.[8]

Teachers may be negatively affected by overcrowding as well. Poor facilities, including overcrowding, have been shown to affect teacher performance and effectiveness and, therefore, also affect student performance.[9] Overcrowding also makes keeping classroom order a significant challenge for teachers and can lead to quicker burnout.

Another potential negative effect of overcrowding in classes pertains to carbon dioxide levels in the classroom. Carbon dioxide levels in a room are directly related to the number of occupants, unless the ventilation system maintains sufficient ventilation to prevent an increase in carbon dioxide levels. Carbon dioxide levels above the recommended target of 500 ppm have been shown to result in decreased decision-making ability and, if elevated further, to drowsiness in the students, consequently decreasing their ability to learn.[10,11]

In addition, there have been studies showing a positive relationship between smaller school size and academic achievement. Smaller schools (high schools with less than 500 students, elementary schools with 100-200 students), tend to have higher academic achievement, especially for low-income, inner-city students.[12,13] Other studies have shown that the rates of vandalism and other serious student misconduct is less in smaller schools.[14] A smaller school may allow students to feel an increased sense of belonging and encourage feelings of personal responsibility and cooperation that may improve learning and academic achievement.[11]

Achieving the optimal school and classroom size is a challenge in many overcrowded school districts. Some methods to overcome these issues may be to design facilities that can be divided into smaller units, with features such as a separate entrance that allows students and staff to feel as though they are part of a smaller school. Furniture can be arranged differently to alleviate crowded conditions and give a sense of more personal space (ie, small clusters of chairs as opposed to rows of chairs, reduced classroom clutter and noise to alleviate over-stimulation). Students can also be given a choice of a "personal space" in the classroom for such activities such as reading, or be allowed to choose the desk in the location of their choice to decrease the effects overcrowding may have on them.

Lighting

Because children depend heavily on light in their learning process, the lighting quality in the school should be optimal. In addition to affecting our ability to see, good lighting also improves our mood and general well-being, increases energy efficiency, and decreases crime and vandalism.

In 1999, the Hechong Mahone Group (HMG), a consulting group that designs energy-efficient buildings, conducted a definitive analysis of classroom daylighting (diffuse sunlight) conditions in more than 2000 classrooms. They showed that the students with the most daylighting progressed 20% faster on math tests and 26% in reading tests over 1 year than those with the least daylighting. Furthermore, students in classrooms where windows could be opened to provide natural ventilation had a 7% to 18% faster educational progress than those with fixed windows.[15] In addition, the HMG Group showed that if a view is available out of a window, students also performed better on tests of mental function and memory recall. Problems with lighting, such as glare from direct sunlight or fluorescent light, unbalanced or insufficient lighting, or even noisy sounds from the lighting system have been found to negatively affect vision and learning. Flicker from fluorescent lighting can cause headaches and stress or even trigger seizures in people with photosensitive epilepsy.

The Illuminating Engineering Society of North America, the organization that sets industry standards and recommendations for lighting, recommends not only lighting above a desk but also the illumination of walls and other vertical surfaces and the overall balance of light in an area.[16] Lighting design in schools should be flexible, with low-glare lighting that incorporates natural light from windows and skylights integrated with electric lighting. It should also be energy-efficient, allow for manual control of settings and seasonal adjustments, and require little maintenance. Light-emitting diode lighting is preferred to maximize both lighting quality and energy efficiency.

Noise

The main factors that affect classroom acoustics are reverberation, ambient (background) noise levels, signal-to-noise ratio, and the pitch and loudness of speech. Reverberation time measures the amount of echo in a room and is the amount of time it takes for a sound/noise to decay to 60 dB once the sound has been turned off. It can be affected by the shape/size of a room, the amount of sound-absorbing material in the room, and the number of people in the room. Ambient noise can be from within the school/classroom, such as fluorescent lighting or heating/cooling systems, or noise from adjacent rooms or outside the school, such as from nearby airports, train tracks, or highways. The signal-to-noise ratio is the difference in decibels between the teacher's voice and the background noise. The American National Standards Institute's acoustical guidelines for schools (ANSI 2010) recommend maximum 0.6 to 0.7 seconds of reverberation time (depending on classroom size), a maximum ambient classroom noise level of 35 dBA, and signal-to-noise ratio of 15 to 20 dB to optimize speech understanding and learning.[17]

Noisy classrooms are extremely common. In 2002, researchers in Ohio evaluated the extent of the problem of noise and reverberation in schools and measured reverberation times and background noise levels in 32 different unoccupied elementary classrooms in 8 public school buildings. Results indicated that most classrooms were not in compliance with American National Standards Institute (ANSI) noise and reverberation standards.[18]

Noise can affect learning in many ways. Besides directly affecting how students can hear their teacher, it can affect their academic achievement through effects on attention, memory, and motivation, as well as on levels of stress directly affecting their health, such as elevated blood pressure and heart rate. Multiple studies have shown that there is a negative relationship between noise levels and student behavioral and performance variables. For example, in a well-regarded study in New York City, 2nd through 6th graders facing a noisy elevated train track had reading scores 3 to 11 months behind those students on the quieter side of the school.[19] Another study, which analyzed aircraft noise exposures in schools near airports in the Netherlands, Spain, and United Kingdom, showed a linear association with aircraft noise exposure and impaired reading comprehension.[20] Students whose first language is not English, hearing impaired students, or those with attention problems or developmental disabilities (ADHD, autism spectrum disorders) experience even more challenges in navigating a noisy school environment.

Classroom noise can also affect teacher well-being and effectiveness. If a teacher has to talk louder because of poor classroom acoustics, the strain on his or her voice increases significantly. Teachers lose valuable instruction time when they are required to repeat instructions or their lessons are interrupted because of noise.

Lastly, although noise in the classroom can affect learning most, noise in other areas of the school building, such as hallways, gymnasiums, cafeteria, and music practice rooms can also contribute to an overall noisy learning environment.

To control noise in the classroom and school, building designers need to anticipate all sources of noise and minimize the effects[21] by carefully considering the function of the room, building materials, mechanical systems, the use of sound-absorbing material, and location of classrooms with more noisy areas (eg, cafeterias, gymnasiums). In addition, methods to decrease noise in the classroom can include the use of voice amplification systems, visual aides to reinforce oral lessons, seating arrangements to accommodate learning in small groups, and scheduling of noisy activities (music practice) during nonpeak learning times.

Temperature and Humidity

Room temperature, humidity, and air movement affect the thermal comfort of the school environment.

Temperature has been shown to affect performance in the workplace as well as schools. Harner's analysis of research studying thermal temperature in schools showed that reading and mathematics skills were negatively affected by classroom temperatures higher than 74°F and that the optimal temperature for learning is between 68°F and 74°F.[22] Optimal temperatures in the school also depend on how a particular room is being used; for instance, a gymnasium requires lower temperatures because of the level of physical activity and/or the type of clothing typically worn, typically different from that of the classroom.

Besides the surrounding outdoor humidity, increased humidity can result from malfunctioning heating, ventilation, and air conditioning equipment, leaks, kitchens, humidifiers, damp carpets, and bathrooms. Optimal air humidity is 40% to 60%. When humidity consistently increases to more than 50%, particularly in warm environments, mold is more likely to grow. Asthma exacerbations, allergic reactions, or other respiratory problems are associated with exposure to mold.[23,24] Lower humidity can decrease the incidence of upper respiratory infections but can also cause erosion of paper or textiles, which can increase dust and other particulate matter in the air.

Indoor Air Quality

Air movement affects more than thermal comfort and humidity. Air movement controls ventilation so that odors are diluted, airborne pollutants (eg, dust, smoke, volatile organic compounds) are reduced, and humidity is controlled. Air movement is usually delivered by mechanical systems that may also heat/cool/dehumidify an area but may also be achieved by natural ventilation, such as open windows.

Adequate air exchange is vital to maintaining the health of students, staff, and visitors alike. Appropriate ventilation can mitigate or prevent the consequences of carbon dioxide accumulation and the use of various volatile substances that occurs regularly within the school (such as cleaning, photocopying, use of erasable white-board markers, for example). Ventilation systems should meet or exceed the minimum standards for airflow and fresh air intake, as specified by the most recent update of ASHRAE Standard 62.1, which has also been adopted by the ANSI.

The quality of air intake must be maintained, as well. Intake of air containing vehicular exhaust fumes from nearby idling vehicles is unsuitable for health. Air containing exhaust from nearby industrial plants obviously is also unsuitable. Care must be taken to locate fresh air intakes in suitable locations and to ensure that these locations remain appropriate for fresh air intake.

Vehicular idling policies should be established and enforced, to prevent accumulation of vehicular exhaust in the vicinity of any building entrances or locations frequented by students. Such vehicular idling policies must apply to all vehicles, including school vehicles and those used by vendors, parents, staff, and visitors alike.

Schools should also be tested for radon levels. Radon is emitted from underground sources on a natural basis and is more likely to be elevated in areas with granite bedrock. Radon accumulation in a building can lead to an increase in the long-term risk of lung cancer. Where elevated indoor radon levels are found, they can be effectively lowered by a combination of covering entry points and/or creating ventilation below the foundation of the building that exhausts the radon outdoors, a process often referred to as "sub-slab ventilation." This is a relatively inexpensive intervention that is essential to protecting student and staff long-term well-being. The US map of radon zones, available from the US Environmental Protection Agency (EPA) Web site at **http://www.epa. gov/sites/production/files/2015-07/documents/zonemapcolor.pdf**, should not be substituted for testing each school facility for radon at least once.

Chemical Safety

School settings pose a risk of injury from chemicals in use, in storage, and in transit. Some chemicals used in chemistry laboratories are strong acids or strong bases, and others pose risks from their irritant potential. Chemicals should be stored only in secure storage areas, carefully separating chemicals with the potential to adversely interact with one another if a leak or spill occurs. Chemical storage areas ideally should have controlled ventilation, which exhausts air from that area directly to the outdoors without reintroducing it into the general school air circulation. The selection of chemicals for inclusion in a school should take the potential hazards of each chemical into mind during the selection process.

Periodically, each school should reexamine its chemicals on site and safely dispose of those no longer needed or with containers that are damaged or leaking. The US EPA and many state environment agencies can assist with this assessment and disposal of school chemicals, using resources such as the US EPA Chemical Cleanout program.

Elemental mercury continues to be a frequent exposure, often from mercury brought into the school by a student. Best practice calls for complete elimination of elemental mercury from the school setting and prohibiting students and teachers from bringing it onto school vehicles and school property.

Chemical exposure in school settings also occurs from materials used for interior painting, furnishing, and cleaning. Low- or zero-volatile organic compound paints and interiors are preferred to optimize indoor air quality in school buildings. Furniture, flooring, and other interior materials lacking chemicals of concern, including formaldehyde, halogenated flame retardants, perfluorinated compounds, and polyvinyl chloride, are preferred. An integrated pest management plan should be developed to minimize the use of toxic chemical pesticides. Finally, unscented products are preferred, including unscented plain soap and water for hand hygiene.

Cleaning Chemicals

Some children may be more sensitive than others to inhaling or touching the residue of chemicals using in cleaning or maintenance. The selection of chemicals should consider not only the effectiveness of the product in its intended use and its price, but should also assess the potential for affecting students and staff during use and during the drying period. Best practices call for floor maintenance (including buffing and waxing) to occur outside of classroom hours and preferably allowing drying time overnight before school occupancy the following morning. Chemical-free floor maintenance practices should be considered and preferred.

Current best practice calls for using cleaning products with the least environmental effects that also retain appropriate cleaning properties. Additional details are discussed in the EPA "Design for the Environment" program.

Several independent organizations evaluate cleaning products and assess their environmental effects and cleaning performance. Cleaning chemicals that are "GreenSeal" or "EcoLogo" certified are preferred. For many applications, chemical-free products, such as unscented soap and water or dilute white vinegar, are preferred.

Facility Safety

Certain features within the school building may pose special concerns. Bathrooms, for example, must be readily accessible to students, staff, and visitors during all times the school is occupied. Bathrooms should have appropriate toilets for the size of the potential occupants, as well as any individuals needing accommodation under the Americans with Disabilities Act. They should constantly be stocked with toilet paper and soap and should have both warm and cold running water. Privacy in bathrooms must be balanced against an increased risk of mischief or assault in a hidden space; an optimal choice requires continuous monitoring or keeping the space open by use of entries that provide barrier-free access without compromising privacy.[2]

School environments may inadvertently pose an unnecessary risk of injury on school grounds.[25] Inadequate path or stair lighting contributes to an increased risk of tripping or falling, leading to injury.

Renovation activities are common in school settings. Ideally, these should take place outside of class time, either during breaks between sessions or over weekends or holidays. Because this is not always possible, areas under renovation should be placed off-limits to students, and staff not directly involved in the renovation. Dust and debris generated in the work area should be contained and prevented from entering the general ventilation of the school.

Failure to exclude students and staff from areas under renovation also can contribute to avoidable trip and fall injuries, and exposures to the fumes, dust, possible asbestos, and other toxicants often generated during construction activities. Best practices call for the development of a safety plan before the onset of renovation that addresses areas of potential impact, including dust and debris, noise, emergency egress, and traffic flow. A multidisciplinary committee should monitor the effectiveness of the plan and have the authority to implement any changes needed to address concerns that may develop.

The risk of injury at school can be mitigated by carefully designed policies and effective implementation of these policies. Safety policies should include preestablished evacuation procedures and lockdown procedures and the circumstances that should lead to these. Effective communication within the school and its outdoor spaces should be tested at least annually, ensuring that all individuals within the school's perimeter will be alerted when necessary. Evacuation and lockdown should be practiced by each class at the beginning of each school year, at a minimum.

Administrative staff should be trained in the decision processes created to respond to emergencies. At least one administrator able to lead an emergency response should be on site at all times that the school is occupied.

Sports Facilities

Sports facilities within the school boundaries also should be assessed to minimize injury potential. Surfaces should be relatively level, without sudden dips in the terrain posing trip hazards. Protruding obstacles in walk and play areas should be eliminated whenever possible, and if not able to be eliminated, should be well-marked and set off from the usual path and play areas.

The decision between using natural turf and artificial turf on sports fields is complex, involving at least considerations about local climate considerations, cost, and athlete safety. If natural turf is chosen, the maintenance of the natural turf should be carried out in consideration of the likelihood of skin contact by children with the turf. Therefore, fertilizer, herbicide, and insecticide use should be used only when necessary and well-marked immediately after application. Children should be excluded from the treated areas until the application has completely dried and preferably until the treatment has been absorbed into the turf. The product applicator and the chemical manufacturer can assist in providing specific guidance on the appropriate timeline.

Artificial turf has evolved since its introduction into the marketplace more than 4 decades ago. Various studies of the relative injury risk of playing on artificial turf as compared with natural turf most often show an increased risk of joint injuries while playing on artificial turf, although some studies have arrived at opposite conclusions.[26-30] These varying results may be confounded by use of difficult footwear designs and artificial turf products of differing age and design.

Studies of the environmental health effects of the recycled materials incorporated into artificial turf suggest that they account for less than 0.1% of the overall risk of cancer or other adverse effects.[31,32]

Playgrounds

Playgrounds are another site of injury risk. Best practices call for the use of impact-absorbing materials below climbing apparatus. Avoidance of sharp edges on all play devices is essential. All equipment should be frequently checked for proper function, and devices repaired or removed as appropriate if they are not in proper working order.

Play settings that maintain natural features may be more interesting and further stimulate the extent of vigorous activity as well as children's learning and creativity, as compared with a play space using only manufactured equipment in a sterile, paved area.[33,34] More vigorous play activity can reduce the risk of elevated childhood body mass index.[35] Play in natural settings can mitigate symptoms of ADHD,[36] anxiety, and depression[37,38] as well as contribute to offset the effects of environmental health disparities on children living in such adverse circumstances.[39] Boring play spaces that do not challenge children's creativity have been associated with higher injury risk in some studies.[33]

Injuries at Play

Playground injuries are a leading cause of injury to elementary and junior high students ages 5 to 14 years while at school.[33] On the basis of published studies, the US Office of Technology Assessment concluded[25] that the most common settings for unintentional school injuries were playgrounds, gymnasiums, and athletic fields. As described in Table 8.2.1 and Table 8.2.2, injuries associated with playgrounds were the most prevalent and accounted for 30% to 45% of unintentional school injuries. Falls, thus, present the greatest risk to children using playground equipment and account for a disproportionate number of severe injuries.

Efforts specifically targeted at reducing playground deaths should emphasize 3 areas: appropriate clothing without protruding cords, adherence to the Consumer Product Safety Commission guidelines regarding playground equipment and the surfaces below the equipment, and good maintenance of equipment.[33]

Table 8.2.1. Playground Injury Data[a]

- Injuries associated with playgrounds accounted for 30% to 45% of all unintentional school injuries.
- 205,850 playground-equipment injuries were treated in US hospital emergency departments during the year November 1998-October 1999 (National Electronic Injury Surveillance System).
- Playground equipment at school was associated with 45% of these injuries.
- Of injuries occurring on playgrounds, 72% involved only 1 child.
- A fall was the mechanism of injury in 79% of these school playground injuries.

Table 8.2.2. Playground Injuries by Injury Type[a]

Injury	Percentage of Total	Comments
Fracture(s)	39%	80% involved elbow, lower arm, or wrist
Laceration(s)	22%	
Contusion(s)/abrasion(s)	20%	
Strain(s)/sprain(s)	11%	

[a]Geller RJ, Rubin IL, Nodvin JT, Teague WG, Frumkin H. Safe and healthy school environments. *Pediatr Clin North Am.* 2007;54(2):351-373.

Ergonomics for Students and Staff

Ergonomics is the science that studies equipment design to maximize productivity by reducing fatigue and discomfort. It strives to provide "a good fit" between a person and the equipment he or she uses and the tasks he or she performs. Recently, increased attention has been placed on improving ergonomics in the school setting to optimize learning as well as to provide a safe, healthy environment for students.[40]

Furniture, especially seating, tables, and desks, is especially important as most students spend the majority of their time at school in a sitting position. Furniture should allow for differences in the anthropometrics of students and be available in various sizes or be adjustable as much as possible. Students should be encouraged to take regular stretch breaks and avoid sitting in the same position for prolonged periods of time. As computer use in the classroom is increasing, similar considerations need to be taken into account for the computer working stations. Frequent breaks should also be taken to minimize eyestrain and to prevent musculoskeletal disorders such as carpal tunnel syndrome.

School bags, including backpacks, computer bags, and athletic bags, are another major area of concern in school ergonomics. The American Academy of Pediatrics (AAP) recommends using bags with wide, padded straps and that both straps are used together. The AAP also recommends limiting the weight to no more than 10% to 20% of the child's body weight. Rolling bags may be a good option for some students, but the need to lift them up and down stairs or through uneven surfaces (snow) should be considered.[41]

Ergonomics for the school staff is also important to consider, because classrooms are often built for smaller-sized students and require teachers to squat, stoop, and bend frequently. Teachers have recently been receiving more training in ergonomics as well, and as they begin practicing what they learn, they may be able to better serve as role models of good ergonomic practices for their students.

Educating students and parents about the importance of ergonomics is also important so that healthy habits are carried out beyond school, at home. Resources, such as Cornell University's Ergonomics at School Guide and the United Kingdom-based Institute of Ergonomics and Human Factors, provide useful, practical information.

Animal Safety

Animals are often kept in school as "class pets." They are also used in science laboratories and as service animals or are visitors to the school. Although they can provide valuable opportunities for learning, there is a risk of injury or illness to students as well as the animal itself. The time and resources needed to properly care for the animal must be carefully considered. Younger students who may still have developing immune systems and may also be more likely to insert their hands or other items into their mouths, are especially at risk of contracting a zoonotic illness, most commonly *Salmonella* infection, *Escherichia coli* O157:H7 infection, and others that cause vomiting, diarrhea, fever, and abdominal cramping. There have also been cases of infectious outbreaks from animal products, such as owl pellets, for dissection. The Centers for Disease Control and Prevention general guidelines to reduce the risk of illness include[42]:

- Always wash hands after handling animals, their food, and/or their habitats. Also always wash hands after using the bathroom, before eating/drinking, before preparing food/drinks, and after removing soiled clothes or shoes. Wash hands as soon as possible at these times.

- Adults should always supervise hand washing in young children.
- Running water and soap are best. Use hand sanitizers if running water and soap are not available.
- Never allow young children to put their hands or objects in their mouth while interacting with animals.
- Adults should supervise human-animal contact, especially with children younger than 5 years.
- Avoid inherently dangerous animals, nonhuman primates (monkeys), mammals at high risk of transmitting rabies (bats), aggressive/unpredictable wild/domestic animals, stray animals with unknown vaccination history, venomous or toxin-producing spiders, insects, reptiles, and amphibians.
- Animals that should not be allowed in schools and child care centers with children younger than 5 years include reptiles, amphibians, live poultry, and ferrets.

In the school setting, there may be students who are immunocompromised because of conditions such as sickle cell disease, diabetes, HIV/AIDS, chemotherapy, or chronic steroid use. Some children may also be affected by allergies and asthma associated with certain animals, most commonly cats and dogs. Pest infestation is a problem in some schools; mouse and cockroach allergens have been found to be even higher than in homes in some communities.[43] Interestingly, a recent study in Baltimore found that mouse allergen is more strongly and consistently associated with poor asthma outcome than cockroach allergens.[44] Schools should adopt a school integrated pest management program to minimize use of pesticides while still maintaining an environment appropriately free of pests (see **http://www2.epa.gov/managing-pests-schools**).

Children with pet allergies may not need direct contact with the specific animal but may react to other students bringing allergens of their pets at home to school. These children may also take these allergens back to their home from school and be symptomatic at home as well.[45]

Another issue concerning animals in schools involves the issue of the rights of students with disabilities. The Individuals with Disabilities Education Act (IDEA) was enacted to allow children with disabilities free, appropriate public education designed to meet their unique educational needs. Conditions considered to be disabilities within IDEA most commonly include intellectual disabilities, speech/language impairment, and hearing or visual impairments, but also include "other health impairments," such as severe allergies. Thus, a visually impaired student has the right to have a service animal at school, but at the same time, the student with severe allergies to animals has a right to be in an animal-free setting. Accommodating both students within the same school could pose a significant challenge.

Relocatable Classrooms/Portables

In some areas of the United States, particularly urban areas, rapid student population growth and decreasing school budgets have made the use of relocatable classrooms, or "portables," increasingly common to alleviate problems with limited space and overcrowding. Many portables are also used as temporary classrooms while older schools are being renovated. The physical conditions of these structures need to be at the same standards as those of the main school building, as discussed previously, but this is often not the case. In California, in 2004, issues most prevalent in portable classrooms at several hundred schools in the state included[46]: inadequate ventilation, excessive classroom noise, poor thermal comfort, moisture problems, and inadequate lighting. In addition, many portables had high indoor formaldehyde levels from the widely used formaldehyde-containing building material/furnishings and inadequate ventilation. Investigators also found lead, arsenic, and pesticide residues in the floor dust, most likely that were tracked in from dirt outside and pesticides used inside or around the building.[22] Potential problems need to identified early and proactively and then be addressed in a timely manner to prevent serious harm to students.

Recommendations for Pediatricians

When assessing a patient's well-being, it is important for pediatricians to inquire about academic performance but also about how school conditions may be related to their health and school performance. When a child, or especially multiple children, complain about symptoms such as headaches, respiratory symptoms, or eye/nose/skin irritation when at school, on the playground, or at times when the school is undergoing renovation, it is important for the pediatrician to consider something in the school environment as a cause of these symptoms. It may be helpful to contact the school nurse or even other pediatricians in the community for more information.

Pediatricians can become involved to optimize their patients' school environment by working as a consultant to the school, providing in-service training of school staff on relevant health topics, directly communicating with schools on a specific student's medical condition, or advocating for patients through activities such as being members of school advisory councils and school boards.

Pediatricians can also emphasize how environmentally responsible schools can be great models of sustainability and provide teaching opportunities to engage students as well as the surrounding community.

Although experience in environmental health may be helpful, there are many excellent resources for pediatric health care providers without that background to advocate and improve the conditions of the schools.

Pediatric environmental health specialty units are a network of experts across the United States, Canada, and Mexico that are dedicated to increasing knowledge about environmental factors affecting children by providing education/training to pediatricians, primary care physicians, and other health professionals as well as parents, teachers, and community groups so that environmental risks that lead to ill health can be mitigated or prevented. They also work with federal, state, and local agencies to address children's environmental health issues in homes, schools, and communities.

Recommendations for Program Directors and Trainees

Although children are more vulnerable to the effects of toxins in the environment, there has been little emphasis on environmental health, especially school environmental health, in pediatric training programs.

The *Training Manual on Pediatric Environmental Health: Putting It Into Practice* has been designed by the Children's Environmental Health Network specifically to assist program directors in incorporating pediatric environmental health into their teaching program. Modules include case studies, discussion questions, and suggested assignments that can be used to teach pediatric environmental health to students, residents, or colleagues and are available online. Reference texts may be useful sources of additional information.[2] If a rotation solely in environmental health is not possible, combining experience in a school setting with other rotations such as community health may be practical. Learning how the environment plays such a significant role in a child's health, academic performance, and general well-being can be useful in all areas of pediatrics and should be encouraged for all trainees.

The school environment can be an excellent training field for public health students majoring in environmental health. Pediatric residents should always be acutely aware of how the environment can affect their patients. Because children spend a great portion of their day at school, the effects of the school environment should be considered in addition to any factors in the home. Within the school environment, there are many factors that need to be considered. Pediatric residents should understand the great opportunity available to them throughout their career to remediate conditions negatively affecting their patients' health and how their efforts could improve their patients' chances of academic success. Students may not always have a strong voice in improving conditions at their school, but pediatricians can and should be strong advocates for students' safety and well-being. The school environment could be an excellent area of exploration for a pediatric resident who is looking for a quality-improvement project to work on during his or her residency training. This allows meeting the competencies of practice-based learning and improvement and systems-based practice.

Take-Home Points

- Children spend a large majority of their time daily at school. Thus, the quality of the physical environment of their school can greatly impact their health as well as their academic success.
- Factors affecting the quality of the school environment, which include school/class size, lighting, noise control, temperature/humidity, and air quality, are suboptimal in many US schools.
- Assessments of school performance and the school environment of patients can provide pediatricians with valuable information about a child's health and should be routinely performed at all well-child visits for school-aged children and adolescents.
- The pediatrician should encourage school authorities to adopt a comprehensive, holistic school environmental health program. This program should address all of the issues discussed in this chapter. A model guideline for school leaders to use is available from the EPA.
- Pediatricians have many opportunities to influence and improve the quality of their community's school environment. These may include serving as consultants to the school or on school advisory councils/boards, providing health training to school staff, and communicating with the school on a specific child's medical condition.
- The pediatrician can affect the child's school performance, if the school environment is interfering with his or her school performance, by advocating for improving the school's environment as a whole or at least for the student's placement in a classroom with a better environment.

> **Resources**
>
> For additional school health related resources, visit www.aap.org/ schoolhealthmanual.

References

1. Alexander D, Lewis L. *Condition of America's Public School Facilities: 2012–13* (NCES-2014-022). US Department of Education. Washington, DC: National Center for Education Statistics. Available at: http://nces.ed.gov/pubs2014/2014022.pdf. Accessed April 13, 2015

2. Frumkin H, Geller RJ, Rubin IL, eds. *Safe and Healthy School Environments*. New York, NY: Oxford University Press; 2006

3. Geller RJ, Rubin IL, Nodvin JT, Teague W.G, Frumkin H. Safe and healthy school environments. *Pediatr Clin North Am.* 2007;54(2):351–373

4. Lewis L, Snow K, Farris E, et al. *Condition of America's Public School Facilities: 1999* (NCES 2000-032). Washington, DC: US Department of Education, National Center for Education Statistics; 2000. Available at: http://nces.ed.gov/surveys/frss/publications/ 2000032/. Accessed April 13, 2015

5. US General Accounting Office. *School Facilities: Condition of America's Schools 1995.* Washington, DC: Health, Education, and Human Services Division; 1995. Available at: www.gao.gov/products/HEHS-95-61. Accessed April 13, 2015

6. Evans GW, Saegert S, Harris R. Residential density and psychological health among children in low-income families. *Environ Behav.* 2001;33(2):165–180

7. Maxwell LE. Crowding, class size and school size. In: Frumkin H, Geller RJ, Rubin IL, Nodvin J, eds. *Safe and Healthy School Environments*. New York, NY: Oxford University Press; 2006:13–19

8. Finn JD, Achilles CM. Tennessee's class size study: findings, implications, misconceptions. *Educational Evaluation and Policy Analysis.* 1999;21(2):97–109

9. Earthman GI. *School Facility Conditions and Student Academic Achievement.* Williams Watch Series: Investigating the Claims of Williams v. State of California. Los Angeles, CA: UCLA Institute for Democracy, Education, and Access; October 2002. Available at: http://escholarship.org/uc/item/5sw56439. Accessed April 13, 2015

10. Satish U, Mendell MJ, Shekhar K, et al. Is CO_2 an indoor pollutant? Direct effects of low-to-moderate CO_2 concentrations on human decision-making performance. *Environ Health Perspect.* 2012;120(12):1671–1677

11. Tillett T. Don't hold your breath: indoor CO_2 exposure and impaired decision making. *Environ Health Perspect.* 2012;120(12):A475

12. Summers AA, Wolfe BL. Do schools make a difference? *American Economic Review.* 1977;67:639–652

13. Fowler WJ. What Do We Know About School Size? What Should We Know? Paper presented at: Annual Meeting of the American Educational Research Association; San Francisco, CA; April 20-24, 1992

14. Garbarino J. Some thoughts on school size and its effects on adolescent development. *J Youth Adolesc.* 1980;9:19–31

15. HMG (Heschong Mahone Group). Daylighting in Schools: An Investigation Into the Relationship Between Daylighting and Human Performance. HMG Project No. 9803. San Francisco: Pacific Gas and Electric, on behalf of the California Board for Energy Efficiency Third Party Program; 1999

16. Illuminating Engineering Society of North America. *Guide for Educational Facilities Lighting*. Document No. IESNA RP-3-00. New York: Illuminating Engineering Society of North America; May 19, 2000

17. ANSI (American National Standards Institute). *Acoustical Performance Criteria, Design Requirements, and Guidelines for Schools*. Melville, NY: Acoustical Society of America; 2002

18. Knecht HA, Nelson PB, Whitelaw GM, Feth LL. Background noise levels and reverberation times in unoccupied classrooms: predictions and measurements. *Am J Audiol.* 2002;11(2):65–71

19. Bonzcraft AL, McCarthy DP. The effect of elevated train noise on reading ability. *Environ Behav.* 1975;7(4):517–527

20. Clark C, Martin R, van Kempen E, et al. Exposure-effect relations between aircraft and road traffic noise exposure at school and reading comprehension: the RANCH project. *Am J Epidemiol.* 2006;163(1):27–37

21. Technical Committee on Architectural Acoustics of the Acoustical Society of America. Classroom Acoustics - A Resource for Creating Learning Environments With Desirable Listening Conditions. Melville, NY: Acoustical Society of America; August 2000

22. Harner DP. Effects of thermal environment on learning skills. *CEFP Journal.* 1974;29(4):25–30

23. Sahakian NM, White SK, Park JH, Cox-Ganser JM, Kreiss K. Identification of mold and dampness-associated respiratory morbidity in 2 schools: comparison of questionnaire survey responses to national data. *J Sch Health.* 2008;78(1):32–37

24. Borràs-Santos A, Jacobs JH, Täubel M, et al. Dampness and mould in schools and respiratory symptoms in children: the HITEA study. *Occup Environ Med.* 2013;70(10):681–687

25. U.S. Congress, Office of Technology Assessment, *Risks to Students in School*, OTA-ENV-633. Washington, DC: U.S. Government Printing Office, September 1995.\ http://ota.fas.org/reports/9538.pdf. Accessed November 19, 2015.

26. Drakos MC, Taylor SA, Frabicant PD, Haleem AM. Synthetic playing surfaces and athlete health. *J Am Acad Orthop Surg.* 2013;21(5):293–302

27. Ekstrand J, Hagglund M, Fuller CW. Comparison of injuries sustained on artificial turf and grass by male and female elite football players. *Scand J Med Sci Sports.* 2011;21(6):824–832

28. Iacovelli JN, Yang J, Thomas G, et al. The effect of field condition and shoe type on lower extremity injuries in American Football. *Br J Sports Med.* 2013;47(12):789–793

29. Dragoo JL, Braun HJ, Harris AH. The effect of playing surface on the incidence of ACL injuries in National Collegiate Athletic Association American Football. *Knee.* 2013;20(3):191–195

30. Meyers MC. Incidence, mechanisms, and severity of match-related collegiate women's soccer injuries on FieldTurf and natural grass surfaces. *Am J Sports Med.* 2013;41(10):2409–2420

31. Schiliro T, Traversi D, Degan R, et al. Artificial turf football fields: environmental and mutagenicity assessment. *Arch Environ Contam Toxicol.* 2013;64(1):1–11

32. Ruffino B, Fiore S, Zanetti MC. Environmental–sanitary risk analysis procedure applied to artificial turf sports fields. *Environ Sci Pollut Res.* 2013;20(7):4980–4992

33. Moore R. Playgrounds: a 150 year-old model. In: Frumkin H, Geller RJ, Rubin IL, eds. *Safe and Healthy School Environments*. New York, NY: Oxford University Press; 2006:86–103

34. Dyment JE, Bell AC. Grounds for movement: green school grounds as sites for promoting physical activity. *Health Educ Res.* 2008;23(6):952–962

35. Bell JF, Wilson JS, Liu GC. Neighborhood greenness and 2-year changes in body mass index of children and youth. *Am J Prev Med.* 2008;35(6):547–533

36. Maas J, Verheij RA, de Vries S, et al. Morbidity is related to a green living environment. *J Epidemiol Community Health.* 2009;63(12):967–973

37. Taylor AF, Kuo FE, Sullivan WC. Coping with ADD: the surprising connection to green play settings. *Environ Behav.* 2001;33(1):54–77

38. Rao A, Ross CL. Health impact assessment and healthy schools. *J Planning Educ Res.* 2014;34(2):141–152

39. Mitchell R, Popham F. Effect of exposure to natural environment on health inequalities: an observational population study. *Lancet.* 2008;372(9650):1655–1660

40. Legg S, Bennett C. *Ergonomics in Schools.* New York: Taylor and Francis; 2007

41. Backpack Safety. HealthyChildren.org Web site. Available at: http://www.healthychildren.org/English/safety-prevention/at-play/Pages/Backpack-Safety.aspx. Accessed April 13, 2015

42. Centers for Disease Control and Prevention. Animals in Schools and Daycare Settings. Available at: http://www.cdc.gov/Features/AnimalsInSchools/. Accessed April 13, 2015

43. Permaul P, Hoffman E, Fu C, et al. Allergens in urban schools and homes of children with asthma. *Pediatr Allergy Immunol.* 2012;23(6):543–549

44. Ahluwalia SK, Peng RD, Breysse PN, et al. Mouse allergen is the major allergen of public health relevance in Baltimore City. *J Allergy Clin Immunol.* 2013;132(4): 830–835

45. Epstein BL. Childhood asthma and indoor allergens: the classroom may be a culprit. *J Sch Nurs.* 2001;17(5):253–257

46. California Air Resources Board, California Environmental Protection Agency, California Department of Health Services. *Environmental Health Conditions in California's Portable Classrooms.* November 2004. Available at: http://www.arb.ca.gov/research/indoor/pcs/leg_rpt/leg_rpt.htm. Accessed April 13, 2015

School Climate

Susan P. Limber, PhD, MA, MLS
CAPT Stephanie Bryn, MPH
Weijun Wang, PhD, MA

Background

Educators have long recognized the importance of school climate,[1] but it wasn't until the 1950s that researchers began to systematically study the phenomenon. Since this time, research has increased dramatically on the nature of school climate, differences in perceptions of school climate among students and adults within a school setting, and implications of school climate for students' well-being, safety, and academic success.[2] In this chapter, this literature is reviewed, efforts and resources to improve school climate are described, and recommendations for pediatricians are provided.

> School climate generally refers to the quality and character of school life[1,2] and involves the social, emotional, and academic experiences of students, their family members, and school personnel.

What Is School Climate?

Although there is no single universally agreed-on definition, school climate generally refers to the quality and character of school life[1,2] and involves the social, emotional, and academic experiences of students, their family members, and school personnel. Although practitioners and educators have used various terms to describe school climate (such as atmosphere, culture, tone, setting, and milieu), there is agreement that school climate is more than an individual experience. It is a group phenomenon—the collective beliefs, values, and attitudes that prevail at school.[2-4] Researchers also agree that school climate is a multidimensional construct that includes interpersonal, organizational, and instructional elements.[5] Cohen et al[1] highlight 4 essential dimensions of school climate:

 a. Safety (including clear and consistent rules, the extent to which individuals feel physically safe, attitudes about violence and bullying);
 b. Teaching and learning (such as the quality of instruction, the extent to which social-emotional and academic learning are valued, whether professional development is systematic and ongoing);
 c. Relationships (including respect for diversity, a sense of connectedness among members of the school community, a pattern of positive relationships between and among students, educators, and families); and
 d. Environmental (including cleanliness, order, and appeal of the facilities; adequate resources).[6]

Individual Characteristics Related to Perceptions of School Climate

Researchers have observed that some individual characteristics are related to students' perceptions of school climate. Many have found that *student age* is negatively associated with students' positive perceptions of school climate and that declines are particularly noteworthy and concerning in the middle school grades.[7] For example, Wang et al[8] followed 677 students from 6th through 8th grades and found that the percentage of boys and girls who perceived a positive school climate decreased throughout the middle school years. Similarly, Way and colleagues[7] found that students' ratings of 4 specific dimensions of school climate (teacher support, peer support, student autonomy in the classroom, and clarity and consistency of school rules) decreased significantly throughout the middle school years. Research that has focused specifically on school connectedness has also documented that as students age, they feel less attached to school.[9,10] Parents of younger children are also more satisfied with the school climate than are the parents of older students.[11]

Others have examined *gender difference* in students' reports of school climate. On many dimensions, it appears that girls have more positive perceptions of school climate than boys.[3,10,12] For example, girls have been found to report more consistency and fairness among school rules,[7,12,13] have a higher sense of relatedness with teachers,[14] feel greater belonging to school,[15] and perceive more support from teachers[7,13,16,17] and support from peers[7] than boys. Others have suggested that there may be interactions between age and gender on dimensions of school climate, such as school connectedness. For example, whereas girls have been found to report greater school attachment in middle schools, boys have reported greater attachment and connectedness than girls in high school.[18]

Researchers have also examined the relationship between students' perceptions of school climate and socioeconomic status (SES) and related variables such as parental education and single-parent family status.[7,13,19] Fan and colleagues[13] found that students with more highly educated parents tended to have more positive perceptions of school order, safety, and discipline and feel more connected to school. Way et al[7] also observed that students of lower SES perceived that school rules were less clear and consistent than did students of higher SES; they also indicated that they felt less peer support. On the other hand, students of lower SES reported higher levels of teacher support.

Although there is evidence that students of racial minorities generally perceive less positive school climate than white students,[3,12,19] it also is clear that students from different racial or ethnic groups appear to perceive different aspects of school climate in different ways.[13,20] For example, Fan et al[13] found that Hispanic and Asian students had less positive perceptions of school order, safety, and discipline than students of other races, and students who were Hawaiian, Native American, multiracial, or of other races reported less positive perceptions of the teacher-student relationship.

Research has also indicated that students who experience chronic illness, mental illness or learning disability may hold more negative perceptions of school climate.[21-23] For example, students with emotional disturbance and mild intellectual disability reported less closeness with teachers, compared with students without disabilities or with other disabilities.[21] Those with emotional disturbance also indicated that they felt less connected to their schools and felt more dissatisfied with relationships with their teachers.[21]

> Students and teachers may perceive school climate somewhat differently.

Researchers have also found that students who are at risk of being marginalized because they are bullied by peers or because of their real or perceived sexual orientation have poorer perceptions of school climate. Bullying involves unwanted aggressive behavior that involves an observed or perceived imbalance in power and is often repeated over time.[24] Bullying behaviors may include oral or written communication, such as taunting, teasing, or verbal threats; physical force, such as shoving or tripping; or relational bullying, such as rumor-spreading, social isolation, and various forms of cyberbullying, such as posting derogatory comments or pictures online.[24] Students who are bullied by peers (physically, verbally, or relationally) report lower school connectedness than nonbullied students.[25] Bullied students (particularly those who are bullied and also bully others) are also significantly more likely to indicate that they dislike school.[26] Youth who identify themselves as lesbian, gay, bisexual, or transgender (LGBT), those who may be questioning their sexuality, or those who may be perceived as LGBT may experience significant bullying by their peers[27-29] and report negative school climate.[30] For example, in a survey of 8584 US students 13 to 20 years of age who identified themselves as LGBT or who were questioning their sexual identity, 92% had been verbally harassed in the last year, 21% had been assaulted at school, 64% had been sexually harassed at school, 90% felt deliberately excluded or left out by other students, and 32% indicated that they missed at least 1 day of school in the previous month because they felt unsafe or uncomfortable.[30]

A variety of academic and behavioral factors related to students' perceptions of school climate have been investigated. In a large-scale national survey of students in the United States, researchers found that students who were held back a grade and those who had behavior problems at school had less positive perceptions of teacher-student relationships.[13] Having behavior problems at school and having siblings who dropped out of high school were negatively related to students' perceptions of school order, safety, and discipline.[13] Others have found that students who get higher grades, do not skip school, and take part in extracurricular activities are more attached to school.[9]

School-Level and Classroom-Level Factors Related to School Climate

In addition to the individual-level factors that are related to students' perceptions of school climate, researchers have also examined school-level factors that are associated with school climate, including school size,[9,13,31,32] school sector (eg, private vs public),[33] student mobility,[3,12] student-teacher ratio,[12,30] and staff turnover.[3] Findings regarding school size have been mixed, with some researchers finding that larger enrollments are negatively associated with aspects of school climate[3,9] and others finding no such relationships.[13,33] Findings are also not clear with regard to private versus public school students' perceptions of school climate. Some researchers have found that students perceive a more positive school climate in private versus public schools,[13] while others have reported no difference in private versus public school students' perceptions of a sense of community within the school.[33] Research suggests that a high student-teacher ratio[12], high principal turnover,[3] and high student mobility[12] are negatively related to students' positive perceptions of school climate.

Although relatively little research has focused on the relationship between classroom-level factors and students' perceptions of school climate, having a high percentage of students in a class who are disruptive is associated with more negative perceptions of school climate.[3,12] Interactions between class size and teacher experience have also been found with regard to students' perceptions of aspects of school climate. Students in larger classes with more experienced teachers viewed the school environment as less safe than students in smaller classes with experienced teachers, but students in larger classes with less experienced teachers perceived the school environment as more safe than those in smaller classes with less experienced teachers.[3]

School climate is significantly related to various aspects of students' academic well-being.[1] For example, researchers[34-36] have found that school connectedness is associated with students' academic self-efficacy, task orientation, mastery,[35] educational aspirations,[36] intrinsic motivation, grades, test scores,[34,35] school drop-out,[36] and school attendance.

Students' and Adults' Perceptions of School Climate

There is evidence that students and teachers may perceive school climate somewhat differently. For example, in their study of fifth grade students and teachers, Mitchell and colleagues[12] found that teachers' perceptions of school climate were more influenced by classroom-level factors, such as poor classroom management and the proportion of students with disruptive behavior, and that students' perceptions of school climate were more influenced by school-level factors, such as the percentage of students who move in and out of the school within a school year, student-teacher ratio, and a change in the principal. These findings suggest that efforts to improve perceptions of school climate may need to focus on somewhat different issues for teachers (eg, training to improve classroom management) versus students (eg, reducing the student-teacher ratio or reducing turnover of principals).

Relationship Between School Climate and Student Well-Being, Safety, and Academic Success

Students' perceptions of school climate are related to their academic outcomes, emotional well-being, and engagement in risky and violent behavior.

Academics

School climate is significantly related to various aspects of students' academic well-being.[1] For example, researchers[34-36] have found that school connectedness is associated with students' academic self-efficacy, task orientation, mastery,[35] educational aspirations,[36] intrinsic motivation, grades, test scores,[34,35] school drop-out,[36] and school attendance. Research has also indicated that children who are bullied at school are more likely than nonbullied peers to want to avoid going to school and have somewhat lower academic achievement.[37] Recent longitudinal research has suggested a causal relationship between being bullied and later academic challenges (see Table 8.3.1 for a listing of academic, social, and mental health consequences of bullying).

Table 8.3.1. The Effects of Bullying on Children and Youth

Children and youth who are bullied are more likely than non-bullied peers to develop:
• Depression[a,b]
• Anxiety[c]
• Panic disorder[c]
• Psychosomatic problems (headaches, stomach pain, sleep problems, poor appetite)[d]
• School avoidance and lower academic achievement[e]
• Problems with alcohol and other drugs[f]

• Children who bully others are more likely than nonbullying peers to:
  – Become involved in later antisocial and criminal behavior[g,h,i]
  – Sexually harass others[j]

[a] Ttofi MM, Farrington DP, Lösel F, Loeber R. Do the victims of school bullies tend to become depressed later in life? A systematic review and meta-analysis of longitudinal studies. *J Aggression Conflict Peace Res.*2011;3(2):63–73

[b] Faris R Felmlee D. Status struggles: network centrality and gender segregation in same- and cross-gender aggression. *Am Sociol Rev.* 2011;76(1):48–73

[c] Copeland WE, Wolke D, Angold A, Costello EJ. Adult psychiatric outcomes of bullying and being bullied by peers in childhood and adolescence. *JAMA Psychiatry.* 2013;70(4):419–426

[d] Gini G, Pozzoli T. Bullied children and psychosomatic problems: a meta-analysis. *Pediatrics.* 2013;132(4):720–729

[e] Buhs ES, Ladd GW, Herald-Brown SL. Victimization and exclusion: links to peer rejection, classroom engagement, and achievement. In: Jimerson SR, Swearer SM, Espelage DL, eds. *The Handbook of School Bullying: An International Perspective.* New York, NY: Routledge. 2010:163–172

[f] Institute of Medicine and National Research Council. *Building Capacity to Reduce Bullying: Workshop Summary.* Washington, DC: The National Academies Press; 2014

[g] Olweus D. *Bullying at School: What We Know and What We Can Do.* New York, NY: Blackwell; 1993

[h] Sourander A, Jensen P, Rönning JA, et al. Childhood bullies and victims and their risk of criminality in late adolescence: the Finnish From a Boy to a Man study. *Arch Pediatr Adolesc Med.* 2007;161(6):546–552

[i] Ttofi MM, Farrington DP, Lösel F, Loeber R. The predictive efficiency of school bullying versus later offending: a systematic/meta-analysis of longitudinal studies. *Crim Behav Ment Health.* 2011;21(2):80–89

[j] Espelage DL, Basile KC, Hamburger ME. Bullying perpetration and subsequent sexual violence perpetration among middle school students. *J Adolesc Health.* 2012;50(1):60–65

Social and Emotional Competence

Students' experiences of school as a place of community are also positively related to areas of social and emotional competence. For example, adolescents' sense of community in school is positively related to self-efficacy (ie, an individual's confidence that he or she will be able to solve a problem or achieve a goal).[38,39] School connectedness also positively affects boys' levels of empathy and ability to take perspectives of others.[40]

Mental Health

Research has found that ratings of school climate by students are positively related to life satisfaction[41] and negatively related to emotional distress, depression, and suicidality.[2,41-44] For example, in a study of high school students, Suldo and colleagues[41] found that students' perceptions of 6 dimensions of school climate (sharing of resources, order and discipline, parent involvement, school building appearance, student interpersonal relations, and student-teacher relations) accounted for 15% to 22% of the variance in indicators of their mental health (as measured by ratings of global life satisfaction and internalizing problems, such as anxiety, somatic complaints, and depression). Parent involvement was the most consistent predictor of students' mental health. More negative perceptions of peer interpersonal relations, sharing of school resources, and physical appearance of the school building predicted more internalizing problems among the students. School climate was more highly associated with girls' mental health than boys' mental health.

Other researchers have also highlighted the relationship between school connectedness and aspects of students' mental health. Studies indicate that students who feel that they belong and are bonded to one's school are less likely to experience emotional distress, suicidality, eating disorders, and depression.[36,43-46] Longitudinal research suggests that school connectedness may serve a protective function against low mood.[43]

Finally, children who are bullied at school are more likely than other children to suffer from low self-esteem, loneliness, anxiety and depression.[47,48] Bullied students also are more likely than their peers to have high levels of suicidal thoughts and to have attempted suicide.[48-51] As illustrated in Table 8.3.1, being bullied is also associated with the development of later mental health problems such as depression, anxiety, panic disorder, and psychosomatic disorders.

> Students who feel that they belong and are bonded to one's school are less likely to experience emotional distress, suicidality, eating disorders, and depression.[36,43-46]

Antisocial, Delinquent, and High-Risk Behaviors

Not only are students' perceptions of school climate related to their mental health, but they also have been found to be associated with the likelihood of their engagement in aggressive, delinquent, antisocial, and high-risk behavior. In fact, The Institute of Medicine[52] noted that "in some situations, a healthful psychosocial environment [at school] may be as important—or even more important—than classroom health education in keeping students away from drugs, alcohol, violence, risky sexual behavior, and the rest of today's social morbidities."[9] For example, researchers have found that aspects of school climate (such as having fair rules and respect for other students) are related to current misconduct and offending[32,53] and they also predict future behavior problems (such as theft, weapon-carrying, skipping school).[8]

Connectedness to school appears to be particularly related to antisocial and high-risk behavior. Students who feel less connected to school are more likely to engage in delinquency, substance use, violent behavior, and early sexual activity; experience unintentional injury; and become pregnant.[9,36,54-57]

Efforts to Promote Positive School Climate

Given the significant effects that school climate can have on the well-being of children and youth, researchers, educators, and policy makers have highlighted the need to support efforts to promote positive school climate. A comprehensive review of such efforts is beyond the scope of this chapter, but several examples are provided.

Standards for Promoting Positive School Climate

The National School Climate Center,[58] with support from a number of educational, mental health, and other national organizations, established 5 standards that support positive school climate:

❶ Develop a shared vision and plan for promoting, enhancing, and sustaining a positive school climate.

❷ Develop policies that promote social, emotional, ethical, civic, and intellectual learning as well as systems that address barriers to learning.

❸ Advance practices that promote the learning and positive social, emotional, ethical, and civic development of students and student engagement as well as addressing barriers to learning.

❹ Create an environment where all members are welcomed, supported, and feel safe in school: socially, emotionally, intellectually, and physically.

❺ Develop meaningful and engaging practices, activities and norms that promote social and civic responsibilities and a commitment to social justice.

Promoting Positive Relationships: Improving School Connectedness

Others have focused on development of research-based efforts to promote specific aspects of school climate. For example, the Centers for Disease Control and Prevention[36] outlined 6 strategies to increase the extent to which students feel connected to school:

❶ Create decision-making processes to facilitate student, family, and community engagement; academic achievement; and staff empowerment.

❷ Promote education and opportunities to enable families to be actively involved in their children's academic and school life.

❸ Provide students with the academic, emotional, and social skills necessary to be actively engaged in school.

❹ Use effective classroom management and teaching methods to foster a positive learning environment.

❺ Provide professional development and support for teachers and other school staff to enable them to meet the diverse cognitive, emotional, and social needs of children and adolescents.

❻ Create trusting and caring relationships that promote open communication among administrators, teachers, staff, students, families, and communities.

Promoting Students' Perceptions of Safety: Best Practices in Bullying Prevention and Response

Recognizing the effects that bullying can have on students and the broader school climate, the Federal Partners in Bullying Prevention[59] have amassed online information and tools to help prevent and address bullying (including cyberbullying). Included in these resources is a description of 10 principles of best practices in prevention of bullying and effective responses to bullying:

❶ Focus on the social climate.

❷ Conduct community-wide bullying assessments.

❸ Seek out support for bullying prevention.

❹ Coordinate and integrate prevention efforts.

❺ Provide training in bullying prevention and response.

❻ Set policies and rules that address bullying.

❼ Increase adult supervision.

⑧ Respond consistently and appropriately when bullying happens.
⑨ Spend time talking with children and youth about bullying.
⑩ Continue efforts over time.

How to Work With Schools

There are several ways that pediatricians can be resources to their local schools to improve school climate.

■ **Talk with school leaders** (building-level principals, superintendents, and school board members). Many schools are concerned with promoting a positive school climate and currently implement bullying or violence prevention programs, programs to address online safety and civility, and initiatives to promote students' social and emotional learning or increase students' connectedness to school. Administrators and school personnel often welcome engagement in and support of these efforts by community leaders. Other schools without such initiatives could benefit from pediatricians' expertise (eg, knowledge about child development, effects of bullying on children and youth) and advocacy to promote initiatives to promote a healthy school climate.[60]

■ **Talk to parent-teacher associations/organizations.** Talk to leaders in parent organizations and offer to provide resources for family members about factors that affect school climate (such as bullying, violence, school connectedness, and social and emotional learning), and community-based counseling and treatment resources.

■ **Engage children and youth** in discussions about bullying, violence, and youth safety at school, online, and in the community; encourage youth-led dialogue and support groups.

Recommendations for Pediatricians

Consistent with the recommendations of the American Academy of Pediatrics Committee on Injury, Violence, and Poison Prevention in its policy statement "Role of the Pediatrician in Youth Violence Prevention,"[61] (**http://pediatrics. aappublications.org/content/124/1/393**) there are several domains in which pediatricians can use their skills and influence to improve school climate and the well-being of school-aged children and youth: (1) clinical practice, (2) advocacy, (3) education, and (4) research.

Clinical Practice

Promote early detection of potential problems and effective intervention.

- During wellness examinations and patient visits, ask screening questions, such as:
  - *How is school going?*
  - *How many good friends do you have?*
  - *Do you ever feel afraid to go to school? Why?*
  - *Do other kids ever bully or tease you at school, in your neighborhood, or online? Who? When and where does it happen? What do they say or do?*[60]

- Gently probe about possible problems at school if a child exhibits signs of school phobia, attention problems, or psychosomatic conditions or if a child has risk factors for involvement in violence or bullying. Pay particular attention to special populations (eg, children with disabilities; those who have special health needs; children who are obese; those who are LGBT or who are questioning their sexual identity) who are at high risk of being bullied, being the victim of violence at school, or of experiencing social or academic difficulties.[60]

- Maintain an accurate database of community-based counseling and treatment resources.[61]

- Provide appropriate and timely treatment and/or referral for violence-related problems, difficulties relating with peers or adults at school, and other areas of concern.

- Provide resource materials to parents on bullying, violence, school connectedness, online safety and civility, and other factors that affect students' well-being at school and beyond.

Advocacy

Join with colleagues to advocate for:

- Adequate community-based behavioral health services[61] and funding for school-based mental health professionals.

- Increased awareness on the part of policy makers, administrators, school personnel, and family members about the importance of school climate to the well-being of children and youth.

- Increased awareness of parents, and children about bullying, violence, and other factors that affect school climate.

- Implementation of evidence-based school policies, programs and practices that improve school climate by improving: safety, the quality of instruction, social and emotional learning, school connectedness, student-teacher relationships, peer relations, and the physical environment of the school.
- Content related to youth violence/bullying prevention in electronic health records, including screen prompts and links to educational materials for parents.[61]

Education

Pediatricians should take advantage of every opportunity to learn more about issues such as online and in-person bullying, violence, and other factors that affect school climate and child well-being and educate others through:

- Continuing medical education or professional development opportunities;
- Coursework or rotation work in medical school or postgraduate training; and
- Assessment of community resources for children, youth, and families.[61]

Research

Pediatricians can promote needed research by:

- Participating in and advocating for research on youth violence, bullying, school connectedness and other aspects of school climate, and for evaluations of efforts to improve school climate; and
- Contributing data to existing injury surveillance systems.

Recommendations for Program Directors and Trainees

Recognizing the importance of increasing pediatricians' understanding of factors that affect school climate and the importance of school climate for the academic, physical, and emotional well-being of children and youth, program directors are encouraged to provide opportunities for trainees to learn more about issues such as bullying, violence, and other factors that affect school climate and child well-being in their coursework or rotation work. Discussions about these issues may be integrated into the residency didactic curriculum, continuity clinic experience, community experiences, and developmental-behavioral rotation activities. Systems-based practice and/or advocacy or community-based projects are opportunities for individual residents to focus on school climate.

Take-Home Points

■ School climate refers to the quality and character of school life and involves the social, emotional, and academic experiences of students, their family members, and school personnel.

■ Key dimensions of school climate include: (1) safety (eg, clear and consistent rules, perceptions of safety, experiences with bullying and violence); (2) teaching and learning (eg, the extent to which social-emotional and academic learning are valued); (3) relationships (eg, a sense of connectedness among members of the school community); and (4) environment (eg, cleanliness and order, adequate resources).

■ Individual characteristics (such as age, gender, socioeconomic status, race or ethnicity, LGBT status, academic and behavioral problems, or presence of chronic illness, mental illness or learning disability) as well as school-level and classroom-level factors have been found to be related to students' perceptions of school climate.

■ Students' perceptions of school climate are related to their academic well-being, social and emotional competence, mental health, and engagement in antisocial and delinquent and high-risk behaviors.

■ Federal and national organizations have developed standards to support positive school climate, strategies to increase student connectedness to school, and best practices in bullying prevention.

■ Pediatricians can work to improve school climate and the well-being of school-aged children and youth through their clinical practice, advocacy efforts, educational opportunities, and research.

Resources

For additional school health related resources, visit www.aap.org/schoolhealthmanual.

References

1. Cohen J, McCabe L, Michelli NM, Pickeral T. School climate: Research, policy, practice, and teacher education. *The Teachers College Record.* 2009;111(1):180–213
2. Cohen J. Transforming school climate: Educational and psychoanalytic perspectives. *Schools: Studies in Education.* 2009;6(1):99–103
3. Koth CW, Bradshaw CP, Leaf PJ. A multilevel study of predictors of student perceptions of school climate: The effect of classroom-level factors. *Journal of Educational Psychology.* 2008;100(1):96–104

4. Modin B, Östberg V. School climate and psychosomatic health: A multilevel analysis. *School Effectiveness and School Improvement.* 2009;20(4):433–455
5. Loukas A, Suzuki R, Horton KD. Examining school connectedness as a mediator of school climate effects. *J Res Adolesc.* 2006;16(3):491–502
6. The National School Climate Center. School climate: what is school climate and why is it important? http://www.schoolclimate.org/climate/. Accessed April 16, 2015
7. Way N, Reddy R, Rhodes J. Students' perceptions of school climate during the middle school years: association with trajectories of psychological and behavioral adjustment. *Am J Community Psychol.* 2007;40(3–4):194–213
8. Wang MT, Selman RL, Dishion TJ, Stormshak EA. A tobit regression analysis of the covariation between middle school students' perceived school climate and behavioral problems. *J Res Adolesc.* 2010;20(2):274–286
9. McNeely CA, Nonnemaker JM, Blum RW. Promoting school connectedness: Evidence from the National Longitudinal Study of Adolescent Health. *J Sch Health.* 2002;72(4): 138–146
10. Niehaus K, Rudasill KM, Rakes CR. A longitudinal study of school connectedness and academic outcomes across sixth grade. *J Sch Psychol.* 2012;50(4):443–460
11. Waasdorp TE, Bradshaw CP, Duong J. The link between parents' perceptions of the school and their responses to school bullying: Variation by child characteristics and the forms of victimization. *J Educ Psychol.* 2011;103(2):324–335
12. Mitchell MM, Bradshaw CP, Leaf PJ. Student and teacher perceptions of school climate: a multilevel exploration of patterns of discrepancy. *J Sch Health.* 2010;80(6):271–279
13. Fan W, Williams CM, Corkin DM. A multilevel analysis of student perceptions of school climate: The effect of social and academic risk factors. *Psychology in the Schools.* 2011;48(6):632–647
14. Furrer C, Skinner EA. Sense of relatedness as a factor in children's academic engagement and performance. *J Educ Psychol.* 2003;95(1):148–162
15. Diaz JD. School attachment among Latino youth in rural Minnesota. *Hisp J Behav Sci.* 2005;27(3):300–318
16. Rueger SY, Malecki CK, Demaray MK. Relationship between multiple sources of perceived social support and psychological and academic adjustment in early adolescence: comparisons across gender. *J Youth Adolesc.* 2010;39(1):47–61
17. Wentzel K, Battle A, Russell S, Looney L. Social supports from teachers and peers as predictors of academic and social motivation. *Contemp Educ Psychol.* 2010;35(3):193–202
18. Nickerson AB, Hopson LM, Steinke CM. School connectedness in community and residential treatment schools: the influence of gender, grades, and engagement in treatment. *Child and Youth Services Review.* 2011;33(6):829–837
19. Battistich V, Solomon D, Kim D, Watson M, Schaps E. Schools as Communities, Poverty Levels of Student Populations, and Students' Attitudes, Motives, and Performance: A Multilevel Analysis. *Am Educ Res J.* 1995;32(3):627–658
20. Schneider SH, Duran L. School climate in middle schools: a cultural perspective. *J Res Character Education.* 2010;8(2):25–37
21. Murray C, Greenberg MT. Relationships with teachers and bonds with school: Social emotional adjustment correlates for children with and without disabilities. *Psychol in the Schools.* 2001;38(1):25–41
22. Maslow G, Haydon AA, McRee, AL, Halpern CT. Protective connections and educational attainment among young adults with childhood-onset chronic illness. *J Sch Health.* 2012;82(8):364–370
23. Sulkowski M, Demaray M, Lazarus P. Connecting students to schools to support their emotional well-being and academic success. *Communiqué.* 2012;40(7):20–22

24. Institute of Medicine and National Research Council. *Building Capacity to Reduce Bullying: Workshop Summary.* Washington, DC: The National Academies Press; 2014

25. O'Brennan LM, Furlong MJ. Relations between students' perceptions of school connectedness and peer victimization. *Journal of School Violence.* 2010;9(4):375–391

26. Limber SP, Olweus D, Wang W. *Trends in Bullying Over 5 Years: Findings from the National Database of the Olweus Bullying Questionnaire.* Kansas City, MO, USA: Paper Presentation at the 9th Annual International Bullying Prevention Association (IBPA) Conference; 2012

27. Harris Interactive, GLSEN. *From Teasing to Torment: School Climate in America, A Survey of Students and Teachers.* New York, NY: GLSEN; 2005

28. Kosciw JG, Diaz EM, Greytak EA. *The 2007 National School Climate Survey: The Experiences of Lesbian, Gay, Bisexual and Transgender Youth in Our Nation's Schools.* New York, NY: GLSEN; 2008

29. Williams T, Connolly J, Pepler D, Craig W. Questioning and sexual minority adolescents: high school experiences of bullying, sexual harassment and physical abuse. *Can J Commun Ment Health.* 2003;22(2):47–58

30. Kosciw JG, Greytak EA, Diaz EM, Bartkiewicz MJ. *The 2011 National School Climate Survey: The Experiences of Lesbian, Gay, Bisexual and Transgender Youth in our Nation's Schools.* New York, NY: GLSEN; 2012

31. Griffith J. School climate as group evaluation and group consensus: student and parent perceptions of the elementary school environment. *Elementary Sch J.* 2000;101(1):35–61

32. Welsh WN. The effects of school climate on school disorder. *Annals of the American Academy of Political and Social Science.* 2000;567(1):88–107

33. Vieno A, Perkins DD, Smith TM, Santinello M. Democratic school climate and sense of community in school: a multilevel analysis. *AmJ Community Psychol.* 2005;36(3-4):327–341

34. Anderman LH, Freeman T. Students' sense of belonging in school. In: Maehr ML, Pintrich PR, eds. *Advances in Motivation and Achievement, Vol. 13. Motivating Students, Improving Schools: The Legacy of Carol Midgley.* Oxford, UK: Elsevier; 2004:27–63

35. Osher D, Kendziora K, American Institutes for Research. Building conditions for learning and healthy adolescent development: a strategic approach. In: Doll B, Pfohl W, Yoon J, eds. *Handbook of Youth Prevention Science.* New York, NY: Routledge; 2010:121–140

36. Centers for Disease Control and Prevention. *School Connectedness: Strategies for Increasing Protective Factors Among Youth.* Atlanta, GA: U.S. Department of Health and Human Services. 2009. http://www.cdc.gov/healthyyouth/protective/pdf/connectedness.pdf. Accessed April 16, 2015

37. Nakamoto J, Schwartz D. Is peer victimization associated with academic achievement? A meta-analytic review. *Social Development.* 2010:19(2):221–242

38. Osterman K. Students' need for belonging in the school community. *Review of Educational Research.* 2000;70(3):323–367

39. Vieno A, Santinello M, Pastore M, Perkins DD. Social support, sense of community in school, and self-efficacy as resources during early adolescence: an integrative model. *Am J Community Psychol.* 2007;39(1–2):177–190

40. Batanova MD, Loukas A. What are the unique and interacting contributions of school and family factors to early adolescents' empathic concern and perspective taking? *J Youth and Adolesc.* 2012;41(10):1382–1391

41. Suldo SM, McMahan MM, Chappel AM, Loker T. Relationships between perceived school climate and adolescent mental health across genders. *School Mental Health.* 2012;4(2):69–80

42. LaRusso M, Romer D, Selman R. Teachers as builders of respectful school climates: Implications for adolescent drug use norms and depressive symptoms in high school. *J Youth Adolescence.* 2008;37(4):386–398

43. Shochet IM, Dadds MR, Ham D, Montague R. School connectedness is an underemphasized parameter in adolescent mental health: results of a community prediction study. *J Clin Child Adolesc Psychol.* 2006;35(2):170–179

44. Loukas A, Ripperger-Suhler KG, Horton KD. Examining temporal associations between school connectedness and early adolescent adjustment. *J Youth Adolescence.* 2009;38(6): 804–812

45. Millings A, Buck R, Montgomery A, Spears M, Stallard P. School connectedness, peer attachment, and self-esteem as predictors of adolescent depression. *J Adolesc.* 2012;35(4): 1061–1067

46. Resnick MD, Bearman PS, Blum RW, et al. Protecting adolescents from harm: findings from the National Longitudinal Study on Adolescent Health. *JAMA.* 1997;278(10):823–832

47. Cook CR, Williams KR, Guerra NG, Kim TE, Sadek S. Predictors of bullying and victimization in childhood and adolescence: A meta-analytic investigation. *School Psychology Quarterly.* 2010;25(2):65–83

48. Klomek AB, Marrocco F, Kleinman M, Schonfeld M, Gould MS. Bullying depression and suicidality in adolescents. *J Am Acad Child Adolesc Psychiatry.* 2007;46(1):40–49

49. Annenberg Public Policy Center of the University of Pennsylvania. Adolescent and young adult victims of cyberbullying at increased risk of suicide. 2010. www.annenbergpublicpolicycenter.org/Downloads/Releases/ACI/Cyberbullying%20release.pdf. Accessed March 18, 2015

50. Kim YS, Leventhal BL, Koh YJ, Boyce WT. Bullying increased suicide risk: prospective study of Korean adolescents. *Arch Suicide Res.* 2009;13(1):15–30

51. Pranjić N, Bajraktarević A. Depression and suicide ideation among secondary school adolescents involved in school bullying. *Primary Health Care Research & Development.* 2010;11(4):349–362

52. Institute of Medicine. Evolution of school health programs. In: Allensworth D, Lawson E, Nicholson L, Wyche J, eds. *Schools and Health: Our Nation's Investment.* Washington, DC: National Academy Press; 1997:65–66

53. Gottfredson GD, Gottfredson DC, Payne AA, Gottfredson NC. School climate predictors of school disorder: Results from the National Study of Delinquency Prevention in Schools. *Journal of Research in Crime and Delinquency.* 2005;42(4):412–444

54. Catalano RF, Haggerty KP, Oesterie S, Fleming CB, Hawkins JD. The importance of bonding to schools for healthy development: findings from the Social Development Research Group. *J Sch Health.* 2004;74(7):252–261

55. Blum R. *School Connectedness: Improving the Lives of Students.* Baltimore, MD: Johns Hopkins Bloomberg School of Public Health; 2005

56. Brookmeyer KA, Fanti KA, Henrich CC. Schools, parents, and youth violence: a multilevel, ecological analysis. *J Clin Child Adolesc Psychol.* 2006;35(4):504–514

57. Resnick MD, Harris LJ, Blum RW. The impact of caring and connectedness on adolescent health and well-being. *J Paediatr Child Health.* 1993;29(suppl1):S3–S9

58. National School Climate Center. National school climate standards: benchmarks to promote effective teaching, learning and comprehensive school improvement. http://www.schoolclimate.org/climate/documents/school-climate-standards-csee.pdf. Accessed April 16,2015

59. Federal Partners in Bullying Prevention. Bullying prevention & response base training module. www.stopbullying.gov/prevention/in-the-community/community-action-planning/prnt_friendly_speaker_notes092112.pdf. Accessed April 16, 2105

60. Federal Partners in Bullying Prevention. Roles for pediatricians in bullying prevention and intervention. http://www.stopbullying.gov/resources-files/roles-for-pediatricians-tipsheet.pdf. Accessed April 16,2015

61. American Academy of Pediatrics, Committee on Injury, Violence, and Poison Prevention. Role of the pediatrician in youth violence prevention. *Pediatrics.* 2009;124(1):393–402

CHAPTER

9

Family and Community Involvement

American Academy of Pediatrics
Division of State Government Affairs
Joyce L. Epstein, PhD

*"It is not enough, however, to work at the individual bedside in the hospital.
In the near or dim future, the pediatrician is to sit in and control school boards,
health departments, and legislatures. He [or she] is a legitimate advisor to the
judge and jury, and a seat for the physician in the councils of the republic is
what the people have a right to demand."*

❧ *Abraham Jacobi, MD, 1904* ❧

Background

Because much of local, state, and federal child health policy is administered through schools and in partnership with families, pediatric school health advocacy plays an important role in child health advocacy. From immunization entry requirements to school nutrition standards to physical and mental health screenings, schools are expected to be the "enforcers" of laws and "communicators," with families directed toward keeping children healthy. Many schools lack the resources to perform well in this role. Schools often are expected to do more with fewer resources. Pediatrician advocates are important partners in ensuring that schools provide safe, healthy learning environments for children and in connecting with families and the community on matters of child health.

Advocacy and the practice of pediatrics have always been intrinsically connected. Indeed, advocacy is such an integral part of pediatric practice that it is now included as a component of pediatric residency training. Advocacy is central to the mission of many nongovernmental organizations and professional organizations such as the American Academy of Pediatrics (AAP). School health advocacy topics present a great learning opportunity to improve trainees' competency in systems-based practice. Four levels of pediatric advocacy work have been identified[1]: individual advocacy, community advocacy, state advocacy, and federal advocacy.

Individual advocacy involves direct care and resources provided to patients every day. An example of individual advocacy is calling an insurance company or contacting a social service agency about abating a home health hazard that is exacerbating a child's asthma. Although pediatricians routinely engage in individual advocacy efforts, individual advocacy is often the first step in broader efforts at the family, school, community, state, and federal levels.

Community advocacy builds on and reaches beyond individual advocacy in that it affects children within the community. A "community" can be defined geographically (as in a neighborhood, school district, or city) or culturally (as an ethnic or racial group or religious cluster.) Community advocacy takes into consideration the environmental and social factors influencing child health and addresses ways in which pediatricians can work with community partners to protect positive health conditions or address issues that negatively affect their patients.

State advocacy efforts by pediatricians focus primarily on the state legislative process. State legislatures play an increasingly important role in health policy and are a prolific source of new laws and regulations. It is estimated that the nation's approximately 7380 state legislators consider more than 150,000 bills every year. Although state legislatures are the primary focus of advocacy on the state level, there are also opportunities for advocacy with the state executive branch through the governor's office, state agencies and regulatory activities, the budget process, and the judicial branch. Pediatricians working with their AAP chapters have had effects on environmental health issues in their states, such as improving indoor air quality by limiting secondhand smoke exposure, improving outdoor air quality by limiting emissions of pollutants, promoting screening for lead poisoning, and many others.

Federal advocacy involves national environmental health issues. For dozens of years, pediatricians have advocated on the federal level about issues such as food safety, toxic chemicals in children's products, climate change, and others that affect children's health. The testimony given by pediatricians during congressional hearings, their briefings for members of Congress, their comments regarding proposed federal regulations, and their engagement in related activities are critical to the success of these efforts in the federal government.

Two additional levels of pediatric advocacy work have been identified in research and development on programs of school, family, and community partnerships.[2] These "close up" or proximate policy levels may be convenient and powerful starting places for advocacy and collaborative actions by pediatricians with immediate or short-term results for improving school health policy and practice.

Family advocacy aims to strengthen parents' and other family members' capacities to support children's health and safety, including physical and mental health and wellness. This may include ensuring that parents understand how to administer a child's prescription, prevent home accidents, and encourage children's learning and development at each age level.

School advocacy refers to the connections pediatricians make with schools and districts in the vicinity of their homes, offices, or hospitals to strengthen the knowledge and skills of teachers and administrators on school health and students' well-being and to share their expertise with students and with families at health-related events at school. If pediatricians have children in school or neighbors with school-aged students, they may find it convenient to focus advocacy efforts on these locations to fit their busy schedules.

How to Work With Schools

A pediatrician may believe that to become involved in advocacy, he or she must know everything about an issue, and about the political or legislative process. The clinical skills a pediatrician already possesses, however, are similar to those needed to be an effective advocate—the ability to translate complex scientific and medical concepts into simple language, to diagnose a problem, and to outline a course of treatment. A good clinician and advocate will listen carefully to understand the views of educators, parents, students, and other community members based on their backgrounds and experiences. Others' views will help build a more pertinent knowledge base and shape the solution to problems.

Identify a health-related problem. Advocacy may begin as soon as a particular problem is identified. The next step is to bring awareness of the issue to decision makers and others who can help to generate a solution. Although one does need a basic understanding of the legislative and policy processes (some of which can be obtained through resources available from the AAP and some from district and school documents), 3 of the most important attributes for success are enthusiasm, a willingness to speak out on behalf of children, and skills working with other stakeholders.

Coordinate a response. Coordination is key to the success of any advocacy effort. By working with and through their AAP chapters, pediatricians can take full advantage of the resources and information available from the AAP, the state chapter, and its coalition partners.

Broadening support, either with the participation of other pediatricians or by seeking partnerships with other organizations that share similar goals and priorities, is critical for successful advocacy efforts. A broad base of support will demonstrate to community leaders and elected officials that there are many people who care about school health issues and that those people are working together and taking action to create positive change.

Pediatricians may use media to promote their advocacy efforts. The 6 levels of advocacy can be enhanced by using school, local, regional, and national media to spotlight the issues through such activities as letters to the editor, opinion/editorial pieces, calling attention to the issue through news stories, or getting editorial support. Also, enhancing understanding of an issue using social media can result in a magnifying effect. Pediatricians know that having the media on one's side when talking with legislators and education leaders can make a difference in ensuring a successful policy outcome. Conversely, media opposition can make advocacy an uphill struggle.

When working on issues as important as school health, it may be hard to imagine that others would not support a pediatrician's efforts or even oppose them. However, pediatricians' advocacy priorities will nearly always compete with those of other groups over resources and funding or reflect different points of view. It often is helpful to bring several pediatricians and key stakeholders to the table (eg, school principals, district superintendents, school psychologists, social workers) to underscore the importance of a particular issue to decision makers as they consider positions of differing interests.

How to Make a Difference in Students' Health

School, Family, and Community Partnerships

Family and school advocacy enables individual pediatricians to serve as important local resources for school health, even if they are not able to participate at the state and national levels. By working directly as partners with a local school or district, pediatricians may zero in on issues that affect the patients they see in their offices or hospitals and observe the effects of their efforts in the short term.

Why Is This Important?

Many studies confirm that healthy students who attend school every day are more likely to achieve academically than are students who are frequently absent from school. When students feel healthy, safe, and cared for in school, they are better able to concentrate on instruction and schoolwork. Other studies show that family and community engagement in students' health help to improve student behavior, social skills, eating habits, and greater likelihood of on-time high school graduation—all important student outcomes. At the school level, studies show that attention to health policies and practices leads to safer schools and more health services for students.[3]

Roles and Topics

A pediatrician is a community partner whose expertise will increase the knowledge of teachers, parents, and students and support positive change in the health of schools, students, and families. The following are a few of many ways that pediatricians can advocate for good health in school-based partnership programs.

- *Provide information* to parents, students, and teachers on nutrition in school lunches and family meals; childhood diseases; the connection of childhood obesity with diabetes; and common childhood conditions such as asthma, allergies, and vision and hearing problems.
- Give *guest-lectures or participate in forums* at school on age-appropriate topics such as strengthening children's self-esteem; connecting good health, good attendance, and high achievement; preventing risky behaviors such as drug, alcohol, and tobacco use and early sexual behavior; eliminating bullying; preventing teen suicide; encouraging safe driving; reducing students' school stress; reducing parents' stress; and limiting other behaviors that can derail progress and success in school.
- *Work with teachers on special topics,* such as how to welcome a student back to school after cancer treatment or other serious hospitalizations; teen pregnancy and teen parenthood; and supporting lesbian, gay, bisexual, and transgender students.
- *Dedicate office space* to reading, math, puzzle, and game corners for students to use while they wait for an appointment. Collaborate with a public library to provide students with summer reading lists by reading level and interest areas that families can pick up when they bring their children for office visits.

- *Conduct professional development sessions* for school and district staff members on health and safety topics that they select, such as preventing school sports injuries and developing school emergency and security plans.
- *Make career awareness presentations* to middle and high school students on the various positions in the field of medicine and the education required for those positions. Retired pediatricians also may be valuable presenters and mentors to students who will be the next generation of doctors, nurses, technicians, and others in the health professions.
- *Advise district or school leaders on wellness surveys* or health topics of interest for teachers, parents, and students.

Information and presentations for teachers, parents, and students must be in clear lay language and may require translators to include all families.

Applying the Framework of 6 Types of Involvement

In some schools, educators wait for pediatricians to volunteer to improve student health in the ways listed above. Other schools, particularly those that develop research-based partnership programs with the National Network of Partnership Schools at Johns Hopkins University, recruit and welcome family and community partners to work with teachers on important goals for student success—including health.[2]

Many studies by National Network of Partnership Schools researchers contributed to the development of a framework of 6 types of involvement that enable school-based action teams for partnerships to select, design, and implement activities that engage all families in different ways and different locations (at home, at school, and in the community). In brief, the 6 types of involvement are: (1) *parenting*—help all families understand child and adolescent development and help all schools understand their children's families; (2) *communicating*—establish 2-way exchanges about school programs and children's progress; (3) *volunteering*—recruit and organize parents' assistance at school, home, or in other locations, (4) *learning at home*—provide information and ideas to families about how to help students with homework and other curriculum-related activities; (5) *decision making*—have parents from all backgrounds and community partners serve as representatives and leaders on school committees and advocates for their own children; and (6) *collaborating with the community*—identify and integrate resources and services from the community to strengthen school programs and students' experiences and enable students and families to contribute to their communities.[2]

Action teams for partnerships choose among hundreds of practices or design new activities for each type of involvement and solve inevitable challenges (eg, different technologies or languages to communicate with families). Each type of involvement requires 2-way connections for educators and families to exchange information as they share responsibilities for children's education. Each activity selected in a program of partnerships is linked to specific goals for students, such as academic goals in specific school subjects (eg, improve reading, math, science) and behavioral goals (eg, improve attendance, good behavior, health). Activities also contribute to the school's welcoming climate—as a partnership place. Using the framework in this way, partnership activities are purposeful—not random—and contribute to goals for student success.

Here are a few examples of activities that pediatricians may conduct to share their expertise and advocate for health and wellness in school-based programs of family and community engagement. The activities may be adapted to any school or grade level.

Type 1: Parenting. Advocate for school breakfasts and lunches during the school year, on weekends, and in the summer to ensure that poor students have healthy food to eat whether school is in or out of session. Conduct or participate in workshops for parents on healthy snacks, preventing bullying, Internet safety, and other topics of interest to parents on child and adolescent development.

Type 2: Communicating. Contribute articles to school or district newsletters or Web sites with clear information on age-appropriate topics such as exercise, safety in sports, required sleep, preventing risky behaviors, and other topics. Advocate for physical education classes every year from preschool through high school for all students, not just a semester, and not just for those on sports teams.

Type 3: Volunteering. Visit classrooms or join assemblies to give talks and hands-on demonstrations to students and/or families on science and health topics in the curriculum by grade level. Join and assist with walkathons for children and families.

Type 4: Learning at Home. Partner with science and health teachers to develop homework for students to show parents what they are learning in class and to interview parents on health topics that affect their everyday life.

Type 5: Decision Making and Advocacy. Join a school's action team for partnerships as a representative of the medical community. As a team member, a pediatrician may work with others to advocate for school health policies, school-friendly schedules of doctors and dentists in the community so that students do not leave class, healthy foods for children's lunches, and other school and district decisions that affect student and family health.

Type 6: Collaborating With the Community. Sponsor a booth at a school-community health fair individually or with other doctors and nurses to provide free immunizations and other screenings (eg, blood pressure, heart rate, eye and ear tests) for children and families. Support a high school student internship at the doctor's office or hospital as a summer experience in medicine.

(See many other examples of health, wellness, and safety activities on the Web site of *Promising Partnership Practices* at **www.partnershipschools.org**.)

Recommendations for Pediatricians

The success of pediatric school health advocacy ultimately rests with the volunteer efforts of individual pediatricians. The national AAP, along with many of its state chapters, has lobbyists and other public policy staff who help to shape laws and regulations on behalf of children. However, the work of professional lobbying staff alone is not enough. The unique perspective and credibility of pediatricians propel some issues forward in a way that a lobbyist alone cannot. Further, health issues that affect the schools, students, and families in the area where pediatricians live and work require up-close and personal attention by partners in education.

Some pediatricians will get involved at the state, national, and community levels as advocates for broad health policies. Others may have time only to participate in their own children's schools or with schools near their offices or hospitals. The proximal places for participation are particularly important for taking positive actions to improve students' physical and mental health, which, in turn, will increase students' academic success at the preschool, elementary, middle, and high school levels.

The pediatrician's voice is critical in helping create the social and political change needed to make lasting advancements in environmental and child health policy, school health programs, and programs of school, family, and community partnerships that increase individual students' success in school.

Recommendations for Program Directors and Trainees

Training program directors in general pediatrics or any of its subspecialties should consider weaving important school health-related advocacy efforts and opportunities as an important teaching tool of developing the trainees' milestones in advocacy at any of the policy levels discussed. This can be done through classroom discussions, small action research projects, letter writing, and media awareness.

For more information on advocacy by pediatricians and how pediatricians can have an effect on school health and child health policy, see the AAP advocacy guide[1] from which much of this material is drawn.

For more information on advocacy to improve school health in local programs of school, family, and community partnerships and examples from diverse communities, see Epstein et al, 2009[2] and the section on "Success Stories" on the Web site of the National Network of Partnership Schools at Johns Hopkins University (**www.partnershipschools.org**).

Resources

For additional school health related resources, visit www.aap.org/schoolhealthmanual.

References

1. American Academy of Pediatrics. *Advocacy Guide: Pointing You in the Right Direction to Become and Effective Advocate.* Elk Grove Village, IL: American Academy of Pediatrics; 2009.
2. Epstein JL, Sanders MG, Sheldon SB, et al. *School, Family, and Community Partnerships: Your Handbook for Action.* 3rd ed. Thousand Oaks, CA: Corwin Press; 2009
3. Centers for Disease Control and Prevention. *Parent Engagement: Strategies for Involving Parents in School Health.* Atlanta, GA: US Department of Health and Human Services; 2012

CHAPTER

10

Staff Wellness

Joy A. Osterhout, MS, MCHES

The United States' K-12 public education system has experienced tremendous historical growth in employment, according to the US Department of Education's National Center for Education Statistics. Between 1950 and 2009, the number of full-time equivalent school employees grew 386%. Of those personnel, teachers' numbers increased 252%, and administrators and other staff experienced growth of 702%. Today, our public education system employs almost 7 million people—teachers, school administrators, support staff, and other professionals who manage the schools, transport and feed our children, and ensure that the school buildings and grounds are safe and well maintained.[1] This large workforce has one of the most important jobs in the world—preparing our children to become healthy, successful, and productive adults.

An abundance of information has been written about strategies for addressing students' health, but less has been written about strategies for addressing school staff health. Historically, school districts addressed disease prevention and health promotion for students and identified teachers as agents for showing students how to adopt and maintain healthy behaviors. However, teachers who lack wellness cannot be healthy role models for students. Additionally, many actions and conditions that affect the health of school staff also influence the health and learning of students. The physical and mental health of school staff is integral to promoting and protecting the health of our students and ensuring their academic success. The Whole School, Whole Community, Whole Child model, a framework for planning and coordinating school health activities recommended by the Centers for Disease Control and Prevention (CDC), points out the importance of staff wellness by including it as one of the 10 components. Several nationwide organizations have also recognized the importance of school staff wellness. The American School Health Association passed a resolution promoting the design and implementation of school-site

> The physical and mental health of school staff is integral to promoting and protecting the health of our students and ensuring their academic success.

health promotion programs; the American Association of School Administrators devoted a chapter on school employee wellness programs in its *Promoting Health Education in America;* the Health Insurance Association of American developed and distributed a manual entitled *Wellness at the School Worksite;* and most recently, the Directors of Health Promotion and Education, with funding from CDC, published *School Employee Wellness: A Guide for Protecting the Assets of Our Nation's Schools,* which provides a process for developing a school staff wellness program, as well as other practical tools and resources.[2]

School districts and schools are also recognizing the importance of staff wellness programs and the role they play in staff and student health and academic success. The School Health Policies and Programs Study (2000) conducted by the CDC found that 41.7% of districts and 93.5% of schools provided some type of health-promotion activities or services for their employees. The activities ranged from making announcements or posting flyers about health-related topics to offering wellness activities, such as sponsoring competitions between groups, giving release time, awarding prizes, and providing financial incentives for staff to participate in health-promotion activities.[3]

School districts, like businesses in the private sector, incur employee-related expenses, such as the cost of absenteeism, health care costs, workers' compensation, lost productivity, and disability. A number of studies have shown that staff wellness programs can directly affect these employee-rated costs and provide other benefits. School staff wellness programs have reported that participating staff increased the intake of low-fat foods, quit smoking, and lowered their cholesterol, thus, changing behaviors that contribute greatly to most illnesses and deaths. Staff wellness programs that emphasize physical activity, stress management, and nutrition increase teacher morale, reduce absenteeism, and result in higher levels of general well-being and the ability of teachers' to handle job stress.[4-6] A couple of brief success stories of school staff wellness programs (from *School Employee Wellness: A Guide to Protecting the Assets of our Nation's Schools)* are below.

Dallas Independent School District, Texas: In a 10-week health-promotion program for staff that focused on exercise and physical fitness, 44% of teachers said they changed their overall lifestyle, 69% changed their diet, 25% who were initially sedentary started a regular program of vigorous exercise, and 18% quit smoking. Other benefits of the program included a reduction in absenteeism—exercising teachers had an average of 1.25 days less of absenteeism than non-exercising teachers—which led to a savings of $149,578 for the district in costs for substitute teachers.[4,7]

Washoe County School District, Nevada: In 2001, the district offered 11 different wellness programs to encourage school staff to engage in healthy lifestyles. Programs focused on brushing and flossing teeth, sensible eating during holidays, the importance of water, reducing TV time, getting the right amount of sleep, exercising for life, seatbelt safety, brain functioning, and fitness challenges. Results indicated that nonparticipants had higher rates (20% higher) of illness-related absenteeism than did participators. A cost-benefits analysis revealed that the district saved $15.60 for every dollar spent on the wellness programs. The program saved the district $2.5 million dollars in 2 years, and employees enjoyed dramatically improved health and quality of life.[8,9]

School districts with staff wellness programs have also found potential new staff are more interested in their school districts because of the focus on staff wellness, and existing staff are more loyal.[10] They have also found that school staff interested in their own wellness are more likely to take an interest in the health of their students, and in turn, students are more likely to engage in healthy behaviors and activities when school staff are modeling such behaviors and activities. Table 10.1 presents a list of the potential benefits of staff wellness programs.

Staff wellness programs should be a systematic approach to improving the health of school staff as well as positively affecting students and schools. Staff wellness programs can promote health, reduce health risk behaviors of staff, identify and correct conditions at the school site that can negatively affect the health of school staff, reduce their levels of productivity, impede student success, and contribute to escalating health care costs.

Table 10.1. Potential Benefits of Staff Wellness Programs

- Decreased staff absenteeism
- Lower health care and insurance costs
- Increased staff retention
- Improved staff morale
- Fewer work-related injuries
- Fewer worker compensation and disability claims
- Increased staff productivity
- Increased motivation to practice healthy behaviors
- Healthy role model for students

The elements of a comprehensive school staff wellness program outlined in *School Employee Wellness: A Guide to Protecting the Assets of Our Nation's Schools* and adapted from Healthy People 2010 and Partnerships for a Healthy Workforce are:

1 Health education and health-promoting activities that focus on skill development and lifestyle behavior change along with awareness building, information dissemination, and access to facilities and are preferably tailored to staff needs and interests;

2 Safe, supportive social and physical environments, including organizational expectations about healthy behaviors and implementation of policies that promote health and safety and reduce the risk of disease;

3 Integration of the worksite program into the school or district structure;

4 Linkage to related programs such as employee assistance programs, emergency care, and programs that help staff balance work and family life;

5 Worksite screening programs, which ideally are linked to medical care to ensure follow-up and appropriate treatment as necessary;

6 Individual follow-up interventions to support behavior change;

7 Education and resources to help staff make decisions about health care; and

8 And evaluation and improvement process to help enhance the wellness program's effectiveness and efficiency.[9]

School Employee Wellness – A Guide for Protecting the Assets of Our National's Schools developed by the Directors of Health Promotion and Education, proposes a 9-step process for establishing a school staff wellness program, as seen in Table 10.2. For more details about establishing a school employee wellness program, the guide can be downloaded at **www.dhpe.org**.

Table 10.2. Steps For Establishing A School Employee Wellness Program

Step 1: Obtain administrative support
Step 2: Identify resources
Step 3: Identify a leader
Step 4: Organize a committee
Step 5: Gather and analyze data
Step 6: Develop a plan
Step 7: Implement a plan
Step 8: Evaluate and adapt the program
Step 9: Sustain the program

Many successful school staff wellness programs rely on physicians, nurses, physician assistants, audiologists, physical therapists, health educators, psychologists, social workers, registered dietitians, and other health professionals in their communities as partners. Health professionals can provide many valuable resources and/or services to staff wellness programs, such as:

- Becoming a member of the staff wellness committee (step 4);
- Helping the staff wellness committee identify health issues of their staff and identifying resources available in the community to support wellness programming (step 5);
- Providing immunizations, such as influenza vaccines for school staff;
- Conducting health screenings and assessments;
- Providing health information and materials;
- Conducting educational workshops on healthy eating, weight management, stress management, medical self-care, cardiopulmonary resuscitation (CPR) and first aid, etc.

Recommendations for Pediatricians

- Find out if your local school has a staff wellness program.
- Be a resource for schools that have staff wellness programs by being part of their planning committees, providing educational sessions, assisting with health screenings and assessments, and linking them with other resources in your system or in the community for the delivery of a staff wellness program.
- Provide educational sessions to the school administration on children's health issues as well as other resources available in the community for children's health issues.

Recommendations for Program Directors and Trainees

Staff wellness programs in schools can be an excellent educational opportunity for family medicine residents, combined medicine-pediatrics residents, or public health students. Program directors should take advantage of these opportunities to enhance the educational experience of their students or residents in staff wellness through the following suggested activities:

Participating in the implementation and design of a staff wellness program at a school or school district.

Using the staff wellness programs as models for quality improvement projects.

Participation in the provision of care or screening to school staff through cooperative agreements between the school district and the training program or through a school health rotation focused on staff wellness.

Staff wellness programs can serve as an excellent field experience and/or internship for public health and nursing students.

The school staff plays an integral part in improving the health and academic success of children. Therefore, it is important that school districts focus on the quality of life and health of their school staff, and work to maintain and improve it. Staff wellness programs are an important tool that can help school districts maintain the health of their employees, and to be successful, they need to utilize partnerships in the community with health professionals and health institutions.

Take-Home Points

- Staff wellness programs can help schools promote a healthy work environment by focusing on staff quality of life, health, and well-being.
- Adults are role models for students. Staff wellness programs can help staff learn about the role they play in modeling healthy habits and choices for their students.
- Investing in a staff wellness program has demonstrated a high return on investment for school districts through decreasing staff absenteeism, improving staff morale, increasing staff retention, and having a positive impact on new staff recruitment.
- Staff wellness can present an excellent educational opportunity for trainees.

Resources

For additional school health related resources, visit www.aap.org/schoolhealthmanual.

References
1. US Department of Education, National Center for Education Statistics. *Digest of Education Statistics Tables and Figures.* Washington, DC: US Department of Education; 2005. Available at: http://nces.ed.gov/programs/digest/d05/tables/dt05_001.asp. Accessed April 13, 2015
2. Blair SN, Tritsch L, Kutsch S. Worksite health promotion for school faculty and staff. *J Sch Health.* 1987;57(10):469–473
3. Grunbaum JA, Rutman SJ, Sathrum PR. Faculty and staff health promotion: results from the School Health Policies and Programs Study 2000. *J Sch Health.* 2001;71(7):335–339
4. Blair SN, Collingwood TR, Reynolds R, Smith M, Hagan RD, Sterling CL. Health promotion for educators: impact on health behaviors, satisfaction, and general well-being. *Am J Public Health.* 1984;74(2):147–149
5. Oxreider A. Our school wellness program cut staff absenteeism and might save lives. *American School Board Journal.* 1987;174(6):29
6. Allegrante JP, Michela JL. Impact of a school-based workplace health promotion program on morale of inner-city teachers. *J Sch Health.* 1990;60(1):25–28
7. Blair SN, Smith M, Collingwood TR, Reynolds R, Prentice MC, Sterling CJ. Health promotion for educators: impact of absenteeism. *Prev Med.* 1986;15(2):166–175
8. Aldana SG, Merrill RM, Price K, Hardy A, Hager R. Financial impact of a comprehensive workplace health promotion program. *Prev Med.* 2005;40(2):131–137
9. Partnership for Prevention. *Healthy Workforce 2010: An Essential Health Promotion Sourcebook for Employers, Large and Small.* Washington, DC: Partnership for Prevention; 2001
10. Bogden JF. *Fit, Healthy, and Ready to Learn: A School Health Policy Guide.* Alexandria, VA: National Association of State Boards of Education; 2000

CHAPTER

11

Global School Health

Thomas L. Young, MD, FAAP
Janeth Ceballos Osorio, MD, FAAP

"Some of the most common health conditions of school-age children affect their education. Malaria and worm infections can reduce enrollment and increase absenteeism, while hunger and anemia can affect cognition and learning, thus exacerbating the problems of even those children who do go to school. The pain associated with tooth decay, and the diarrhea and respiratory disease associated with poor hygiene, may also affect both attendance and learning. These are not rare problems. The major health conditions that affect children's education are highly prevalent among poor schoolchildren. It is estimated that in low-income countries, worms infect some 169 million school-age children, each of whom loses some 3.75 IQ points as a consequence. Some 300 million schoolchildren have iron-deficiency anemia, causing them to lose some 6 IQ points per child. Hunger affects learning and attention: some 66 million schoolchildren go to school hungry. All of these conditions translate into the equivalent of between 200 million and 500 million days of school lost to ill health in low-income countries each year."[1]*

Background

. . . .

History of Global School Health

Children's health has been addressed at school globally for more than a century.[2] It is known that poor health and malnutrition are important underlying factors for low school enrollment, absenteeism, poor classroom performance, and early school dropout.[1] However, the application of health promotion at schools is a newer concept that started over the last 30 years and is associated with the development of health promotion policy.[3] In 1978, the Declaration of Alma-Ata called for multisectoral approaches to health promotion and for public participation in developing and providing health programs.[4]

In 1986, the World Health Organization (WHO) Regional Office for Europe, guided by the Ottawa Charter for Health Promotion, developed the concept of the health-promoting school (HPS)[2,5]; an application of, at the time, developing a theoretical model of health promotion to the setting of the school. The original HPS model consisted of 3 main elements: curriculum, school culture and environment, and health and caring services.[6] To the present, this concept has spread gradually from its European origins to many parts of the word, including Australia, New Zealand, Hong Kong, and South Africa.[2,3] In Europe, the HPS model has been implemented and organized under the Schools for Health in Europe Network (SHE Network), led by the Dutch Institute for Health Promotion and Disease Prevention, a WHO collaborating center.[7]

In the United States, the coordinated school health program (CSHP) was developed in the early 1980s. This model added elements, including school health programs for staff and integrated school and community health promotion efforts. The CSHP has evolved over time and is the model implemented by the Centers for Disease Control and Prevention's (CDC's) Coordinated School Health Program.[6]

In 1995, the WHO launched its Global School Health Initiative, with the goal to increase the number of schools than can truly be called "health-promoting schools." Among the initiative's strategies are: research to improve school health programs; generation of technical documents to consolidate the research and expert opinion about the nature, scope, and effectiveness of school health programs; strengthening the collaboration between health and education agencies; and creating networks and alliances for the development of health-promoting schools.[8]

Parallel to the health-promotion movements, the United Nations Educational, Scientific, and Cultural Organization (UNESCO) led in the early 1990s Education for All, a movement in education promoting the important link between health and education.[1,6] Ten years later, UNESCO and WHO prepared together the 10-year retrospective "Thematic Study: School Health and Nutrition," presented and discussed at the Education for All (EFA) World Education Forum in Dakar, Senegal, in April 2000.[6,9] At that forum, major United Nations (UN) agencies agreed to harmonize actions around common elements of their models on school health, such as the HPS model and child-friendly schools. The report stimulated UNESCO, UNICEF, WHO, the World Bank, and nongovernmental organizations to launch together the Focusing Resources on Effective School Health (FRESH) framework.[10,11] Other international agencies have joined as FRESH partners, including the Education Development Center (EDC), Education International (EI), Partnership for Child Development (PCD), Save the Children, and World Food Programme (WFP).[6,9,12]

Other international initiatives also address school health, such as EFAIDS (Education for ALL and HIV/AIDS education)[13]; IATT (UNAIDS Inter-Agency Task Team on Education), convened by the UNESCO in 2002 to support the education sector in HIV and AIDS[14]; IUHPE (International Union on Health Promotion and Education); and the SCN (United Nations Standing Committee on Nutrition),[15] among others.

More than a decade after the launch of FRESH, international agencies continue to push for the development of school health promotion. The school sections at the 18th IUHPE World Conference on Health Promotion and Education in 2004 in Melbourne, the 6th Global Conference on Health Promotion in 2005 in Bangkok, as well as the FRESH partners meeting in 2006 in Paris all have called for mechanisms and processes to coordinate efforts and share resources and experiences for making further progress on school health promotion. Also in 2006, World Health Assembly called for immediate action to address the underlying socioeconomic causes of poor health in schools, and in 2007, WHO, in collaboration with other United Nations Agencies and WHO Collaborating Centers, held in Vancouver, Canada, a Technical Meeting on School Health, Building School Partnership for Health, Education Achievements, and Development.[12]

School-Aged and Adolescent Global Health Issues

School-aged and adolescent students represent 25% of the world's population. Although considered a relatively healthy age group, there is ample opportunity to improve the current health of children and adolescents and help prevent future health problems through school health interventions.

Morbidity and mortality risk are different depending on resource levels of countries and regions in which youth live. A recent analysis of global burden of disease by Gore et al described cause-specific disability-adjusted life-years (DALYs) by age, region, and level of resources for youth 10 to 24 years of age in the countries and region (Tables 11.1 and 11.2).[16] DALYs for youth in Africa were 2.5 times higher than for youth in high-income countries. Globally, the 3 main causes for years lost to disability (YLDs) for youth 10 to 24 years of age (Figure 11.1) were neuropsychiatric disorders (45%), unintentional injuries (12%), and infectious and parasitic diseases (10%).The major risk factors for this age group were alcohol use, unsafe sex, iron deficiency, lack of contraception, and illicit drug use.

It is interesting to note that:

- 10- to 14-year-olds have the lowest risk and DALYs.
- High-income countries have lowest risk.
- Neuropsychiatric risk is similar between income levels and regions of the world.
- Asia and Africa have the highest risk for DALYs with infectious diseases.

Table 11.1. DALYs per 1000 Population by Country Income for Youth Ages 10-24 Years

DALYs 10-24 years	Male	Female	Both
High-income countries	85	78	82
Low- and middle-income countries			
Africa	184	232	208
Americas	143	109	126
Southeast Asia	140	170	154
Eastern Mediterranean	147	144	145

Abbreviation: DALY; disability-adjusted life-years.
Reproduced with permission. Gore FM, Bloem PJ, Patton GC, et al. Global burden of disease in young people aged 10-24 years: a systematic analysis. *Lancet.* 2011;377(9783):2095. ©2011 Elsevier.[16]

Table 11.2. Main Causes of DALYs for 10- to 24-Year-Olds and for 5-Year Age Groups

	Males		Females		Total	
Cause	Cause	Total DALYs (100,000s) (%)	Cause	Total DALYs (100,000s) (%)	Cause	Total DALYs (100,000s) (%)
10-24 years						
1	Road traffic accidents	93 (7.8%)	Unipolar depressive disorders	115 (9.8%)	Unipolar depressive disorders	193 (8.2%)
2	Unipolar depressive disorders	78 (6.6%)	Schizophrenia	46 (4.0%)	Road traffic accidents	127 (5.4%)
3	Violence	69 (5.8%)	Bipolar disorder	44 (3.7%)	Schizophrenia	96 (4.1%)
4	Alcohol use	62 (5.3%)	Abortion	43 (3.7%)	Bipolar disorder	88 (3.8%)
5	Schizophrenia	50 (4.2%)	HIV/AIDS	38 (3.2%)	Violence	81 (3.5%)
6	Bipolar disorder	45 (3.8%)	Road traffic accidents	34 (2.9%)	Alcohol use	71 (3.0%)
7	Self-inflicted injuries	35 (3.0%)	Self-inflicted injuries	32 (2.7%)	HIV/AIDS	70 (3.0%)
8	HIV/AIDS	32 (2.7%)	Maternal sepsis	32 (2.7%)	Self-inflicted injuries	67 (2.8%)
9	Tuberculosis	32 (2.7%)	Lower respiratory infections	30 (2.6%)	Tuberculosis	60 (2.6%)
10	Asthma	32 (2.7%)	Panic disorder	30 (2.6%)	Lower respiratory infections	60 (2.6%)

DALY indicates disability-adjusted life-years. Reproduced with permission. Gore FM, Bloem PJ, Patton GC, et al. Global burden of disease in young people aged 10-24 years: a systematic analysis. *Lancet.* 2011;377(9783):2097. ©2011 Elsevier.[16]

Table 11.2. Main Causes of DALYs for 10- to 24-Year-Olds and for 5-Year Age Groups *(continued)*

Males		Females		Total	
Cause	Total DALYs (100,000s) (%)	Cause	Total DALYs (100,000s) (%)	Cause	Total DALYs (100,000s) (%)
10–14 years					
1 Road traffic accidents	15 (6.0%)	Lower respiratory infections	15 (6.3%)	Unipolar depressive disorders	28 (5.7%)
2 Unipolar depressive disorders	14 (5.4%)	Unipolar depressive disorders	14 (6.1%)	Lower respiratory infections	28 (5.6%)
3 Lower respiratory infections	13 (4.9%)	Asthma	12 (5.1%)	Road traffic accidents	26 (5.2%)
4 Asthma	10 (4.1%)	Migraine	11 (4.8%)	Asthma	23 (4.6%)
5 Drownings	10 (3.8%)	Road traffic accidents	10 (4.2%)	Refractive errors	19 (3.8%)
6 Refractive errors	10 (3.7%)	Refractive errors	9 (3.8%)	Iron-deficiency anemia	17 (3.4%)
7 Falls	9 (3.4%)	Iron-deficiency anemia	8 (3.5%)	Falls	16 (3.2%)
8 Iron-deficiency anemia	9 (3.4%)	Falls	7 (2.9%)	Migraine	16 (3.2%)
9 Schizophrenia	6 (2.5%)	Diarrheal diseases	6 (2.7%)	Drownings	14 (2.9%)
10 Lymphatic filariasis	6 (2.5%)	Fires	6 (2.5%)	Diarrheal diseases	12 (2.4%)

Reproduced with permission. Gore FM, Bloem PJ, Patton GC, et al. Global burden of disease in young people aged 10–24 years: a systematic analysis. *Lancet.* 2011;377(9783):2097. ©2011 Elsevier.[16]

Table 11.2. Main Causes of DALYs for 10- to 24-Year-Olds and for 5-Year Age Groups *(continued)*

	Males		Females		Total	
Cause	Cause	Total DALYs (100,000s) (%)	Cause	Total DALYs (100,000s) (%)	Cause	Total DALYs (100,000s) (%)
15-19 years						
1	Unipolar depressive disorders	34 (8.0%)	Unipolar depressive disorders	53 (11.7%)	Unipolar depressive disorders	86 (9.9%)
2	Road traffic accidents	33 (7.8%)	Schizophrenia	23 (5.2%)	Schizophrenia	46 (5.3%)
3	Alcohol use	30 (7.2%)	Bipolar disorder	22 (4.9%)	Road traffic accidents	46 (5.3%)
4	Schizophrenia	23 (5.4%)	Abortion	17 (3.8%)	Bipolar disorder	44 (5.1%)
5	Bipolar disorder	23 (5.3%)	Panic disorder	16 (3.5%)	Alcohol use	34 (4.0%)
6	Violence	21 (5.1%)	Maternal sepsis	14 (3.1%)	Violence	26 (3.0%)
7	Drug misuse	11 (2.6%)	Self-inflicted injuries	13 (3.0%)	Self-inflicted injuries	24 (2.8%)
8	Asthma	11 (2.6%)	Road traffic accidents	13 (2.9%)	Panic disorder	23 (2.7%)
9	Self-inflicted injuries	11 (2.5%)	Chlamydia	10 (2.3%)	Asthma	18 (2.0%)
10	Drownings	10 (2.5 %)	Iron-deficiency anemia	9 (2.1%)	HIV/AIDS	17 (2.0%)

Reproduced with permission. Gore FM, Bloem PJ, Patton GC, et al. Global burden of disease in young people aged 10-24 years: a systematic analysis. *Lancet.* 2011;377(9783):2097. ©2011 Elsevier.[16]

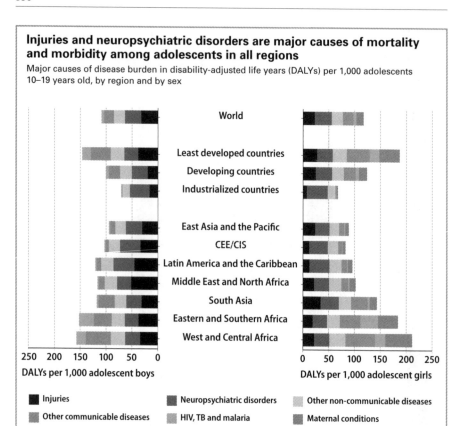

Injuries and neuropsychiatric disorders are major causes of mortality and morbidity among adolescents in all regions

Major causes of disease burden in disability-adjusted life years (DALYs) per 1,000 adolescents 10–19 years old, by region and by sex

World

Least developed countries
Developing countries
Industrialized countries

East Asia and the Pacific
CEE/CIS
Latin America and the Caribbean
Middle East and North Africa
South Asia
Eastern and Southern Africa
West and Central Africa

250 200 150 100 50 0   0 50 100 150 200 250
DALYs per 1,000 adolescent boys   DALYs per 1,000 adolescent girls

■ Injuries   ■ Neuropsychiatric disorders   ▨ Other non-communicable diseases
▨ Other communicable diseases   ▨ HIV, TB and malaria   ▨ Maternal conditions

Note: Neuropsychiatric disorders include depression, bipolar disorder, anxiety/panic disorders (including post-traumatic stress disorder and obsessive-compulsive disorder), psychotic disorders (including schizophrenia), seizure disorders (including epilepsy and Parkinson's disease) and alcohol and drug-use disorders.

Disability-adjusted life years (DALYs) are a summary measure combining years of life lost because of premature mortality (YLLs) and years lost because of disability (YLDs) for incident cases of the disease or injury. One DALY represents the loss of the equivalent of one year of full health. Population data are for the year 2004. The data have been recalculated according to UNICEF regional classification.

Source: WHO, The Global Burden of Disease: 2004 update, 2008, and United Nations Department of Economic and Social Affairs, Population Division, World Population Prospects: The 2010 revision, CD-ROM edition, 2011.

Figure 11.1. Main causes of DALYs[16]
Reproduced with permission. United Nations Children's Fund (UNICEF). Progress for Children: A Report Card for Adolescents, Number 10, April 2012. New York, NY: UNICEF; 2012.

Figures 11.2 and 11.3 on the pages that follow demonstrate mortality by age group in Africa, a low-resource continent.

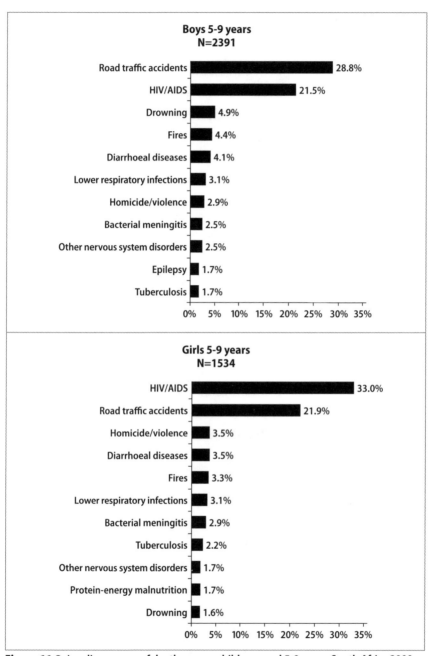

Figure 11.2. Leading causes of death among children aged 5-9 years, South Africa 2000.
Reproduced with permission. Bradshaw D, Bourne D, Nannan N. What are the leading causes of death among South African children? *MRC Policy Brief No 3*. Cape Town, South Africa: Medical Research Council; 2003. Available at: http://www.unicef.org/southafrica/SAF_publications_mrc.pdf. ©2003 Medical Research Council.

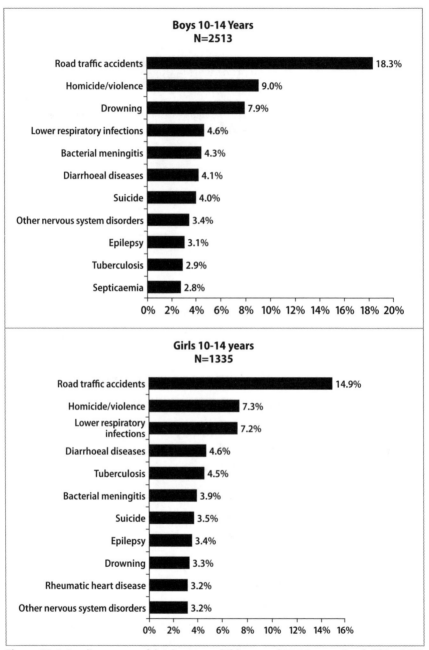

Figure 11.3. Leading causes of death among children aged 10-14 years, South Africa 2000.
Reproduced with permission. Bradshaw D, Bourne D, Nannan N. What are the leading causes of death among South African children? *MRC Policy Brief No 3*. Cape Town, South Africa: Medical Research Council; 2003. Available at: http://www.unicef.org/southafrica/SAF_publications_mrc.pdf. ©2003 Medical Research Council.

It is clear that school health interventions need to address the specific risk of youth on the basis of health risk factors in their country, resources available, and age groups that are targeted. Figure 11.4 displays major risk factors affecting the DALYs by age and region of the world. This information will be useful in targeting school health prevention programs.

HEALTH ISSUES IN SCHOOL CHILDREN BY COUNTRY RESOURCE LEVEL

Low-Resource Communities
- Diarrhea, anemia, parasites, pneumonia, safe water, HIV/AIDS, mental health

Medium-Resource Communities
- Injuries, violence, unsafe sex, substance abuse, smoking, anemia, infections, mental health

High-Resource Communities
- Injuries, obesity, smoking, substance abuse, suicide prevention, mental health

Following are recommended targeted health interventions based on age group, region, and resource level of countries.

Low-resource countries and regions, such as some countries in Africa, India.

- 5- to 10-year age group: quality nutrition and micronutrients, especially anemia; safe water and hygiene; sanitation; parasite prevention and treatment; and malaria prevention.
- 10- to 20-year age group: mental health, injury prevention, HIV/AIDS education and prevention, violence prevention, and nutrition education.

Medium-resource countries and regions, such as South America.

- 5- to 10-year age group: nutrition education, obesity prevention, smoking and substance abuse prevention, and malaria prevention.
- 10- to 20-year age group: injury prevention, violence prevention, mental health, HIV/AIDS education and prevention, and suicide prevention.

High-resource countries and regions, such as the United States, Europe, and Australia.

- 5- to 10-year age group: obesity prevention, nutrition education, smoking and substance abuse prevention
- 10- to 20-year age group: mental health, smoking and substance abuse prevention, injury prevention, suicide prevention, and HIV/AIDS prevention.

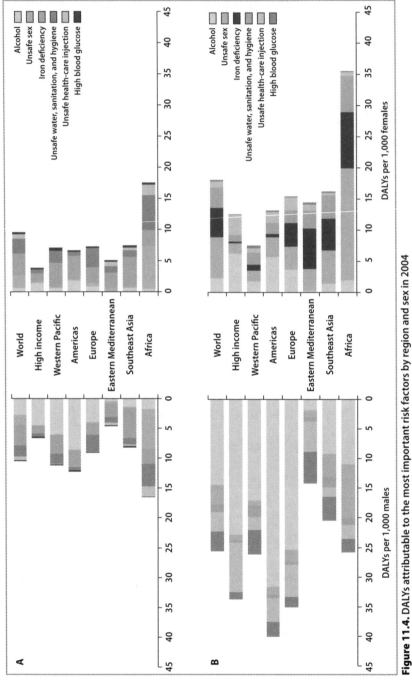

Figure 11.4. DALYs attributable to the most important risk factors by region and sex in 2004

(**A**) 10–14-year-olds. (**B**) 15–24-year-olds. DALY=disability-adjusted life-year. Physical injuries refer to unintentional injuries resulting from occupational risks. Reproduced with permission. Gore FM, Bloem PJ, Patton GC, et al. Global burden of disease in young people aged 10-24 years: a systematic analysis. *Lancet.* 2011;377(9783):2099. ©2011 Elsevier.[16]

Global School Health Models

Focusing Resources on Effective School Health

The FRESH framework was born at the World Education Forum in Dakar, Senegal, in April, 2000. The forum was jointly organized by WHO, UNESCO, UNICEF, and the World Bank as strategy session aiming at raising the education sector's awareness of the value of implementing an effective school health, hygiene, and nutrition program as major strategy to achieve education for all.[10] The FRESH framework targets interventions feasible to implement even in the most resource-poor schools and in hard-to-reach rural areas as well as in accessible urban areas and that promote learning through improved health and nutrition. The basic FRESH framework has 4 components that are the starting point to developing an effective child-friendly school health program. Each individual country can develop its own strategy to match local needs based on the framework. The 4 core components of the FRESH framework are[11]:

- **Health-related school policies,** including skills-based health education and the provision of health services, and also policies that ensure a safe and secure physical environment and a positive psychosocial environment, and that address issues such as abuse of students, sexual harassment, school violence, corporal punishment, and bullying. The policies need involvement of different levels, including the national level, and teachers, children, and parents at the school level.
- **Provision of safe water and sanitation,** reinforcing health and hygiene messages to both students and the wider community. For example, construction policies will help ensure that facilities address issues such as gender access and privacy. Separate facilities for girls, particularly adolescent girls, are an important contributing factor to reducing dropout at menses.
- **Skills-based health education,** focusing on the development of knowledge, attitudes, values, and life skills needed to make and act on the most appropriate and positive health-related decisions. The development of attitudes related to gender equity and respect between girls and boys and of skills such as dealing with peer pressure is central to effective skills-based health education and positive psychosocial environments.
- **School-based health and nutrition services,** addressing problems that are prevalent and recognized as important within the community. For example, micronutrient deficiencies and worm infections may be effectively dealt with by infrequent (6 monthly or annual) oral treatment.

The FRESH framework also describes different strategies to support its implementation. The strategies are[11]:

- *Effective partnerships between teachers and health workers and between the education and health sectors.* The success of school health programs demands an effective partnership between Ministries of Education and Health and between teachers and health workers. These sectors need to identify respective responsibilities and present coordinated action to improve health and learning outcomes for children.
- *Effective community partnerships.* The involvement of the broader community (eg, the private sector, community organizations, and women's groups) can enhance and reinforce school health promotion and resources. These partnerships, which should work together to make schools more child friendly, can jointly identify health issues that need to be addressed through the school and then help design and manage activities to address such issues.
- *Pupil awareness and participation.* Children who participate in health policy development and implementation are involved in efforts to create a safer and more sanitary environment; in health promotion aimed at their parents, other children, and community members; and in school health services, learning about health by doing.

Whole School, Whole Community, Whole Child

The Whole School, Whole Community, Whole Child (WSCC) model was developed by the CDC to address a broad range of health problems of youth in schools. The CDC developed the WSCC model to coordinate the many parts of school health into a systematic approach.[17,18] This approach can enable schools to:

- Eliminate gaps and reduce redundancies across the many initiatives and funding streams.
- Build partnerships and teamwork among school health and education professionals in the school.
- Build collaboration and enhance communication among public health, school health, and other education and health professionals in the community.
- Focus efforts on helping students engage in protective, health-enhancing behaviors and avoid risk behaviors.

The following are working descriptions of the components of coordinated school health[18]:

❶ Health Education: Health education provides students with opportunities to acquire the knowledge, attitudes, and skills necessary for making health-promoting decisions, achieving health literacy, adopting health-enhancing behaviors, and promoting the health of others. Comprehensive school health education includes courses of study (curricula) for students in pre-K through grade 12 that address a variety of topics such as alcohol and other drug use and abuse, healthy eating/nutrition, mental and emotional health, personal health and wellness, physical activity, safety and injury prevention, sexual health, tobacco use, and violence prevention. Health education curricula should address the National Health Education Standards (NHES) and incorporate the characteristics of an effective health education curriculum. Health education assists students in living healthier lives. Qualified, trained teachers teach health education.

❷ Physical Education: Physical education is a school-based instructional opportunity for students to gain the necessary skills and knowledge for lifelong participation in physical activity. Physical education is characterized by a planned, sequential K-12 curriculum (course of study) that provides cognitive content and learning experiences in a variety of activity areas. Quality physical education programs assist students in achieving the national standards for K-12 physical education. The outcome of a quality physical education program is a physically educated person who has the knowledge, skills, and confidence to enjoy a lifetime of healthful physical activity. Qualified, trained teachers teach physical education.

❸ Health Services: These services are designed to ensure access or referral to primary health care services or both, foster appropriate use of primary health care services, prevent and control communicable disease and other health problems, provide emergency care for illness or injury, promote and provide optimum sanitary conditions for a safe school facility and school environment, and provide educational and counseling opportunities for promoting and maintaining individual, family, and community health. Qualified professionals such as physicians, nurses, dentists, health educators, and other allied health personnel provide these services.

❹ **Nutrition Services:** Schools should provide access to a variety of nutritious and appealing meals that accommodate the health and nutrition needs of all students. School nutrition programs reflect the US Dietary Guidelines for Americans and other criteria to achieve nutrition integrity. The school nutrition services offer students a learning laboratory for classroom nutrition and health education and serve as a resource for linkages with nutrition-related community services. Qualified child nutrition professionals provide these services.

❺ **Counseling, Psychological, and Social Services:** These services are provided to improve students' mental, emotional, and social health and include individual and group assessments, interventions, and referrals. Organizational assessment and consultation skills of counselors and psychologists contribute not only to the health of students but also to the health of the school environment. Professionals such as certified school counselors, psychologists, and social workers provide these services.

❻ **Healthy and Safe School Environment:** A healthy and safe school environment includes the physical and aesthetic surroundings and the psychosocial climate and culture of the school. Factors that influence the physical environment include the school building and the area surrounding it, any biological or chemical agents that are detrimental to health, and physical conditions such as temperature, noise, and lighting. The psychosocial environment includes the physical, emotional, and social conditions that affect the well-being of students and staff.

❼ **Health Promotion for Staff:** Schools can provide opportunities for school staff members to improve their health status through activities such as health assessments, health education, and health-related fitness activities. These opportunities encourage staff members to pursue a healthy lifestyle that contributes to their improved health status, improved morale, and a greater personal commitment to the school's overall coordinated health program. This personal commitment often transfers into greater commitment to the health of students and creates positive role modeling. Health-promotion activities have improved productivity, decreased absenteeism, and reduced health insurance costs. The publication "School Employee Wellness: A Guide for Protecting the Assets of Our Nation's Schools" is a comprehensive guide that provides information, practical tools, and resources for school employee wellness programs.[19]

8 **Family/Community Involvement:** An integrated school, parent, and community approach can enhance the health and well-being of students. School health advisory councils, coalitions, and broadly based constituencies for school health can build support for school health program efforts. Schools actively solicit parent involvement and engage community resources and services to respond more effectively to the health-related needs of students. The publication "Parent Engagement: Strategies for Involving Parents in School Health" describes strategies and actions schools can take to increase parent engagement in promoting positive health behaviors among students.[20]

The Goals of WSCC are[18]:

- increase health knowledge, attitudes, and skills;
- increase positive health behaviors and health outcomes;
- improve education outcomes; and
- improve social outcomes.

Although the WSCC model is widely used in the United States, it has also been adopted and used in school health programs in other regions of the world. The CDC Web site, **http://www.cdc.gov/HealthyYouth/cshp/**, offers a number of strategies to implement WSCC programs as well as the School Health Index, a specific model addressing obesity, smoking, injury prevention, and asthma. The American Cancer Society has also published an excellent guide on how communities can develop a Community School Health Council.[21]

Health-Promoting Schools

The health promoting schools (HPS) model is a global concept to achieve health and education for all. It is based on the social model of health and emphasizes the entire organization of the school.[22] This model was developed at the European WHO symposium titled "The Health-Promoting School" at Peebles, Scotland, in 1986.[5,6] The HPS model is used extensively throughout Europe embedded within the educational curriculum of schools. Its implementation is organized by the SHE Network, established in 1992. Because the HPS model works on interrelated areas within the school environment, it is most effective in producing long-term changes to students' attitudes.

The HPS model has 6 components: **healthy school policies, the school's physical environment, the school's social environment, individuals' health skills and action competencies, community links, and health services.**[22-24] *Healthy school policies* are those that are clearly defined in documents or in accepted practices that promote health and well-being (eg, policies that enable healthy food choices at school; policies that discourage bullying). *The school's physical environment* refers to the buildings, grounds, and equipment in and surrounding the school, such as: the building design and location; the provision of natural light and adequate shade; the creation of space for physical activity; and facilities for learning and healthy eating. *The school's social environment* is a combination of the quality of the relationships among and between staff and students. It is influenced by the relationships with parents and the wider community. *Individuals' health skills and action competencies* refer to both the formal and informal curriculum and associated activities, where students gain age-related knowledge, understanding, skills, and experiences that enable them to build competencies in taking action to improve the health and well-being of themselves and others in their community and that enhance their learning outcomes. *Community links* are the connections between the school and the students' families, plus the connection between the school and key local groups and individuals. Those enhance the HPS and provide students and staff with a context and support for their actions. *Health services* are the local and regional school-based or school-linked services that have a responsibility for child and adolescent health care and promotion through the provision of direct services to students including those with special needs. An example of an HPS model on healthy eating could include the following features[23]:

- ensuring healthy school food is available at breakfast or lunch time;
- providing an attractive environment for food consumption that takes students' wishes into account;
- developing a policy on snack provision, including vending machines.
- ensuring fresh water is available in schools;
- encouraging students to develop skills in food cultivation, preparation, and purchase with involvement of parents and local food organizations;
- making provision for related physical activity initiatives, such as safe and active routes to schools or secure bicycle storage; and
- making links with associated issues, such as mental and emotional health, the cultural role of food, and the role of the media in marketing food.

There is enough evidence of success of the HPS model.[3,23] Among the most effective programs are those that promote healthy eating, physical activity, and mental health; however, its implementation can have some drawbacks, and the school communities need structured assistance implementing the HPS framework.[22]

Essential Package Model

The Essential Package model is based on the FRESH model described in this chapter. UNICEF and the World Feeding Program (WFP) are collaborating to improve the health and education on children in resource-poor communities. The benefits of this package include cost-effectiveness, enhancement of other child development initiatives, ensuring better educational outcomes, and improving social equality. By addressing both education and health in the same model, the Essential Package takes a holistic view of improving the future of children.[25] The 12 components of the package are:

1. Basic education
2. Food for education
3. Promotion of girl's education
4. Potable water and sanitary latrines
5. Health, nutrition, and hygiene education
6. Systemic deworming
7. Micronutrient supplementation
8. HIV and AIDS education
9. Psychosocial support
10. Malaria prevention
11. School gardens
12. Improved stoves

Nutrition-Friendly Schools Initiative

The Nutrition-Friendly Schools Initiative (NFSI) was developed by the WHO to specifically target the double burden of nutrition problems of malnutrition and obesity that are cooccurring in many countries now as resources improve (Table 11.3). There are 5 components to this model[26]:

1. Having a written nutrition-friendly schools policy
2. Enhancing awareness and capacity building of the school community
3. Developing a nutrition and health-promoting school curriculum
4. Creating a supportive school environment
5. Providing supportive school nutrition and health services

Table 11.3. Nutrition Friendly School Initiatives.

	FRESH (Focusing Resources on Effective School Health)	Health-Promoting Schools (HPS)	Child-Friendly Schools (CFS)	Essential Package (EP)	NFSI
Partners	UNESCO, UNICEF, WHO, World Bank, others	WHO	UNICEF	UNICEF-WFP	EDC, FAO, SCN, UNESCO, UNICEF, World Bank, WFP, others
Year	2000	1995	1995	2002	2006
Goal	Improve learning outcomes through health	Health promotion according to context	Rights-based quality basic education in a healthy environment	Improve learning through health (focus on undernutrition)	Address the double burden of nutrition related ill health
Content	4 basic components 1. Health-related school policies 2. W&S, healthy school environment 3. Skills-based health education 4. Health and nutrition services 3 strategies 1. Partnerships between teachers and health workers 2. Community partnerships 3. Pupil participation	6 strategies regarding 1. Engagement of staff, students, parents, and communities 2. Safe and healthy environment 3. Skills-based health education 4. Health services 5. Health promoting policies and practices 6. Focus on community health concerns	13 characteristics 1. Children's rights 2. Whole child 3. Child centered 4. Gender-sensitive 5. Quality learning 6. Reality education 7. Flexibility, diversity 8. Inclusion 9. Mental and physical health 10. Affordable and accessible 11. Teacher capacity 12. Family focused 13. Community based	12 cost-effective interventions to improve the health and nutrition of school-age children, including basic education, food for education, W&S, health education, deworming, MN supplementation, etc.	5 key components with 22 essential criteria regarding nutrition-friendly schools policy awareness and capacity building of the school community, nutrition and health-promoting school curriculum, supportive school environment, and school nutrition health services

Department of Nutrition for Health and Development. *Nutrition-Friendly Schools Initiative (NFSI). A School-Based Programme to Address the Double Burden of Malnutrition.* Available at: http://www.who.int/nutrition/topics/NFSI_Briefing_presentation.pdf. Accessed November 24, 2015.

Other School Health Models

Child Friendly Schools is another UNICEF model for a comprehensive school model including a healthy environment and health services.[27,28] *Water, Sanitation, and Hygiene in Schools* (WASH) is yet another UNICEF program for schools focusing on safe water and sanitation.[29]

School Health Program Examples by Country Economy

School health programs have vastly developed over the last decade after the FRESH framework was launched. In 2000, a survey of 36 countries in Sub-Saharan Africa suggested that only 8% implemented a school health and nutrition program that met the criteria for equity and effectiveness. By 2007, 44% of these countries had fully compliant programs, and many of the remainder were well on their way to achieving a comprehensive approach.[1] The following are examples of school health programs around the world by country economy.

Low-Income Country Economy

Kenya: Action-Oriented and Participatory Health Education in Primary Schools. This school health program was implemented in 9 primary schools in the Bondo District, western Kenya, from 1999 to 2002. The program was initiated after initial research showed high prevalence of intestinal helminth infections among school-aged children. The program consisted on health education focused on geohelminth and schistosomiasis infections.

The school health education program consisted of 3 interventions:

❶ The use of flip charts as an interactive tool in the school's health education.
❷ Establishment of an extracurricular health club.
❸ In-service training in the form of continual professional support.

The interventions addressed 2 elements of the health-promoting school concept: a healthy school environment (physical and psychosocial) and outreach to families and community. The health club had the greatest effect on students' competence and knowledge. The intervention with greatest effect was the combination of health clubs with flip charts.

Remarkable changes were achieved in the students' personal and environmental hygiene choices such as placement of hand-wash facilities next to the pit latrines in schools, establishment of compost heaps and rubbish pits, and placement of dish racks for drying utensils at the students' homes. Teachers reported that children took action to manage their health, for example, burning and selling charcoal to get money to buy shoes to be neat as well as to avoid hookworm infection.

The action-oriented and participatory health education strategies had an effect on the students and their community (commitment, participation, and knowledge of worm transmission and prevention).

Middle-Income Country Economy

Brazil: Addressing the Social Determinants of Health: The Experience of a Municipal School in Rio de Janeiro.[6]

The ABC & Art Project is a participative school management and health promotion initiative in the Municipal School Alexandre de Gusmão in Rio de Janeiro. The school is located in a low-income neighborhood where drug trafficking is the most attractive income-generating alternative for young people. The project started in 2000 and is still progressing. The school team partnered with a local hospital to provide training of teachers and volunteer mothers on how to protect and promote oral health at school age and to create a health post, responsible for emergencies in the area, with a nurse designated to be the liaison with the school and a referral system for students to access oral and mental health services. The project also used art and literature as tools for mobilizing children and families in a health-promoting and empowering experience. Other strategies of the project are creating a council with community activists and investing in musical instruments to set up workshops on drama, guitar, percussion, and fold dances. This project was implemented in the context of an HPS model that reflected the characteristics and identity of the city. The program emphasizes the strengthening of 3 critical axes: participation management, popular education, and intersectorial action.

High-Income Country Economy

Germany: Anschub.de – "Alliance for Sustainable School Health and Education."[6]

The Anschub.de is an alliance for sustainable health and education in Germany. It was established in 2002 and planned as a nationwide program. The core target groups of the program are students, teachers, and parents and also the responsible bodies for schools in the community, in the educational and health ministries, and in the administration.

Anschub.de has created a national alliance of supporting organizations and experts in school health promotion and education, and a new concept for school health promotion in Germany, the concept of the "good and healthy school." Anschub.de also has created a communication strategy to overcome barriers inside and outside the school; more than 10 new modules for heads of schools, for classroom teachers, and for parents to support them in building up a good and healthy school and healthy learning and teaching; a fan-fold document and a brochure that inform the target audiences and the general public about the good and healthy school concept, values, principles and strategies; and networks of schools supported by local or regional governmental organizations and nongovernmental organizations.

Challenges and Opportunities in Global School Health: Immunization Model

One of the most significant challenges in developing school health programs is funding. Who should pay for school health services? Collaboration between public health and school systems is essential and can greatly enhance stable funding for school health services. One model to build on could be school-based immunization programs. Immunizations clearly improve the health of children—immunized children are healthier, have higher attendance rates, and provide protection to other students through herd immunity. There are challenges to school-based immunization programs, and WHO has developed a School Vaccination Readiness Assessment Tool[30] to help communities assess their readiness and prioritize strategies to implement plans for school immunizations. Funding is always a challenge, but the opportunity for public health and education systems to work together in planning and shared funding can lead to both systems accomplishing their goals of healthy and successful students.

How to Work With Schools

Pediatricians are logical partners in improving the health and education of children. Pediatricians can serve as school consultants, advisors, members of school health councils, or direct providers. By approaching the school with the goal of improving school performance by improving the health of children, we become natural partners. Being informed and advocating for one of the above school health models, we can build a strong collaboration for all children.

Recommendations for Pediatricians

- Pediatricians involved in global health should visit local schools in their community to be aware of local health issues of school-aged children, school health policies, and resources available at the schools.
- Pediatricians interested in global health should consider working with one of the global school health models presented in this chapter.
- Looking at successful global school health programs can serve as an excellent guide for planning new programs to improve school health.
- Advocate for children with special health care needs in schools in global communities in which you work.

Recommendations for Program Directors and Trainees

- Global school health models can serve as an excellent format to discuss frameworks for global interventions in improving the health of school-aged children and adolescents.
- Programs with pediatric global health tracks should consider interventions in schools and study the different school health models described in this chapter.
- Residency programs should encourage residents to visit community school health programs to see how they might apply to global school health needs.
- Trainees interested in global health should consider the various global health models presented here and target the school health components that address the health needs of the community they plan to serve.
- Trainees should visit local school health programs to develop an understanding of different methods to address health of school-aged children.

Take-Home Points

- There are a number of well-developed global school health models to address improving the health of school-aged children and adolescents.
- Reviewing successful school health programs and models in the region in which you are interested in working can help you implement a successful school health program.
- Components of a global school health model should address the unique health problems of the community you are serving and the resources available.
- Global school health programs have been successful at addressing important health needs of school-aged children and adolescents.

Resources

For additional school health related resources, visit www.aap.org/
schoolhealthmanual.

References

1. Bundy D. *Rethinking School Health a Key Component of Education for All.* Washington, DC: The World Bank; 2011:1-336
2. Young I. Health promotion in schools: a historical perspective. *Health Promotion and Education.* 2005;12(3-4):111-117
3. Stewart-Brown S. *What is the Evidence on School Health Promotion in Improving Health or Preventing Disease and, Specifically, What is the Effectiveness of the Health Promoting Schools Approach?* Copenhagen, Denmark: WHO Regional Office for Europe; 2006
4. Young I. *The Health Promoting School. Report of a WHO Symposium.* Edingburgh, Scotland: Scottish Health Education Group/World Health Organization Regional Office for Europe; 1986
5. World Health Organization. *Primary Health Care. Report of the International Conference on Primary Health Care, Alma-Ata, USSR, 6–12 September 1978.* Geneva, Switzerland: World Health Organization; 1978
6. Whitman CV, Aldinger CE, ed. *Case Studies in Global School Health Promotion: From Reseach to Practice.* New York, NY: Springer; 2009
7. Schools For Health in Europe. SHE Network. Available at: http://www.schoolsforhealth.eu/. Accessed April 13, 2015
8. World Health Organization. School and Youth Health. Global School Health Initiative. Geneva, Switzerland: World Health Organization; 2012. Available at: http://www.who.int/ school_youth_health/gshi/en/. Accessed April 13, 2015
9. Education World Forum. *The Dakar Framework for Action - Education for All: Meeting our Collective Commitments.* Paris, France: United Nations Educational, Scientific and Cultural Organization; 2000
10. Schoolsandhealth.org. FRESH Focusing Resources on Effective School Health. Available at: http://www.schoolsandhealth.org/FRESH. Accessed November 24, 2015
11. Matsuura K, Bellamy C, Bruntland G, Wolfensohn JD. *Focusing Resources on Effective School Health: a FRESH Start to Enhancing the Quality and Equity of Education.* Dakar, Senegal: UNESCO, UNICEF, WHO, the World Bank; 2000
12. World Health Organization. *Report of the Technical Meeting of Building School Partnership for Health, Education Achievements and Development.* Vancouver, Canada: World Health Organization; 2007
13. Education International. EFAIDS an EI/WHO/EDC Programme. Available at: http://www. ei-ie.org/en/. Accessed April 13, 2015
14. United Nations Educational, Scientific and Cultural Organization. UNAIDS Inter-Agency Task Team on Education. Available at: http://www.unesco.org/new/en/hiv-and-aids/ about-us/unaids-iatt-on-education/. Accessed April 13, 2015
15. United Nations System Standing Committee on Nutrition. Available at: http://www.unscn. org/. Accessed April 13, 2015
16. Gore FM, Bloem PJ, Patton GC, et al. Global burden of disease in young people aged 10-24 years: a systematic analysis. 2011;377(9783):2093-2102
17. Allensworth DD, Kolbe LJ. The comprenhensive school health program: exploring an expanded concept. *J Sch Health.* 1987;57(10):409-412

18. Centers for Disease Control and Prevention. Adolescent and School Health. Available at: http://www.cdc.gov/healthyyouth/cshp/index.htm. Accessed April 13, 2015

19. Centers for Disease Control and Prevention, National Center for Chronic Disease Prevention and Health Promotion. School Employee Wellness: A Guide for Protecting the Assets of Our Nation's Schools. Available at: http://dhpe.site-ym.com/?page=Programs_ SEW. Accessed November 24, 2015

20. Centers for Disease Control and Prevention. Parent Engagement: Strategies for Involving Parents in School Health. 2012. Available at: http://www.cdc.gov/healthyyouth/protective/ parent_engagement.htm. Accessed November 24, 2015

21. Shirer K. Promoting Healthy Youth, School and Communities: A Guide to Community School Health Councils. 2003. Available at: http://www.cancer.org/acs/groups/content/@nho/ documents/document/guidetocommunityschoolhealhcou.pdf. Accessed April 13, 2015

22. Senior E. Becoming a health promoting school: key components of planning. *Global Health Promotion.* 2012;19:23

23. St Leger L, Young I, Blanchard C, Perry M. *Promoting Health in Schools: From Evidence to Action.* Saint Denis Cedex, France: International Union for Health Promotion and Education; 2010

24. The International Union for Health Promotion and Education (IUHPE). Achieving Health Promoting Schools: Guidelines for Promoting Health in Schools. 2nd ed. 2008. Available at: http://www.iuhpe.org. Accessed April 13, 2015

25. World Food Programme and UNICEF. The Essential Package: Twelve Interventions to Improve the Health and Nutrition of School-Age Children. Available at: http://www. un.org/esa/socdev/poverty/PovertyForum/Documents/The%20Essential%20Package.pdf. Accessed April 13, 2015

26. World Health Organization. Nutrition-Friendly Schools Initiative. Available at: http://www. who.int/nutrition/topics/NFSI_Briefing_presentation.pdf. Accessed April 13, 2015

27. UNICEF. Child Friendly Schools. Available at: http://www.unicef.org/education/files/ CFS1Web.pdf. Accessed April 13, 2015

28. UNICEF. Child Friendly Schools Manual. Available at: http://www.unicef.org/publications/ files/Child_Friendly_Schools_Manual_EN_040809.pdf. Accessed April 13, 2015

29. UNICEF. Water, Sanitation and Hygiene (WASH) in Schools. Available at: http://www. unicef.org/publications/files/Child_Friendly_Schools_Manual_EN_040809.pdf. Accessed April 13, 2015

30. World Health Organization. School Vaccination Readiness Assessment Tool. Available at: http://apps.who.int/iris/bitstream/10665/90566/1/WHO_IVB_13.02_eng.pdf. Accessed April 13, 2015

CHAPTER

12

Program Assessment and Evaluation

Catherine N. Rasberry, PhD, MCHES
Seraphine Pitt Barnes, PhD, MPH, CHES

Background

What Is Program Evaluation?

Evaluation can be defined as the systematic assessment of a program's worth, merit, or significance.[1,2] (In this chapter, the term "program" is used broadly to refer to any specific intervention, policy, practice, or service.) In program evaluation, determining the worth, merit, or significance of a program often means determining whether a program is having its intended effect. However, program evaluation can also describe an existing need (and, therefore, provide support for implementing a program) or the manner in which an existing program is being implemented. Evaluations provide information program staff can use for making decisions about the need for a program, whether a given program works, why a program is or is not working, and ways to improve a program.[2,3]

Most people use evaluation routinely in all aspects of life—both personal and professional. Physicians regularly use evaluation and research data to inform clinical decisions. For example, a physician would not prescribe a new drug for a patient before being confident that research supports its safety and effectiveness. In the same way, it is important to collect data to inform decisions about school health programs of all types—from basic vision and hearing screenings to more comprehensive and complex programs that help students better manage chronic conditions, such as diabetes or asthma. By asking the right questions and then systematically collecting the right data, evaluators can make assessments of the worth, merit, significance, or condition of a program to make decisions and provide recommendations for improvement.

Who Are the Evaluators?

There is no hard and fast rule for who should evaluate a program. Usually when school health programs are being evaluated, the evaluation is led by program staff, an external evaluator brought in as a consultant, or a staff member at the district level who has evaluation expertise. Regardless of who leads the evaluation, it is critical for program staff to be involved.

Why Is Program Evaluation Important?

Program evaluation is a critical tool for use in selecting, implementing, improving, and justifying health-related programs. Without program evaluation, it would be difficult for program staff to identify what effects their programs had on participants. Not only does evaluation provide information on whether a program is working, it can also be used before a program is implemented to identify the need for a program and provide context about the audience, need, and setting that can help the program staff select the most appropriate program to use and determine the best strategies for implementation. Once a program is implemented, program evaluation can help determine whether a program is being implemented correctly, whether a program is having its intended effects, whether it is cost-effective, and how it can be improved.

Types of Evaluation

Evaluations can be classified into 2 broad categories: *formative* and *summative*. Within those 2 categories, there are several specific types of evaluations that can be further defined.

Formative Evaluation

Formative evaluation produces information that can form or shape the program being evaluated. These evaluations are often conducted before or during program implementation. Three of the most common types of formative evaluations are *evaluability assessments*, *needs assessments*, and *implementation* (or *process*) *evaluations*.[2-4]

Evaluability Assessments

Evaluability assessments systematically identify whether a program is justified, feasible, and likely to provide useful results.[2,5] Evaluators often engage in this exploratory evaluation process to determine whether an existing program is ready for evaluation. Key considerations for determining evaluation readiness include having a sound and logical program design, well-defined and plausible program goals, feasible program implementation with the intended audience, program implementation with fidelity, sufficient resources for program implementation, capacity for data collection on outcomes, and agreement among stakeholders regarding the use of findings.[5] The results of an evaluability assessment may reveal 1 of 2 conclusions: the program is ready for evaluation, or the program is not ready for evaluation. If a program is ready for evaluation, the program design is sound and logical (often reflected in a comprehensive logic model), the program is being implemented as intended, the capacity for data collection exists, and there is agreement on how data will be used. Furthermore, it may be that the evaluability assessment determines parameters for the evaluation (eg, the type of data that can be collected or what the focus of the evaluation should be). If a program is not ready for evaluation, it may be that the program design is flawed and unlikely to produce the expected outcomes. An evaluability assessment may suggest that program stakeholders revisit the program design and expected outcomes and make modifications to the program or to the outcomes.

Needs Assessments

Needs assessments are used to determine the need for a program, better understand the nature and scope of the existing need, and make some initial assessments of what might help meet the need.[2] In some cases, evaluators use needs assessments to help prioritize program topics or interventions. For example, a school health services coordinator might conduct a needs assessment with school health staff to determine the focus and content of professional development activities. By reviewing existing data (eg, program records, suggestion box entries, e-mails from students and staff) and/or administering surveys to, interviewing, or conducting focus groups with staff, the coordinator could determine content areas in which staff need additional training and support. In addition, such an assessment might help the coordinator identify different training priorities for different types of staff. For example, school counselors might need training on making referrals for health services, but school-based health clinic office staff might be better served with training on creating a welcoming environment for students.

Implementation Evaluations

Implementation evaluations (sometimes called process evaluations) are used to explore how programs are provided, including delivery and/or program fidelity and to identify areas of strength or weakness (eg, in a program's delivery approach, facilitator effectiveness, fidelity, or content) to improve the program.[2-4] Evaluators can use these evaluations to help program staff examine program operations to explain why programs are or are not successful. Questions might include: Did the program reach the desired audience? Did participants enjoy the program? In what aspects of the program did people participate?[3] For example, if school nurses were delivering a diabetes education program to students with diabetes, an implementation or process evaluation could be used to see if the lessons were well attended, offered to the correct students, enjoyable for students, and taught as intended (with the correct content, using the correct methods, in the correct sequence, and for the correct amount of time).

Summative Evaluation

Summative evaluation produces information that describes the effects or outcomes of the program being evaluated. Although the word summative implies that this type of evaluation happens only at the very end of a program, the evaluation process should begin as the program is taking shape. It is not realistic to expect a program to be fully refined and polished before evaluating it; in fact, the evaluation process should be part of a continuous cycle of program improvement that consistently helps refine and strengthen a program. Two common types of summative evaluations are *outcome evaluations* (sometimes referred to as *impact evaluations*) and *cost-related evaluations*.[2]

Outcome Evaluations

Outcome evaluations are used to determine whether the program had the intended effects on target outcomes.[2-4] Evaluators often use these evaluations to determine whether a program worked, and they can provide valuable data for selecting programmatic approaches and justifying effective programs. For example, if an evaluation of an asthma management program found that asthma control improved for students who received both classroom education on asthma basics and 1-on-1 assistance with medication inhalation technique compared with students who received only classroom education, the program staff might decide to incorporate the one-on-one assistance with medication inhalation technique into its program approach.

Cost-Related Evaluations

Cost-related evaluations are used to determine the relative costs for achieving the outcomes of the program. Cost-effectiveness analysis compares costs of the program to nonmonetary outcomes; findings are often expressed as cost per life-year saved or quality-adjusted life year saved. Cost-benefit analysis compares costs to the related benefits, and both are expressed in terms of money.[6,7] Cost-benefit analysis can describe the return on investment associated with implementing a program, and because all measures are expressed in monetary terms, it provides a common metric for comparing different types of programs (eg, health and nonhealth programs).[8] Both types of cost analyses provide information that can be used to justify a program or make decisions about the most efficient and affordable approaches to achieve desired results.[3]

TYPES OF EVALUATIONS

There are a variety of ways to describe different types of evaluations. Some evaluators like the terms formative and summative, others do not. Some evaluators use outcome evaluation and impact evaluation interchangeably, and others have specific and distinct definitions for each. The types of evaluations presented here are intended to offer a feel for the different forms evaluations can take—not to support one type of terminology over another. In the end, the most important part of any evaluation is the *process* used to conduct the evaluation—not the label used to describe it.

Steps in Evaluation

Evaluation does not have to be elaborate, but it should be systematic. In 1999, the Centers for Disease Control and Prevention (CDC) published a *Framework for Program Evaluation in Public Health* that can serve as a useful guide for pediatricians, school health coordinators, other school staff, and stakeholders involved in evaluating school health programs. It outlines 6 steps and defines 4 standards that are essential for effective evaluation.[1] Although the steps are presented in a designated order here, the circular shape of the model reflects an often cyclical approach to evaluation, whereby steps can be revisited and refined. Some of the steps (eg, engaging stakeholders) will occur multiple times over the course of an evaluation. A more detailed description of the 6 evaluation steps is provided in the government report.

Standards for Effective Evaluation

In addition to highlighting 6 steps of evaluation, the CDC *Framework for Program Evaluation in Public Health* identifies 4 standards that should guide all evaluations: utility, feasibility, propriety, and accuracy. Utility standards help ensure that the evaluation will meet the needs of the users. Feasibility standards help the evaluators ensure the evaluation will be realistic and practical, politically viable, and cost-effective. Propriety standards are used to ensure all evaluation activities are ethical, legal, and conducted in a manner that protects the participants and those impacted by the evaluation's findings. Accuracy standards are useful to ensure that findings will be correct and adequate to inform decision-making.[1] In addition, the Joint Committee on Standards for Educational Evaluation identified a fifth set of standards, evaluation account-ability standards, that are used to ensure sufficient and complete documenta-tion of an evaluation and support assessing the design, processes, and findings from the evaluation (in essence, evaluating the evaluation).[9]

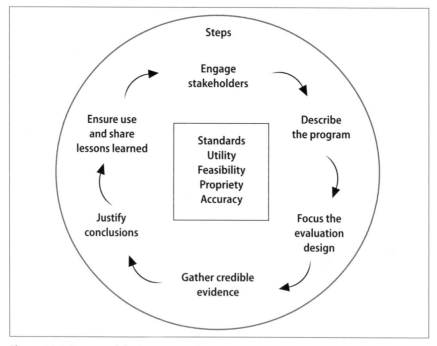

Figure 12.1. Framework for Program Evaluation. Reproduced from Centers for Disease Control and Prevention, Evaluation Working Group. *Framework for Program Evaluation in Public Health.* Atlanta, GA: Centers for Disease Control and Prevention; 1999. Available at: http://www.cdc.gov/eval/framework/.

Step ❶: Engage Stakeholders

The first step in the framework involves engaging stakeholders. To do this, it is important for evaluators to first identify them. Stakeholders in health-related programs usually fall into 1 of 3 groups: the people involved in the operations of the program, the people served or affected by the program, or the people who will use the evaluation findings (ie, those who may be in a position to take some action regarding the program). It is important to engage all groups to have an effective evaluation. By involving these people in the early stages of the evaluation, evaluators can increase the evaluation's credibility and the likelihood that the findings will be used. In addition, the involvement of stakeholders can help enhance cultural competence, protect evaluation participants, and avoid conflicts of interest.[1]

In school health programs, there are a number of people who may be important stakeholders. It is important for evaluators to think broadly about the variety of individuals who may have interest in the program or its evaluation findings. These people might include program staff; funders or sponsors (including external organizations); school board members; district administrators; school nurses; teachers; school counselors; principals; bus drivers; facility, custodial, and maintenance personnel; other school staff; students; parents and family members; local coalitions related to the program; or other community organizations.

Stakeholders can be involved in an evaluation in many ways. By considering who the stakeholders are, what their strengths are, and how they are involved in the program, evaluators can make strategic decisions about the most useful ways to involve them. Stakeholders may help design or conduct the evaluation, review the progress and final results, or provide guidance and feedback throughout the evaluation process.

If the program being evaluated has a large number of stakeholders and it seems ineffective to involve them all in the evaluation, it may be possible to narrow the list of involved stakeholders to those who are most critical to the program. Those who are most critical can be involved in the evaluation more directly, and the larger group of stakeholders can be kept informed of all evaluation activities and progress without extensive involvement in the evaluation. It is rarely necessary or helpful to have every stakeholder involved in every aspect of the evaluation.

Step ❷: Describe the Program

The second step in the framework is describing the program that will be evaluated. This is a key step that helps set the foundation for the evaluation. In describing the program, it is important to articulate:

- the need the program is intended to address;
- the expected effects of the program;
- the activities of the program;
- the resources available to support the program activities;
- the program's current stage of development or maturity; and
- the context in which the program operates.

All of these characteristics shape the program and help inform the focus and methods of the evaluation.[1]

One tool for describing the program is a logic model. A logic model is a visual depiction of the way a program is intended to work. Often displayed as a flow chart or table, the logic model links resources to activities and activities to desired effects.[1] Logic models can be designed with several different elements, but common components often include inputs (eg, resources, staff), activities (eg, teaching students with asthma better medication inhalation techniques), outputs (eg, number of students taught), and outcomes ranging from short-term (eg, students demonstrate better medication inhalation technique) to long-term (eg, students experience fewer asthma exacerbations). By involving stakeholders in the development and refinement of a program's logic model, evaluators can help ensure that all individuals invested in the program share a common understanding of the program's key activities and intended outcomes.

LOGIC MODELS

Logic models not only are excellent tools for program evaluation, they can also be tremendously useful for describing a program to stakeholders or other interested persons both effectively and concisely. There are a number of online resources that provide more detailed information on developing and using logic models.

Step ❸: Focus the Evaluation

The third step in the evaluation framework is focusing the evaluation on what to evaluate and how to frame the evaluation activities. There are 6 key considerations to keep in mind when focusing an evaluation[1]:

- purpose;
- users;
- uses;
- evaluation questions;
- methods; and
- agreements.

Purpose. Evaluations can serve a number of different purposes, and it is important for program evaluators to select the type of evaluation that is best suited to address that specific program. For example, is the purpose of the evaluation to identify a need within a certain population, assess the current state of a program, determine what type of effect a program is having, or assess a program's cost-benefit ratio?

Users and Uses. Once the purpose is decided, focus the evaluation by considering the users of the evaluation findings and the potential uses of the findings and recommendations. The users are the people who will receive the findings of the evaluation and make decisions based on them—those likely to be among the stakeholders identified in step 1. Often, different users are interested in answering different questions. The uses are how evaluation findings will be applied (eg, to improve the program, to advocate for more or continued funding, to build support for introducing the program to other schools). By prioritizing the most important uses and ensuring input and buy-in from key users, the evaluation can be designed with the greatest likelihood of producing meaningful findings to inform decisions and actions.[1]

Evaluation Questions. Selecting evaluation questions is a critical aspect of focusing the evaluation. Evaluation questions define the primary issues to be examined in the evaluation. Evaluators can benefit from brainstorming potential questions with key program stakeholders to determine what questions are most important. The selected evaluation questions should be aligned with the purpose of the evaluation and the priorities identified, of interest to stakeholders, and answerable. Examples of evaluation questions include:

- What are the professional development needs of health services staff for responding to students' asthma exacerbations at school?
- What percentage of students with asthma received training on medication inhalation technique?

■ Did students with asthma who participated in the school-based asthma management program demonstrate better asthma control after the program than before the program?

It is likely that different stakeholders will have different questions they want to answer, but eventually, the goal is to narrow down to a limited number of key questions the evaluation will answer. These questions will serve as the boundaries for the evaluation, so it is important to be clear about what an evaluation will be able to answer and what it will not be able to answer. Getting buy-in from stakeholders at this step of the process can help ensure that all stakeholders understand what can be expected from the results.

Methods. Once evaluation questions have been identified, evaluators should select the most appropriate evaluation methods to answer the questions. Evaluations can have experimental, quasi-experimental, or nonexperimental designs, or they can include a combination of those designs. Each design choice comes with its own set of unique strengths and limitations; there is no single design that is best in every situation. The "best" design is one that allows program staff to answer the evaluation questions with a level of rigor and credibility that is suitable to the users. Four of the standards of effective evaluation—utility, feasibility, propriety, and accuracy—are critical considerations in selecting the evaluation design.

Evaluation Design Options. Evaluators can use several different types of designs to answer evaluation questions. These designs are typically categorized as experimental, quasi-experimental, or nonexperimental.

The designs, in essence, represent a continuum in which experimental designs offer evaluators the greatest ability to detect causal relationships between variables (eg, participation in a program activity led to a change in a health outcome), and nonexperimental designs offer the least ability to detect those types of relationships with certainty.[3,10]

Experimental designs are often considered the gold standard of evaluation designs—they are characterized by random assignment of participants to an intervention condition (ie, participating in the program) or a control condition (ie, not participating in the program).[11] In practice, however, it can be difficult to use this design without significant resources (financial and human) and the flexibility to assert substantial control over both intervention and control conditions.

Like experimental designs, quasi-experimental designs use an intervention and a control condition, but unlike experimental designs, participants are not randomly assigned to a condition.[11] Because random assignment is not required, quasi-experimental designs are often much more practical for program staff to use. Though they cannot account for all differences that might occur between the intervention and control group, a quasi-experimental design will often meet stakeholders' requirements for rigor and provide valuable information on possible program effects.

Nonexperimental designs do not use a control condition. One example is a design that measures outcomes only among program participants at the end of the program (this is called a 1-group post-test–only design).[3,10,11] Because it lacks multiple time points and a comparison group, this design does not allow evaluators to make a statement about one variable (eg, program participation) causing another (eg, an intended behavior). Another nonexperimental design measures a variable of interest both before and after program participation but only measures it among program participants. Even though this type of design (called a 1-group pretest-post-test design) includes more than 1 time point, it still cannot rule out enough possible outside influences to allow an evaluator to say with confidence that it was program participation rather than some other factor that impacted any change in the outcome of interest.[3,10] There are many situations in which limited data, resources, or external factors lead evaluators to appropriately select nonexperimental designs. For example, needs assessment questions (eg, Why are students choosing not to participate in elective health screenings?) may be answered sufficiently with a 1-time survey or data collection.

Agreements. Evaluators use agreements to articulate the roles and responsibilities of different stakeholders in the evaluation and document decisions about the evaluation's purpose, focus, procedures, methods, and safeguards. Although these agreements may be formal or informal, written or spoken, they should always involve the key stakeholders, primary users of the evaluation, individuals involved in conducting the evaluation, and individuals or organizations providing funding or in-kind support.[1]

Step ❹: Gather Credible Evidence

In step 4 of the evaluation framework, gathering credible evidence, the evaluators begin to collect data to answer the questions selected in the previous step. Gathering credible evidence is critical, because it allows for sound judgments and well-supported conclusions and recommendations. The information collected through the evaluation must be both valid and relevant for the findings to be valued and used.[1]

Indicators and Data Sources. Credibility can be impacted by the indicators selected (ie, the key characteristics of a program that are relevant to the evaluation), sources of data, quality of data, quantity of data, and logistics of data collection. Evaluators use indicators to create specific measures to represent the general concepts of the program, as well as its context and expected effects. Indicators can be selected to describe both program activities (eg, program participation rates, client satisfaction, intervention exposure) and program effects (eg, changes in behavior, changes in policy, changes in environment).[1] For example, an evaluator who is trying to determine whether a before-school walking program has helped decrease obesity among students could use key measures such as the number of minutes each student walked (as an indicator of intervention exposure) and each student's body mass index calculated from measures of height and weight (as an indicator of obesity).

Once indicators have been selected, evaluators should identify sources of data to measure each indicator, keeping in mind that indicators can sometimes be measured by more than 1 data source and more than 1 type of data (ie, qualitative and quantitative data).[1] For example, if a school pediatrician was trying to assess the extent to which school staff referred students for health services, he or she could consider several data sources—reports from teachers, students, or students' parents, or records of referrals from school health staff (eg, school nurses, school counselors, school social workers). Use of more than one data source or more than one type of data could increase both the credibility of her evidence and the evaluation's likelihood to provide explanations for what was actually happening in the program.

DATA SOURCES AND METHODS

There are many different sources and methods that evaluators can use to gather information about the operations or impact of their programs. It is important to consider all possible sources and methods. Then, narrow to the ones that are most likely to accurately and efficiently answer the evaluation questions that have been selected.

Data may be gathered from existing documents (eg, e-mails, meeting agendas, training materials, programmatic records), existing databases, students, students' families, community members, school and district administrators and other staff, program staff, and funders.

Possible methods for data collection include document review, surveys, interviews, focus groups, and clinical or other assessments.

Data Quality and Quantity. Other key factors in credibility include the quality and quantity of data. Data quality can be increased by using appropriate and validated data collection instruments, strong evaluation designs, credible (and sometimes multiple) data sources, sound data management practices, accurate coding, and thorough error-checking. Although a data set may never be perfect, the goal is to obtain data that are of high enough quality to meet the stakeholders' criteria for credibility. In terms of quantity, it is important to ensure the evaluation includes enough data to draw conclusions with confidence and provides enough data to detect changes attributable to participating in a program.[1]

One of the challenges in evaluation is that increases in data credibility often come with increased cost. Given that, it is always important to balance increasing the credibility of data with the practical limitations of an evaluation. Sometimes, a lower level of credibility and rigor is still acceptable to the stakeholders and is necessary to stay within resource restraints.

Data Collection Logistics. Logistics involve the "methods, and physical infrastructure for gathering and handling evidence."[1] When conducting evaluations of school health programs, logistics can be particularly challenging. The academic calendar puts limits on data collection timing. Not only does data collection often have to be planned within the shorter school year, it also has to be planned around interruptions such as winter and spring breaks, pep rallies and assemblies, and field trips as well as critical times for teachers and students such as midterms, finals, or standardized testing. In addition, data collection from students requires carefully planned processes for obtaining both student assent and parental consent and ensuring either anonymity or confidentiality of the data. Furthermore, because of the varying reading levels of both students and parents, documents that permit evaluators to collect data such as assent and consent forms, and data collection forms need to be tailored to the reading level of the participants. In many cases, evaluators may need to produce documents in more than 1 language, and in some instances, data collectors may need to read forms and documents to younger children rather than asking the students to complete them on their own. Evaluators will need to obtain appropriate clearances to collect data from education agency staff, students, and parents.

Step ❺: Justify Conclusions

After gathering data, evaluators are ready to move to step 5 of the framework—justifying conclusions. This process involves analyzing and synthesizing data, interpreting findings, considering stakeholder values and making judgments, and offering recommendations.[1] To illustrate this process, consider the example of an evaluation of a program offering breakfast to students in their classrooms each morning in an attempt to increase students' readiness to learn (and by extension, improve academic performance).

Analyzing and Synthesizing Data. The process for analysis and synthesis of the data is driven by the evaluation questions that were selected, the types of data collected, and input from stakeholders.[1] One key question, selected by stakeholders for the classroom breakfast evaluation was "How many students are reached by the program?" To answer that question, as well as the other evaluation questions, the following data were collected: the number of students participating in the program each day, students' responses to a survey about the program, and focus group feedback on the program from teachers. To answer the evaluation question, the evaluator synthesizes data (ie, looks across all the data sources to make a broad statement about what is happening) and determines that participation levels are relatively high—approximately 85% of all students are eating breakfast in their classrooms. In addition, the evaluator analyzes key pieces of data that have particular relevance for answering the evaluation question. In analyzing the survey data from youth, the evaluator discovers that the number 1 reason students reported for not participating in the program was being late to school. Then, the evaluator looks through the qualitative interview data from teachers and finds that teachers reported that when students were late to school, often arriving after the breakfast offerings had been returned to the cafeteria. Furthermore, teachers report that the students who are chronically tardy also tend to be among the students at highest risk of poor academic performance.

Interpreting Findings. Once data have been analyzed and/or synthesized, it is time to interpret the findings. In this example, the evaluator can make sense of the program participation findings and articulate practical significance of the information collected[1]—program participation rates are generally high, but when students are not participating in the breakfast program, it is often because they have missed the distribution of breakfast items because of tardiness.

Considering Stakeholder Values When Making Judgments. The interpretations can then be compared to stakeholder standards, or values, to make judgments about the program. Standards help determine the criteria by which success is defined, and once the stakeholders' standards have been articulated and operationalized, it is possible to examine the data interpretations in the context of what constitutes success, thereby making judgments about the program's worth, merit, or significance.[1] If the stakeholders believe it is important for all students to participate in the program, it may be reasonable to conclude that the program is not reaching its greatest potential for success.

Offering Recommendations. Finally, the evaluators and stakeholders should make recommendations for action based on the evaluation. Recommendations should always be consistent with the evaluation conclusions and in line with stakeholders' values.[1] In this example, the evaluator is likely to recommend that program staff and stakeholders explore options for providing breakfast to students who arrive late to ensure greater program participation among all students—particularly those who may be at increased need.

Step ❻: Ensure Use and Share Lessons Learned

The sixth step of the framework is ensuring use of the evaluation findings and sharing the lessons learned. Although this step is listed last, in reality, preparation for this step begins at the start of the evaluation. There are several critical elements to consider for evaluators to ensure findings will be used[1]:

- design;
- preparation;
- feedback;
- follow-up; and
- dissemination.

When initially designing the evaluation, it is important to make sure that the evaluation questions and methods that are selected will meet the needs of the primary users. As previously mentioned, it is essential for evaluators to select an evaluation design that is appropriate for the evaluation's focus and meets the level of credibility desired by the stakeholders.[1]

In addition, the evaluators can help prepare key stakeholders to use the findings. For example, evaluators could provide key stakeholders with hypothetical data and then lead a discussion about how those data would inform decisions. This is an opportunity for stakeholders and users to build their skills and it allows all people involved in the evaluation to consider the ways that both positive and negative findings could affect the program and future decisions.[1]

Another way to help ensure findings are used is to continually get feedback from stakeholders throughout the evaluation. By sharing proposed methods, data collection instruments, preliminary findings, and draft reports, the evaluators can help ensure that the work they are doing will meet the needs of the stakeholders. It provides multiple opportunities to refocus the work if it seems to be drifting from its original intent or use.[1]

When sharing findings with stakeholders, it is also important that evaluators follow up with them to make sure users have the support they need to accurately interpret the findings. It sometimes helps to remind users of the intended use of the findings and help highlight lessons learned that can inform meaningful decisions and actions. Furthermore, follow-up is key for program staff to also be certain users are not overstating findings, taking them out of context, or misrepresenting the findings to others.[1]

Finally, it is important for evaluators to have a plan for communicating findings. Both stakeholders and primary users can provide particularly valuable input into this plan, and it should take into consideration timing, style, tone, message source, vehicle, and format of products (eg, presentations, summary documents). The plan should also allow for communicating the evaluation's focus and context as well as strength, weaknesses, and limitations. Although findings are often shared through evaluation reports, there are other options that might be more appropriate for certain situations or audiences. For example, oral presentations at stakeholder meetings or short summary documents might be more effective ways to reach certain users and decision makers.

How to Work With Schools

There are a number of key considerations that are important for conducting evaluations with or in schools. Three primary considerations are key stakeholders, permissions and consent requirements, and unique challenges of schools.

Key Stakeholders in Schools

The first step in any evaluation is to engage stakeholders, and when working with schools, it is particularly important to carefully consider the individuals that have interest in or may be affected by the evaluation. For example, before beginning any evaluation in a school district or school or with school staff, it is critical to get the support of key administrators, including the principals, superintendent, and possibly school board members. Framing the value of the evaluation in terms of benefit to the students or staff or in relationship to the factors for which administrators are often held accountable (eg, academic achievement, attendance) can help build support for the evaluation. If the school has a school health team or the district has a school health council, members of these groups could provide valuable input and support for the evaluation. In addition to administrators and school health council or teams, it is important to consider the variety of people who may be affected by or have opportunity to implement recommendations from the evaluation. For example, in implementing recommendations from evaluations of asthma programs, some school districts have engaged maintenance and facilities staff to help improve indoor air quality and bus drivers to reduce asthma triggers caused from buses idling near the students. Other possible stakeholders to consider include teachers, counselors, social workers, administrative assistants, teachers' aides, custodial workers, maintenance and facilities staff, bus drivers, and representatives of parent-teacher organizations. Engaging a variety of stakeholders early and throughout the evaluation ensures that information needs are met and evaluation results will be used.

Permissions and Consent Requirements

Before collecting data from students, staff, or even school records, it is recommended that the evaluators speak with the school district administration to identify any requirements for informing participants about the evaluation and obtaining necessary permissions and/or consent. Many school districts have a research or evaluation office that has guidelines for how data can be collected in schools and how those data can be used. Some districts convene a special board, an Institutional Review Board for the Protection of Human Subjects, to review and approve evaluation and data collection protocols.[12] In addition, school records can be protected by the Family Education Rights and Privacy Act or, in the case of some school-based health clinics, even the Health Insurance Portability and Accountability Act; the district's research or evaluation office can help determine which protections to consider when planning an evaluation.

Unique Challenges of Schools

There can be a number of challenges that are unique to working in school settings. One of the most noticeable challenges, as previously mentioned, is working around the academic calendar. In the process of planning, evaluators should consider scheduling data collection to avoid the summer, winter, and spring breaks as well as high-pressure times such as the weeks leading up to standardized testing. If possible, it can also be helpful to schedule the evaluation so that findings will be analyzed in time to inform programmatic improvements for the following semester or school year and to schedule dissemination plans so that documents communicating key findings will be provided to school board members, district staff, principals, other administrators in advance of related key decisions.

Another challenge in schools comes from the nature of data collection. Data collection from students in schools often happens in classrooms or group settings, and in those types of settings, it is particularly important to ensure that processes are in place to ensure students' privacy. For example, if students are taking surveys, it is important to ensure they have sufficient space or barriers to prevent them from seeing each other's responses. In addition, the process of collecting the data should be examined to ensure it provides maximum privacy for students. For example, if a study is being conducted with all students with diabetes, it would not be appropriate to announce over the intercom that students should report to a certain location to participate in the "diabetes study"; such an approach would inappropriately disclose the participants' condition to others.

When conducting evaluations in schools, it is also important to recognize that the mission of schools is to educate students. As a result, teaching time will be protected and should be respected as much as possible. Data collection will need to be efficient and not intrude on teaching time or be disruptive to learning. In addition, teachers and other staff are often asked to assist or participate in data collection. It is essential to recognize that teachers and other staff face time pressures as well, including part-time schedules, which may pose a challenge to data collection.

Recommendations for Pediatricians

Pediatricians consulting with or working for the school district are well-positioned to support school health programs and evaluation of those programs. Their role is to encourage and enable schools and districts to create environments and conduct programmatic work that enhances the health of their students and staff and to support the evaluations that can improve and justify those programs. Pediatricians can be strong advocates for the value of evaluation findings in continuous program improvement leading to greater benefits for students and staff.

Pediatricians should not, however, feel that they need to be experts in evaluation. Although it is reasonable and appropriate to participate directly in evaluation work if they have relevant expertise, it is also completely appropriate for pediatricians to help the school or district identify an external evaluator—either a paid consultant or a community volunteer—to spearhead the evaluation efforts. Regardless of who is leading the evaluation, pediatricians' science and medical background should allow them to assist program staff and evaluators in thinking critically about which evaluation questions to ask and which stakeholders to engage. In addition, they may have particularly valuable perspectives for interpretation of the findings and resulting recommendations.

HIRING AN EXTERNAL EVALUATOR

In situations where program staff and school district staff are not comfortable with their level of expertise or do not have time to lead an evaluation, it may be desirable to hire an external evaluation consultant to design and lead the evaluation. Tips for hiring an evaluator are provided in a short evaluation brief available at **http://www.cdc.gov/healthyyouth/ evaluation/pdf/brief1.pdf**.

Recommendations for Program Directors and Trainees

It is critical for program directors to instill in trainees a standard of evidence-based programming and continuous improvement that is data-driven. Evaluation can help provide the evidence of effectiveness and data to inform improvements that will help justify and build additional support for programs. Program directors can stress that, even without expertise in formal evaluation, pediatricians can play a vital role in engaging the appropriate stakeholders, identifying and garnering human and fiscal resources for evaluation, asking the right questions, thinking critically and systematically about how to answer those questions, and using the findings to revise or enhance programmatic activities.

Program directors can also remind trainees that sometimes the findings will not be what they expect, and that as pediatricians, they will have an important role in supporting programs that are effective. Program directors can also stress that it is equally valuable to know if a program is not working the way it was intended, and trainees should embrace less than desirable findings and look for ways to use them to revise programs or help inform the selection of other programs that may be better suited for the situation. By using evaluation consistently, trainees will be able to develop and implement the best possible programs with the greatest opportunities for improving the health of the students and staff in their schools and district.

Overall, trainees are in an excellent position to learn more about both health programs in schools and evaluation. They should learn as much as they can about what approaches are most effective in school settings for improving the health of students and staff and work to incorporate what they have learned as they move forward in their careers. In addition, trainees can encourage the schools and other professionals they work with to continually look for evidence of effectiveness and to build evaluation into their programs and activities. Trainees can be leaders in highlighting the usefulness of data—both when the findings are desirable and when they are not—for improving school health work. Working with schools on program evaluation affords the pediatric resident or fellow the opportunity to further develop competence in practice-based learning and improvement and systems-based practice.

Take-Home Points

- Evaluation is the systematic assessment of a program's worth, merit, or significance.
- Program evaluation is a critical tool for use in selecting, implementing, improving, and justifying health-related programs.
- Evaluations can be broadly grouped into 2 main types—formative and summative.
- Common types of formative evaluations include needs assessments and implementation evaluations.
- Common types of summative evaluations include outcome or impact evaluations and cost-related evaluations.
- There are 6 key steps in the evaluation process:
  1. engage stakeholders;
  2. describe the program;
  3. focus the evaluation;
  4. gather credible evidence;
  5. justify conclusions; and
  6. ensure use and share lessons learned.

- Utility, feasibility, propriety, and accuracy are 4 standards that should guide all evaluations.
- It is important to involve program stakeholders in the evaluation process (planning, implementation, and articulating data implications).
- Pediatricians, program directors, and trainees have a responsibility to support health programs, the evaluation of those programs, and the improvement of programs based on the evaluation findings.

Resources

For additional school health related resources, visit www.aap.org/schoolhealthmanual.

References

1. Centers for Disease Control and Prevention. Framework for program evaluation in public health. *MMWR Recomm Rep.* 1999;48(RR-11):1-40
2. Trochim WMK. Introduction to evaluation. Research Methods Knowledge Base Web site. http://www.socialresearchmethods.net/kb/intreval.php. Accessed April 13, 2015
3. Grembowski D. *The Practice of Health Program Evaluation.* Thousand Oaks, CA: Sage Publications; 2001
4. US Government Accountability Office. *Designing Evaluations.* GAO Publication No. GAO-12-208G. Washington, DC: US Government Accountability Office; 2012
5. Wholey JS, Hatry HP, Newcomer K. *Handbook of Practical Program Evaluation.* 3rd ed. San Francisco, CA: Jossey-Bass; 2010
6. Gold MR, Siegel JE, Russell LB, Weinstein MC, eds. *Cost-Effectiveness in Health and Medicine.* New York, NY: Oxford University Press; 1996
7. National Institutes of Health. HTA 101: V. Economic Analysis Methods. Available at: http://www.nlm.nih.gov/nichsr/hta101/ta10107.html. Accessed June 23, 2015
8. Haddix AC, Teutsch SM, Corso PS, eds. *Prevention Effectiveness: A Guide to Decision Analysis and Economic Evaluation.* 2nd ed. New York, NY: Oxford University Press; 2003
9. American Evaluation Association. The program evaluation standards. Available at: http://www.eval.org/p/cm/ld/fid=103. June 23, 2015
10. Steinberg KS, Bringle RG, Williams MJ. *Service-Learning Research Primer.* Scotts Valley, CA: National Service-Learning Clearinghouse; 2010. Available at: http://csl.iupui.edu/doc/service-learning-research-primer.pdf. Accessed June 23, 2015
11. Trochim WMK. Types of designs. Research Methods Knowledge Base Web site. Available at: http://www.socialresearchmethods.net/kb/destypes.php. Accessed April 13, 2015
12. United States Department of Health and Human Services. Institutional Review Boards. Available at: http://www.hhs.gov/ohrp/assurances/irb/index.html. Accessed April 13, 2015

INDEX